Research Ethics Forum

Volume 5

The series, Research Ethics Forum aims to encourage discussion in the field of research ethics and the ethics of research. Volumes included can range from foundational issues to practical issues in research ethics. No disciplinary lines or borders are drawn and submissions are welcome from all disciplines as well as scholars from around the world. We are particularly interested in texts addressing neglected topics in research ethics, as well as those which challenge common practices and beliefs about research ethics. By means of this Series we aim to contribute to the ever important dialogue concerning the ethics of how research is conducted nationally and internationally. Possible topics include: Research Ethics Committees, Clinical trials, International research ethics regulations, Informed consent, Risk-benefit calculations, Conflicts of interest, Industry-funded research, Exploitation, Qualitative research ethics, Social science research ethics, Ghostwriting, Bias, Animal research, Research participants.

More information about this series at http://www.springer.com/series/10602

Henry Silverman
Editor

Research Ethics in the Arab Region

Springer

Editor
Henry Silverman
University of Maryland
Baltimore, MD, USA

ISSN 2212-9529 ISSN 2212-9537 (electronic)
Research Ethics Forum
ISBN 978-3-319-65264-1 ISBN 978-3-319-65266-5 (eBook)
https://doi.org/10.1007/978-3-319-65266-5

Library of Congress Control Number: 2017959191

Printed on acid-free paper

This Springer imprint is published by Springer Nature
The registered company is Springer International Publishing AG
The registered company address is: Gewerbestrasse 11, 6330 Cham, Switzerland

To
My family who continues to inspire me.

Acknowledgments

The publishing of a book about a topic in the Arab region is dependent on the input of many individuals from that area of the world, and as such I am indebted to many colleagues whom I have had the good fortune of having met during the last ten years. These individuals have guided my efforts on many levels and have also become my closest friends. I would like to give special recognition to Professor Nahed Ali, the Associate Editor of this book, who made many useful comments on many chapters and who has given me guidance regarding the Arab culture. I would also like give special thanks to Dr. Hany Sleem at the National Hepatology and Tropical Medicine Institute, who has been unsparingly with his time and efforts and with whom I have been dependent on obtaining information on many apsects of research ethics in Egypt. I am also grateful to other colleagues from Egypt who have become leaders in the field of research ethics and they include Tamer Hifnawy, Azza Saleh, Magdi Shehata, Rehab Abdel Hai, Amal Matar, Hala Mansour, Mohamed Salem, and Maged El-Setouhy. I wish to acknowledge the efforts of a special group of individuals from Sudan who have been pivotal in establishing research ethics programs at their universities, and they include Sara Lavinia-Brair, Shaza Abass, Shahd Osman, and Tahra El Mahdi. From Jordan, I would like to give special thanks to Suhail Al-Amad and Ibrahim Ramahi for the many conversations I have had with them regarding research ethics in Jordan. From Yemen, I would like to recognize the great efforts of Abdulla Bahattab, who is establishing bioethics programs under most difficult circumstances. Ghiath Al Ahmad, originally from Syria, has become a leading bioethicist in the Kingdom of Saudi Arabia. From Morocco, I give thanks to the special efforts of Latifa Adarmouch, Salma Ait Batahar, Bahia Bennani, Chakib Nejjari, and Mohamed Amine. There are many other colleagues and friends from the Arab region whom I have met, too numerous to name, who have made a difference in who I am today as an academic and a person. I would like to give special thanks to many individuals whom I met through the Fogarty International Center (FIC) of the National Institutes of Health with training programs similar to the Middle East Research Ethics Training Initiative (MERETI). They include Douglas Wassenaar, Kaveh Khoshnood, Eric Meslin, Bebe Loff, and Martin Strosberg. I gratefully acknowledge the receipt of continued funding for the MERETI training grant from the FIC/NIH during the past ten plus years that has made the writing of this book possible, with special recognition to tireless efforts of Dr. Barbara Sina in her capacity as the Program Officer at the FIC. Finally, I wish to acknowledge the support and encouragement given by the publishing editors, Christopher Wilby and Floor Oosting, and the helpful comments from an anonymous referee. I am grateful and blessed that I am able to provide such a list of remarkable individuals.

Dr. Nahed Ali served as the Associate Editor for this book. Her broad experiences in the field of ethics helped ensure that the ethical issues discussed in this book are relevant to the Arab region.

She is currently Professor of Forensic Medicine and Toxicology at the School of Medicine, Suez Canal University, Egypt. She is also a Professor of Bioethics in Joint Master of Health Professions Education, a joint program of studies between the Universiteit Maastrich (Netherlands) and Suez Canal University. She received her Bachelor degree in Medicine and Surgery from the School of Medicine, Ain Shams University, Egypt (1980) and her Medical degree in Forensic Medicine and Toxicology at the School of Medicine, Al-Menia University, Egypt (1991). Subsequently, she received a Master of Science in Health Education, Ithaca College, USA (2013). Dr. Ali also serves as the chair of the research ethics committee at Suez Canal University.

Thank you all! Henry Silverman

Contents

Contributors

Shaza Abass Faculty of Dentistry, University of Khartoum, Khartoum, Sudan

Mohamed Elhassan Abdalla College of Medicine, University of Sharjah, Sharjah, UAE

Latifa Adarmouch School of Medicine, Cadi Ayyad University, Marrakesh, Morocco

Mamoun Ahram School of Medicine, The University of Jordan, Amman, Jordan

Office of Research, Jordan University Hospital, The University of Jordan, Amman, Jordan

Amal Al-Omari Office of Scientific Affairs and Research, King Hussein Cancer Center, Amman, Jordan

Nahed M. Ali Suez Canal University, Ismailia, Egypt

Ghiath Alahmad King Abdullah International Medical Research Center, Riyadh, Saudi Arabia

Suhail Al-Amad College of Dental Medicine, University of Sharjah, Sharjah, UAE

Monash University, Melbourne, Australia

Maysa Al-Hussaini Department of Pathology and Laboratory Medicine, King Hussein Cancer Center, Amman, Jordan

Institutional Review Board (IRB), King Hussein Cancer Center, Amman, Jordan

May M. Al Kassar Human Research Protection Program, Weill Cornell Medicine in Qatar, Ar-Rayyan, Qatar

American University of Beirut, Beirut, Lebanon

Master of Science, Population Health, American University of Beirut, Beirut, Lebanon

Aisha Al Khamiri Internal Medicine Resident, Tawam Hospital, Abu Dhabi, UAE

Farida Al Marzooqi Internal Medicine Resident, Tawam Hospital, Abu Dhabi, UAE

Noha Asem Faculty of Medicine, Cairo University, Giza, Egypt

Institutional Review Board, Cairo University, Giza, Egypt

Bilal Azakir Beirut Arab University, Beirut, Lebanon

Martin Boleček QuintilesIMS, Vienna, Austria

Rachel V. Brady QuintilesIMS, Vienna, Austria

Clinical Site Monitoring, Central and Eastern Europe, Middle East and North Africa, Quintiles, Durham, NC, USA

Kirsty Clark Chronic Disease Epidemiology, Yale School of Public Health, New Haven, CT, USA

Violent Conflict & Health, Introduction to Ethics & Public Health, New Haven, CT, USA

Qualitative Analysis of Multi-Level Barriers to HIV Testing among Women in Lebanon, New Haven, CT, USA

Rana Dajani Biology and Biotechnology Department, Hashemite University, Zarqa, Jordan

Samer S. El-Kamary Epidemiology & Public Health, University of Maryland Baltimore, Baltimore, MD, USA

Kaveh Khoshnood Epidemiology of Microbial Diseases, Yale School of Public Health, New Haven, USA

Fogarty International Center/NIH, Bethesda, USA

Farida Lada The City University of New York, New York, NY, USA

Jihad Makhoul Department of Health Promotion and Community Health, Faculty of Health Sciences, American University of Beirut, Beirut, Lebanon

Vladimír Mišík LongTaal, Clinical Trial Analytics, Bratislava, Slovakia

Rima Nakkash Department of Health Promotion and Community Health, Faculty of Health Sciences, American University of Beirut, Beirut, Lebanon

Satish Chandrasekhar Nair Departments of Academic Affairs and Internal Medicine Residency Program, Tawam Hospital in Affiliation with Johns Hopkins Medicine USA, Al Ain, UAE

Shahd Osman Public Health Institute, Federal Ministry of Health, Khartoum, Sudan

Azza Saleh Central Directorate of Research & Health Development, Ministry of Health & Population, Cairo, Egypt

Theodor Bilharz Research Institute, Giza, Egypt

Henry Silverman University of Maryland, Baltimore, MD, USA

Hany M. Sleem Egyptian Network of Research Ethics Committees (ENREC), Cairo, Egypt

National Hepatology and Tropical Medicine Research Institute (NHTMRI), Cairo, Egypt

Cindy Sousa Bryn Mawr College, Graduate School of Social Work and Social Research, Bryn Mawr, PA, USA

Robert Wachbroit Department of Epidemiology and Public Health, University of Maryland, Baltimore, MD, USA

Nadia Zaki Faculty of Medicine, Alexandria University, Alexandria, Egypt

About the Editor

Henry Silverman MD, MA, is Professor of Medicine at the University of Maryland, School of Medicine. He divides his time between caring for patients in the intensive care units, teaching medical ethics to students, residents and faculty, chairing the hospital's ethics committee, directing a training program in research ethics focused in the Middle East, and performing qualitative and quantitative research in research ethics.

Dr. Silverman majored in biomedical engineering at Rensselaer Polytechnic Institute, where he received his B.S. and M.S. degrees in 1974. He then studied medicine at The Johns Hopkins University (MD 1974) followed by a residency in internal medicine and a pulmonary and critical fellowship at The Johns Hopkins Hospital (1983). He then became a faculty member at the University of Maryland, School of Medicine. He received his MA Degree in Bioethics from Georgetown University in 1995. His teaching efforts have been recognized by several teaching awards, including the Senior Resident's Award for Teaching (1988),the Senior Medical Student's Award for Humanism in Medicine (2001), and the Master of Public Health Program Teaching and Mentoring Award (2013).

Introduction

Henry Silverman

Recently, there has been a growth of scholarship in research ethics accompanied by several revisions of international research ethics guidelines highlighting issues pertaining to international collaborative research performed in low and middle income countries (LMICs) (Council for International Organizations of Medical Sciences (CIOMS) and World Health Organization (WHO) 2016; World Medical Association 2013). Several reasons explain for focusing the lens of research ethics on international collaborative research. First and foremost, commentators have expressed concerns regarding inadequate protection of the rights and welfare of research participants leading to unnecessary harms, exploitation, and injustices at both the micro and macro levels (Bhutta 2002; London 2010; Pratt and Loff 2014). Second, oversight mechanisms that exist in LMICs have not been able to respond effectively to the ethical and legal issues that arise from the growth of such research, especially clinical trials (Kirigia et al. 2005; Moodley and Myer 2007). Indeed, many commentators have expressed concerns about the lack of regulatory oversight and the ineffectiveness of ethics review in LMICs (Bhutta 2002; Hyder et al. 2009; Nuffield Council on Bioethics 2002). Third, there is a growing recognition that the local context governed by culture and religion warrant differences in the application of general principles of research ethics, but there is controversy regarding whether such applications of ethics principles respect local diversity or whether they represent inappropriate double standards (Christakis 1992; Landes 2005; Macklin 2004; Tangwa 2004). Finally, studies have demonstrated a disturbing prevalence of research misbehaviors that include data falsification and fabrication, plagiarism, inappropriate authorship practices, and lack of transparency regarding conflicts of interest (Okonta and Rossouw 2013, 2014).

H. Silverman (✉)
University of Maryland, Baltimore, MD, USA
e-mail: hsilverm@medicine.umaryland.edu

H. Silverman (ed.), *Research Ethics in the Arab Region*, Research Ethics Forum 5,
https://doi.org/10.1007/978-3-319-65266-5_1

The Arab region[1] has not been immune to these issues and as such, similar scholarship reflecting these research ethics issues has begun to emerg from this region. Hence, it is time to briefly review the recent growth of research and clinical trials in the Arab region and the status of the regulatory and ethical oversight mechanisms in this region.

The Growth of Research in the Arab Region

There has been a global migration of clinical trials into emerging markets that include low- and middle-income countries (LMICs) throughout the world (Glickman et al. 2009; Normile 2008). For example, in 1995, 94% of the clinical trials was conducted in North America and Western Europe, but this activity decreased to about 79% by 2005 (Glickman et al. 2009). The majority of this shift among the emerging markets went towards Central and Eastern Europe (CEE) and the Commonwealth of Independent States (CIS: includes Russia, Ukraine and some other countries of the former USSR), which captured 41% of the emerging markets patient share, ahead of Latin American, Asia, Africa, and the Middle East and North Africa (MENA) (Misik 2012).

Several reasons account for the growth of research and clinical trials in LMICs. First, in order to improve global health, significant changes are needed to address the inequitable sharing of resources between the Global North and South. For example, the 2000 Global Forum on Health Research 10/90 Report revealed that 90% of global research expenditures target only 10% of the global burden of disease (Global Forum for Health Research 2000). To address this gap, research for health[2] has become an increasingly global endeavor, as witnessed by the participation from both the public and private sectors in international research.

The globalization of research for health has also been fueled by efforts to address diseases that rarely occur in Western countries, such as malaria, dengue fever and tuberculosis as well as diseases that have affected disproportionately LMICs compared to the West (e.g., AIDS epidemic). Additionally, the pharmaceutical industry has increasingly become a leading global actor in research during the past quarter of a century, as witnessed by the global migration of clinical trials into emerging markets that include LMICs throughout the world (Glickman et al. 2009; Normile 2008). Pharmaceutical companies are attracted by the availability of large "naïve" populations (i.e., have not been treated for the disease being studied) who lack access to essential drugs, availability of cheap labor, and the undeveloped regulatory mechanisms in LMICs (Schipper and Weyzig 2008). The pharmaceutical industry

[1] Although the region bounded by the Middle East and North Africa has been referred to by many as the MENA region, we use instead the phrase the "Arab Region", as the content of this book applies to only the Arab countries in the MENA region.

[2] We make a distinction between "health research" and "research for health", as the former phrase refers to the narrower concept of research that investigates biomedical mechanisms, whereas the latter phrase is inclusive of any research that promotes societal health, e.g., health systems research.

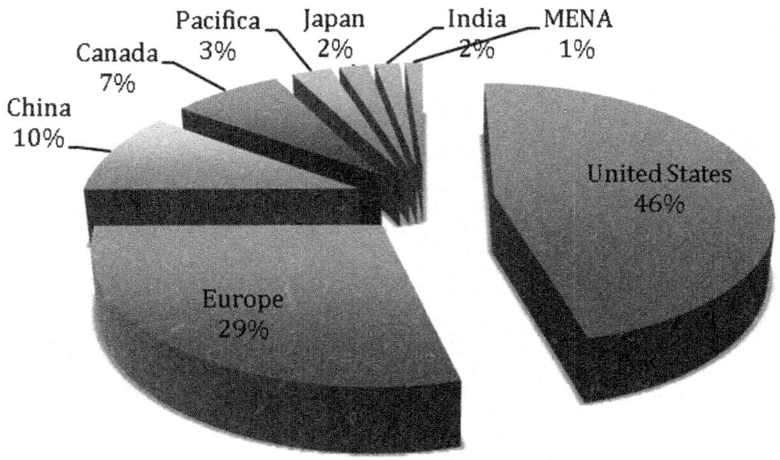

Fig. 1 The distribution of clinical trials around various regions in the world (Source: clinicaltrials.gov Graph by Suhail Al-Amad)

sees an opportunity to enhance their productivity of development by shortening the duration of the clinical trials, e.g., via shorter site start-up times and faster patient enrollment (Emanuel et al. 2003). Also, costs per research participant can be significantly lower due to lower salaries and overheads (Malakoff 2008; Misik 2012). Finally, the conduct of clinical trials in LMICs achieves market objectives in the LMICs, insofar that many drug regulatory authorities in LMICs require domestic testing of drugs that have been approved in Western countries (Nwabueze 2016).

The benefit of introducing a variety of medications and investigational new drugs cannot be overlooked, but exploitation of human participants and violation of their rights cannot be ignored, especially in countries where regulatory and accountability mechanisms are deficient. These concerns and its associated ethical dilemmas have been continuously raised by ethicists and human right activists and will continue to be expressed as long as appropriate actions to protect human research participants are inadequate.

Clinical trials activity in the Arab region has lagged behind when compared to other emerging markets, such as India, China, Russia and Mexico. According to a recent review of the clinicaltrials.gov website (National Institutes of Health 2015), there were 2291 clinical trials registered in the various countries in the Arab region. This represents 1% of all registered clinical trials around the world (Fig. 1, where MENA represents the Arab region). More than half of these clinical trials are confined to only two countries, Saudi Arabia and Egypt (Fig. 2).

While the global proportion of research for the Arab region is low compared with other emerging markets, nonetheless, research in this region has been growing in recent years with better utilization of the region's potentials at the human and financial levels (Adams et al. 2011). Recent data has also shown a noticeable rise in scientific research activities in the Arab region. For example, the UNESCO Science Report shows that between 2008 and 2014 there was an increase of almost 110% in

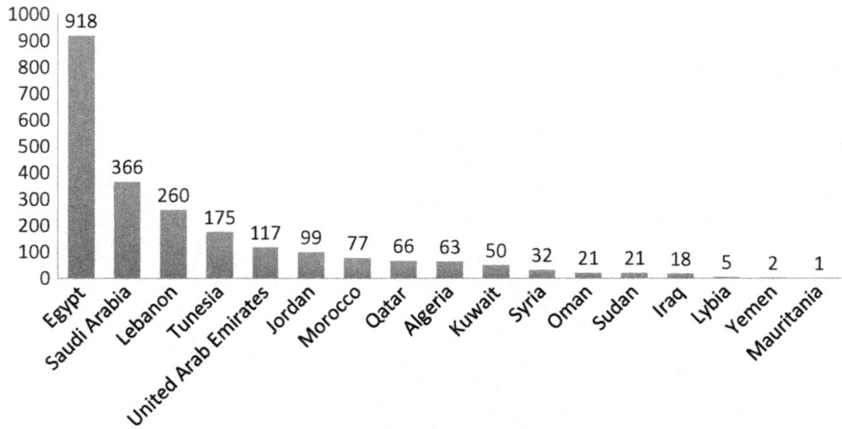

Fig. 2 Number of clinical trials registered in various Arabian countries (Source: *clinicaltrials.gov* Graph created by Suhail Al-Amad)

publications from all countries in the Arab region. By comparison, scientific publications rose by 14% for the UK and the European Union and by 11% for the USA during the same time period (United Nations Educational, Scientific, and Cultural Organizations).

Despite growing political volatility, the Arab region is poised for clinical trials growth. Several factors fuel the interest in conducting clinical trials in this region. First, there is a demand for medications in the region due to high population growth, an increased prevalence of life-style related diseases and non-communicable diseases, and desires to improve life expectancy and lower mortality rates, as well as improve access to treatment. The region's current market for biopharmaceuticals, however, outpaces the volume of clinical trials conducted in the region and will cause governments, regulatory agencies, and other stakeholders to demand conduct of in-country clinical trials to ensure that the currently approved drugs are also applicable to the DNA characteristics of the Arab populations (Gulf Daily News, February 12, 2016).

A second factor that fuels an interest in conducting clinical research in the Arab region stems from the region's high prevalence of certain diseases. For example, the region exhibit the world's second highest prevalence of diabetes, as well as a high prevalence of many genetic diseases due in part to the high percentage of consanguineous marriages (Al-Gazali et al. 2006). The region also has a high prevalence of hepatitis, asthma, cancer, cardiovascular disease, and obesity (Abraham 2011).

The Arab region also possesses other attractive features that include highly centralized healthcare systems, many excellent healthcare facilities, hospitals, investigators interested in conducting clinical trials, governments and institutions focused on attracting clinical research, hospital documents in English or French, and many Western-trained investigators with excellent command of English. Finally, the pharmaceutical industry also see favorable conditions in the Arab region to conduct clinical trials similar to that in other LMICs, which include large "naïve" populations who lack access to essential drugs, undeveloped regulatory drug authorities, and lower salaries and overheads that lead to faster approval of drugs at low costs (Emanuel et al. 2003; Malakoff 2008; Misik 2012).

Status of the Regulatory and Ethical Oversight Mechanisms for the Protection of Research Participants

Associated with the increase in research activity, ethical concerns regarding the performance of research in this area of the world have surfaced for a variety of reasons. First, there are inadequacies in the regulatory oversight mechanisms for research and a lack of or deficiencies in research regulations (Alahmad et al. 2012). Another concern with the growth of clinical trials in the Arab region, similar to what occurs in other LMICs, is that functioning ethics review systems have not increased proportionately with the increase in research activities (Abdur Rab et al. 2008) (Sleem et al. 2010b). For example, Abdur Rab and colleagues showed that 28% of regional researchers did not obtain ethical clearance for research proposals submitted for funding to the WHO's office in Cairo in 2008 and 24% failed to mention plans to obtain informed consent (Abdur Rab et al. 2008). Another study showed that many basic elements of informed consent were omitted from informed consent forms (Abou-Zeid et al. 2006). There are also concerns with the responsible conduct of research in the Arab region, as a recent study documented a significant prevalence of research misbehaviors (Marwan Felaefel 2017). Finally, several survey studies have shown a lack of training in research ethics among investigators and members of research ethics committees (Asem and Silverman 2009; El-Dessouky et al. 2011; Kandeel et al. 2011). All of these deficiencies can lead to inadequate protection of the rights and welfare of research participants.

Due to these concerns with research ethics capacity in the Arab region, this book aims to give a timely review of research ethics concepts and activities occurring in the Arab region and focus particularly on 1) how the local context, in terms of social, cultural, religious, and political forces, have shaped the ethical issues that might differ from other world regions; 2) the current status and gaps of the national regulatory and ethical oversight mechanisms for research, including the functioning of research ethics committees; and 3) current efforts at building capacity in research ethics at the institutional and individual levels. Weaved throughout this book, we provide case studies of regulatory systems, research ethics committees, and clinical trial sites in several countries that can serve as models for the Arab region.

We believe that the targeted audiences for this book include international and regional bioethicists, regulatory agencies (e.g., Ministries of Health and Drug Regulatory Authorities), the pharmaceutical industry, contract research organizations, members of research ethics committees, investigators and members of the research staff, and top officials of universities and research institutes who aim to develop a culture of responsible conduct in research. The authors who have contributed to this volume are predominantly from the Arab region and are currently active in various aspects of research ethics and research oversight in the Arab region. We continue with this introductory chapter by giving a summary of the chapters included in this book.

Summary of Chapters

This book is divided into several Parts that reflect the following aspects of research ethics: ethical issues in the conduct of research; research governance in the Arab region that include the status of national regulations, regulatory oversight mechanisms, research ethics committees, and a final Part devoted to the development of research ethics capacity.

Prior to the presentation of these specific Parts of the book, Nahed Ali and Samer El-Kamary give their insight regarding the contribution of Islamic teachings to the foundation of bioethical thought in the Arab region. The potential importance of Islam emanates from the dominant role it plays in the everyday lives of the majority of the population in the Arab region. To be sure, while Islam recognizes the four principles of bioethics that are similar to those in Western bioethics, the weight given to each of these principles and the application of these principles in the social and cultural contexts that exist in the Arab region will differ from what occurs in the West. This importance of religious values contrasts with the secularization of ethics that has occurred in the West for centuries.[3]

Following this review of Islam and bioethics, Part 1, entitled: "Ethical Issues in Research in the Arab Region", explores the important ethical issues that arise from research involving human participants in the Arab region. This section begins with "What Kind of Research Ethics for the Arab Region", in which I review the controversy regarding whether ethical principles are universal or are relative based on social, cultural, and religious influences. While the resolution of this debate remains unresolved, I present the argument that others have made that the current concept of research ethics is overly reliant on a Western value system that does not overlap fully with value systems of other cultures. As such, when local researchers resist the roll out of universal ethical norms, they may be seeking guidelines that display greater cultural sensitivity. In addition to recognizing the contribution of other ethical values to a concept of research ethics, one should also acknowledge the role of post-colonial influences in the development of a research ethic in the region. Post-colonists theorists recognize that contemporary social relations occur in the aftermath of colonialism. Such a recognition leads to the adoption of a solidarity approach to international collaborative research between international sponsors/researchers on one hand, and research participants/countries, on the other hand. Such an approach should promote social justice as well as enable the "empowerment" of research participants that lead to an "emancipatory" bioethics for international collaborative relationships.

[3] Consideration of Islam's contribution to bioethics should not fail to recognize the important role that culture plays in many of the ethical issues occurring in the Arab region.

Robert Wachbroit next discusses the different concepts of exploitation and its particular relevance to clinical research. He analyzes how the history of colonialism influences a definition of exploitation for international research that is conducted in low- and middle income countries.

The following chapters in Part I explore a range of topics in research ethics that raise particular issues relevant to the Arab region. Nahed Ali analyzes the ethical issues when research involves vulnerable populations and explores how the social, cultural, and political context in the Arab region highlight particular issues regarding vulnerability. Similarly, Shahd Osman next discusses how such contextual issues shape informed consent practices in the Arab region. I next present the special ethical issues that are raised when children participate in research and the existing barriers to their inclusion in research in the Arab region. Mohamed Hassan Abdalla reviews the competing concepts offered to analyze risks and benefits and discusses cultural and social aspects of such an analysis.

The next two chapters review research topics that incorporate ethical issues shaped by cultural and religious aspects in the Arab region. Mamoun Ahram presents issues involved with genetic research and the establishment of biobanks in the Arab region with a particular focus on Jordan's biobanking activities. Rana Dajani discusses the foundation of the ethics of stem cell research in the Arab region as informed by Islamic teachings.

The following three chapters focus on social behavioral research and how the ethical issues of such research is defined by the particular social, economic, and political problems existing in the Arab region. I discuss the general ethical issues raised in social behavioral research and point out how the risks of such research depends on the methodological approaches used in such research as well as on the types of vulnerable populations and the sensitivity of the topics that exist in the Arab region.

After this analysis, Kaveh Khoshnood, Cindy Sousa, and Kirsty Clark discuss the ethical issues when performing research involving vulnerable individuals who live in conflict settings, an issue that has increasingly become more important and extant due to the recent conflicts occurring in this region. This is then followed by Shahd Osman's more formal analysis of the ethical requirements that guide research involving refugees and internally displaced persons.

This section ends with Misik and colleagues exploring the extent of clinical trials being performed in the Arab region by using data from the clinicaltrials.gov website. They show that there is an extraordinary mismatch between the growths of pharmaceutical sales compared with the number of clinical trials being performed in the Arab region. Such a mismatch raises the ethical concern of benefits and risks, as many approved drugs consumed by the Arab populations have not been previously tested in clinical trials involving the local populations. Specifically, the pharmocodynamic properties of drugs tested on other regional populations may not be appropriate for the native Arab populations, as the genetic makeup of the Arab populations may differ sufficiently from the populations in the parts of the world where the clinical trials were initially conducted.

Part II is entitled "Research Governance in the Arab Region" and consists of an introductory chapter where I present a survey of the various types of regulatory models. I also discuss the challenges of governance systems, which include 1) the measures available to ensure compliance with the regulations; 2) the mechanisms to regulate and provide oversight of local research ethics committees in the Arab region; and 3) coordination between the independent roles and responsibilities between national and local research ethics committees on one hand, and the National Regulatory Authorities, on the other hand.

Part III examines the existing national research ethics regulations and the role such regulations play in the regulation and oversight of research. First, Ghiath Alahmad surveys the current landscape regarding the professional codes, national guidelines, and national regulations in the Arab region that provide a framework for research governance for research ethics. His review is based on a survey of 13 countries in the Arab region and he shows that policies regulating bioethical issues in research vary between the different countries in the Arab region. In some counties, research practices are governed by professional guidelines, others have governmental guidelines, while others have developed comprehensive legislative frameworks to regulate research. He performs a critical analysis of these regulations and highlights the contents, the research governance infrastructures, the ethics review process established by the regulations, and their scope of coverage and enforceability. He specifically reports on the national regulations in the United Arab Emirates, Qatar, Bahrain, Kuwait, Saudi Arabia, and Jordan (Alahmad et al. 2012). In countries where regulations do not exist, Alahmad explores the documents that guide research practices. For example, in Egypt and Lebanon, medical professional guidelines as well as ministerial decrees provide guidance for the ethics of research practice. The remaining countries either refer to international guidelines or are silent on research ethics. National regulations are key, as such legal instruments can define the boundaries of appropriate legal and ethical conduct in research. In a study conducted among RECs in Egypt, 92% of the respondents listed the lack of national regulations as one of several challenges to the effective functioning of RECs (Sleem et al. 2010b).

Following this overview, Ghiath Alahmad and Latifa Adarmouch examine in detail the national regulations that exist in Saudi Arabia and Morocco, respectively. Major parts of these regulations can serve as exemplary models for other countries. However, their reviews also reveal that there are real substantive differences between the regulations on several issues in research ethics that warrant further discussion. Efforts are needed to establish more harmonious regulations in this region, especially if there is to be efficient conduct of multi-site clinical trials.

Part IV explores the regulatory and ethical oversight landscape in the Arab region. After I present a short introduction, the ensuing chapters compare in depth the regulatory systems that exist in Jordan, Saudi Arabia, Egypt, Lebanon, and the United Arab Emirates. Such a comparison highlights the different types of regulatory systems that exist in the Arab region. While this review shows deficiencies in several of these regulatory models, it also demonstrates that research governance in several countries has attained a level of sophistication comparable to those existing in other Western countries. As such, it challenges the popular assumption that many countries in the Arab region lack adequate regulatory mechanisms for the oversight of research involving human participants.

Part V focuses on the scope and nature of ethics review in the Arab region. I introduce this Part regarding research ethics committees (RECs) by emphasizing the importance of accountability and transparency mechanisms needed to ensure the public trust in research. Hany Sleem and myself next explore the challenges of RECs in the Arab region that include insufficient member expertise, lack of diverse membership, scarcity of human and capital resources, limited continuing education in research ethics, and lack of national guidelines (Sleem et al. 2010a).

The establishment of RECs is a relatively new phenomenon in the Arab region. Accordingly, Jihad Makhoul and Rima Naklash discuss their research findings, as well as that of other studies performed in the Arab region, regarding the attitudes and beliefs of investigators toward these committees. Following this discussion, I discuss methods to assess the functioning of RECs in the region and review our recent efforts with a self-assessment tool that many RECs have used in the region (Sleem et al. 2010a). Recently, Egypt's Ministry of Health have required RECs in Egypt to use this tool to assess their structures and processes needed for effective functioning.

The next chapters in PartV provide case studies of RECs at two different institutions: Noha Asem discusses the REC at Cairo University and Maysa Al-Hussaini reviews the REC at the King Hussein Cancer Center. Their reviews demonstrate the level of sophistication of the operations of their RECs, both of which can serve as exemplary models for other RECs in the Arab region. Farida Lada concludes this Part by reviewing the important administrative aspects of RECs that can enhance the functioning of RECs.

Part VI reviews capacity-building efforts to enhance the responsible conduct of research in the Arab region. Shaza Abass discusses her experience with the development of training programs in research ethics in Sudan for members of RECs and investigators and the challenges she has encountered in organizing these programs. Suhail Al-Amad next presents an overview of responsible conduct in research (RCR) and reviews specific data regarding the prevalence of research misbehaviors in the region. He discusses causes of research misconduct and how responsible conduct in research can be promoted.

An important aspect in the ethical conduct of clinical trials is the ability of universities and research institutes to develop functioning clinical trial units. As such, Nadia Zaki and Amal Omari discuss their experiences and challenges with establishing their clinical trial centers at their respective institutions. Nadia Zaki reviews the experience with the Clinical Research Center at Alexandria University in Egypt and Amal Al Omari reviews the current operations of the King Hussein Cancer Center in Amman, Jordan. The successes of these two research centers should serve as models for the establishment of other research centers in the Arab region.

In the last chapter, I will say a few concluding remarks about this exploration of research ethics in the Arab region coupled with a final comment regarding a "road map" for the future and what stakeholders need to focus on to institute necessary changes that will enhance research ethics capacity.

References

Abdur Rab, M., A. Abou-Zeid, M. Afzal, and H.J. Silverman. 2008. Ethical practices for health research in the Eastern Mediterranean region of the world health organization: A retrospective data analysis. *PloS One* 3: e2094.

Abou-Zeid, A., M. Afzal, and H.J. Silverman. 2006. *Informed consent as an ethical requirement for health research in the Eastern Mediterranean region of the World Health Organization*. Washington, DC: PRIM&R Conference.

Abraham, R. 2011. MENA: The dawn of a new era: The Middle East and North Africa region has seen a recent increase in clinical trials research. *Applied Clinical Trials*.

Adams, K, C. King, D. Pendlebury, D. Hook, and J. Wilson. 2011. Global research report Middle East. *Thomson Reuters*. Available at: http://sciencewatch.com/sites/sw/files/sw-article/media/globalresearchreport-aptme.pdf

Al-Gazali, L., H. Hamamy, and S. Al-Arrayad. 2006. Genetic disorders in the Arab world. *BMJ* 333: 831–834.

Alahmad, G., M. Al-Jumah, and K. Dierickx. 2012. Review of national research ethics regulations and guidelines in Middle Eastern Arab countries. *BMC Medical Ethics* 13: 34. https://doi.org/10.1186/1472-6939-13-34.

Asem, N., and H.J. Silverman. 2009. *Perspectives of faculty at Cairo Universitiy towards research ethics and informed consent*. Nashville: Abstract Presentation at PRIM&R.

Bhutta, A.Z. 2002. Ethics in international health research: A perspective from the developing world. *Bulletin of the World Health Organization* 80: 114–120.

Christakis, N.A. 1992. Ethics are local: Engaging cross-cultural variation in the ethics for clinical research. *Social Science & Medicine* 35 (9): 1079–1091.

Council for International Organizations of Medical Sciences (CIOMS), and World Health Organization (WHO). 2016. *International ethical guidelines for health-related research involving humans*. Vol. Retrieved from: http://www.cioms.ch/index.php/12-newsflash/400-cioms-inernational-ethical-guidelines

El-Dessouky, H.F., A.M. Abdel-Aziz, C. Ibrahim, M. Moni, R. Abul Fadl, and H. Silverman. 2011. Knowledge, awareness, and attitudes about research ethics among dental faculty in the Middle East: A pilot study. *International Journal of Dentistry* 2011: 694759. https://doi.org/10.1155/2011/694759.

Emanuel, E.J., L.E. Schnipper, D.Y. Kamin, J. Levinson, and A.S. Lichter. 2003. The costs of conducting clinical research. *Journal of Clinical Oncology* 21: 45–50.

Glickman, S.W., J.G. McHutchison, E.D. Peterson, C.B. Cairns, R.A. Harrington, R.M. Califf, and K.A. Schulman. 2009. Ethical and scientific implications of the globalization of clinical research. *The New England Journal of Medicine* 360 (8): 816–823. https://doi.org/10.1056/NEJMsb0803929.

Global Forum for Health Research. 2000. The 10/90 report on health research. Last Accessed 23 Apr 2013 at: http://announcementsfiles.cohred.org/gfhr_pub/assoc/s14791e/s14791e.pdf

Gulf Daily News. 2016. *Clinical trials to be rolled out in Bahrain*. Retrieved from: http://www.tradearabia.com/news/HEAL_300785.html

Hyder, A.A., L. Dawson, A.M. Bachani, and J.V. Lavery. 2009. Moving from research ethics review to research ethics systems in low-income and middle-income countries. *Lancet* 373: 862–865.

Kandeel, N., A. El-Nemer, N.M. Ali, H. Kassem, M. El-Setouhy, M.E. Elgharieb, et al. 2011. A multicenter study of the awareness and attitudes of Egyptian faculty towards research ethics: A pilot study. *Journal of Empirical Research on Human Research Ethics* 6 (4): 99–108. doi:https://doi.org/10.1525/jer.2011.6.4.99.

Kirigia, J.M., C. Wambebe, and A. Baba-Moussal. 2005. Status of national research bioethics committees in the WHO African region. *BMC Medical Ethics* 6: 10.

Landes, M. 2005. Can context justify an ethical double standard for clinical research in developing countries? *Globalization and Health* 1 (1): 11. https://doi.org/10.1186/1744-8603-1-11.

London, A.J. 2010. Justice in the application of science: Beyond fair benefits. *American Journal of Bioethics* 10 (6): 54–56. https://doi.org/10.1080/15265161.2010.483184.

Macklin, R. 2004. *Double standards in medical research in developing countries*. Cambridge: Cambridge University Press.

Malakoff, D. 2008. Clinical trials and tribulations: Spiralng costs threaten gridlock. *Science* 322: 210–213.

Marwan Felaefel, M., M. Salem, R. Jaafar, G. Jassim, H. Edwards, F. Rashid-Doubell, R. Yousri, N. Ali, and H. Silverman. 2017a. A cross-sectional survey study to assess prevalence and attitudes regarding research misconduct among investigators in the Middle East. *Journal of Academic Ethics*: 1–17. https://doi.org/10.1007/s10805-017-9295-9.

Misik, V. 2012. *Expected growth of industry-sponsored clinical trials in the Middle East bencharked on other global regions*. Accessed 12 Jan 2014 at: http://www.quintiles.com/assets/2010/2111/2118/2233/1336/96587bf96585-cb96581e-94982-96588f96589b-bf96632aba99661.pdf

Moodley, K., and L. Myer. 2007. Health research ethics committees in South Africa 12 years into democracy. *BMC Medical Ethics* 8: 1–8.

Normile, D. 2008. The promise and pitfalls of clinical trials overseas. *Science* 322: 214–216.

Nuffield Council on Bioethics. 2002. *The ethics of research related to healthcare in developing countries*. London: Nuffield Council on Bioethics.

Nwabueze, R.N. 2016. *Legal and ethical regulation of biomedical research in developing countries*. New York: Routledge (Taylor & Francis Group).

Okonta, P., and T. Rossouw. 2013. Prevalence of scientific misconduct among a group of researchers in Nigeria. *Developing World Bioethics* 13 (3): 149–157. https://doi.org/10.1111/j.1471-8847.2012.00339.x.

Okonta, P.I., and T. Rossouw. 2014. Misconduct in research: A descriptive survey of attitudes, perceptions and associated factors in a developing country. *BMC Medical Ethics* 15: 25. https://doi.org/10.1186/1472-6939-15-25.

Pratt, B., and B. Loff. 2014. A framework to link international clinical research to the promotion of justice in global health. *Bioethics* 28 (8): 387–396. https://doi.org/10.1111/bioe.12009.

Schipper I, and F. Weyzig. 2008. *Ethics for drug testing in low and middle INcome countries: Considerations for European market authorisation*. Centre for Research on Multinational Corporations (SOMO), Retrieved at: https://www.somo.nl/ethics-for-drugs-testing-in-low-and-middle-income-countries/

Sleem, H., R. Adelhai, I. Al-Abdallat, M. Al-Naif, H. Gabr, E.T. Kehil, et al. 2010a. Development of an accessible self-assessment tool for research ethics committees in developing countries. *Journal of Empirical Research on Human Research Ethics* 6: 85–96.

Sleem, H., S. El-Kamary, and H.J. Silverman. 2010b. Identifying structures, processes, resources and needs of research ethics committees in Egypt. *BMC Medical Ethics* 11: 12.

Tangwa, G.B. 2004. Between universalism and relativism: A conceptual exploration of problems in formulating and applying international biomedical ethical guidelines. *Journal of Medical Ethics* 30 (1): 63–67.

United Nations Educational, Scientific, and Cultural Organizations. n.d. UNESCO science report 2010. *The current status of science around the world*. Available at: http://unesdoc.unesco.org/images/0018/001898/189883E.pdf

World Medical Association. 2013. *Declaration of Helsinki*. Available at: http://www.wma.net/en/30publications/10policies/b3/.

Islam and Bioethics

Nahed M. Ali and Samer S. El-Kamary

For the last several decades, bioethics have progressively developed in the life sciences and health due to rapid progress in research and advanced medical therapeutics coupled with the realization that not all that medicine can do for patients necessarily means that all should be done.

The same line of thinking applies to research, as there are appropriate limits to the harms and wrongs that should occur to research participants, even if "it might be highly advantageous to science" (Bernard 1865). Essentially, there may be a variety of moral costs associated with human progress that should not be borne by individuals and society. This caveat warrants a careful balancing between scientific progress against the protection of the rights and welfare of research participants. As such, national governments and international organizations have developed bioethical principles and guidelines for the ethical conduct of research. This institutionalization of ethics is accomplished in each country based on different social, cultural, economic, and religious contexts. While commentators have stressed the secularization of ethics (Engelhardt 1998), one cannot deny that bioethics in general have been informed by the principles of religious morality. Nowhere is this more evident than in the Arab region, where Islam plays a dominant role in the everyday lives of the majority of the population. As such, one must take into consideration the instances in which religious values contribute to the basis of bioethics.

Acknowledgement of the role that Islamic principles and teachings have in the Arab region contrasts with the secularization of ethics that has occurred in the West for centuries. As such, people in the Arab world might not be comfortable with western-style bioethics and want bioethical considerations to be consistent with

N.M. Ali (✉)
Faculty of Medicine, Suez Canal University, Ismailia, Egypt
e-mail: Ali.nahed@med.suez.edu.eg

S.S. El-Kamary
Epidemiology & Public Health, University of Maryland Baltimore, Baltimore, MD, USA

H. Silverman (ed.), *Research Ethics in the Arab Region*, Research Ethics Forum 5,
https://doi.org/10.1007/978-3-319-65266-5_2

Islamic principles. It should be noted that this conviction is upheld not only by Islam, but is shared by the other monotheistic religions in the region. Indeed, the moral conduct of those who follow the three monotheistic religions are profoundly influenced by the presence of God in their lives, as well as their interpretations of their respective religious texts in determining appropriate behavior and ethical practice, interpretations that might vary considerably among them (Boustany 2011).

Although we acknowledge the existence of all three monotheistic religions in the Middle East and North Africa, since Muslims are in the majority, one must take into consideration how Islamic religious values contribute to the basis of bioethics in the Arab region, especially since there is no prior or contemporary Islamic theory of bioethics that delineates the necessary and sufficient principles by which one can justify bioethical issues (Darwish 2014). Instead, Arab bioethicists, most of whom are religious scholars, appeal to sources of Islamic Law, which we now will attempt to further elucidate.

The Sources of Islamic Law

Islamic Religious Law, commonly known as the Shari'a consists of precepts and principles developed by Muslim scholars and jurists over centuries. While in Western culture the law regulates only some sectors of behavior, the influence of Shari'a is far more extensive in the sphere of the private, social, political and religious life of the believer. For Muslim law, each human act belongs to one of the following five categories: compulsory (fard, wagib), recommended (mandub, mustahabb), free (ja'iz, mubah), reprehensible or unadvised (makruh) and forbidden (haram).

The power of Shari'a to regulate the behavior of Muslims derives from its moral and religious authority. At the basis of the Shari'a there are four "roots of the law" or sources, from which the principles and rules of Muslim law have been drawn and of which the first three are of divine origin (An-Na'im 1990; Atighetchi 2009; Free Online Islamic Course 2016). These roots are as follows:

1. The Holy Qur'an
2. Sunnah and Hadith of the Prophet Muhammad (Peace Be Upon Him-PBUH)
3. Ijma' (unanimous consensus)
4. Qiyas (reasoning by analogy).

The Holy Qur'an

Muslims believe that the Holy Qur'an is the compiled and unchanged words of Allah (the Arabic word for God). To avoid possible alterations over time, a clear distinction was made between the Qur'an and any accompanying explanations or interpretations (which were never included in the Qur'an itself). It is the real foundation on which the entire structure of Islam rests. The Holy Qur'an is the absolute and the final authority in any discussion related to Islamic principles or codes. One could even say that the Holy Qur'an is the only source and that the other two sources are directly or indirectly derived from the Quranic teachings. The Holy Qur'an, however, deals with the **essentials**. It left the **details** to be explained by Prophet Muhammed through the Hadith and Sunnah. Through the process of consensus (Ijma'), Muslim scholars use the principles set forth in the Qur'an, Hadith and Sunnah to formulate contemporary laws and solutions.

The Sunnah and Hadith

After the Holy Qur'an, the most important Islamic textual material is the *Sunnah* and *Hadith* of the Prophet Muhammad. The *Sunnah* represent the practices of the Prophet Muhammad while the *Hadith* encompasses his sayings. If Qur'an and Sunnah is not clear about an issue, then it is obligatory on Muslim scholars to arrive at a proper solution in light of the Qur'an and Hadith.

It must be remembered that there is a clear distinction between the Holy Qur'an and the Hadith; the Holy Qur'an is the Word of Allah. Hadith, on the other hand, is the word of the Prophet Muhammad, as narrated by various persons.

As the Holy Qur'an deals mainly with the broad principles of Islam, the details were frequently supplied by Prophet Muhammad, by his practices and his sayings. Since written communication was not very common in those days, the transmission of the practices and sayings of the Prophet took place from one person to another by the word of mouth.

While the Qur'an was memorized verbatim by Prophet Muhammed and his companions throughout his lifetime, and it was collected and recorded soon after his death, it took almost two centuries to collect, verify, and record the Sunnah. And, because Shari'a is derived from the Sunnah as well as the Qur'an, its development as a comprehensive legal and ethical system had to await the collection and authentication of the Sunnah. The jurists who founded the main schools of Islamic jurisprudence to which the vast majority of modern Muslims follow, did their founding work between the middle of the eighth century and the middle of the ninth century CE, 100–200 years after the Prophet's death. The techniques and methods for the derivation of general principles and specific rules of Shari'a, such as ijma' (consensus) and qiyas (analogy) were not settled until the ninth century.

Ijma' (Unanimous Consensus)

Ijma' refers to the consensus of the community, which is sought when then are questions about appropriate practices (or at least the consensus of the legal scholars within the community). The Prophet Muhammad once said that his community (i.e. the Muslim community) would never agree on an error. Although defined as the third source in order of importance, as there is "continuous and unanimous" agreement of the Muslim scholars, it is considered as a valid source of Law reflecting a position that is inspired by God.

Qiyas (Analogy)

When the first three sources of divine inspiration fail to provide a clear rule of conduct in a given situation, it becomes lawful for the majority of the legal schools and within very varying limits, to have recourse to qiyas or reasoning by analogy and legal precedent to decide new case law. *Qiyas* implies trying to draw a directive for a situation, which is not expressly mentioned in the *Shari'a*, from another situation, which closely resembles it and about which there is an express directive of the *Shari'a*. For instance, 'if a person says that because the affects of taking drugs is comparable to that of consuming liquor, therefore, the punishment for taking drugs should be the same as consuming liquor', the person would be said to have made *Qiyas* (drawn analogy) on the punishment of taking liquor and derived the punishment for taking drugs.

Qiyas (reasoning from analogy) is a kind of *Ijtehad*, which is an Islamic legal term that means "independent reasoning" or the exercise of judgement or "the utmost effort an individual can put forth in an activity." It is recognized as the decision-making process in Islamic law (sharia) through personal effort (jihad) which is completely independent of any school (madhhab) of jurisprudence (fiqh)

The first three sources of the religious law (the Qur'an, Sunnah and ijma') represent the only unquestioned authorities in Islam. However, after the death of the Prophet in 632 CE, it became evident that a mere literal knowledge of the Qur'an and the "sayings" of the Prophet would not be sufficient to provide guidance for conduct on many problems. Hence, the jurists during the early centuries after Muhammad used qiyas with considerable freedom in their effort to "personally" interpret (Ijtehad), explain and comment upon the "roots" of the law, consequently drawing on them for the principles and rules of the Shari'a.

Indeed, Shari'a consists of a vast body of jurisprudence in which individual jurists express their views on the meaning of the Qur'an and Sunnah and the legal implications of those views. Thus, the Shari'a has a considerable capacity of adaptation to situations as they vary: a peculiarity made historically possible as Islam does not have a supreme juridical-religious authority, nor an official teaching capable of guiding the faithful in all the circumstances on which the three sources are lacking in precise and exhaustive directives (Atighetchi 2009). This flexibility was one of the elements that contributed to the expansion of Islam over the centuries to completely different peoples and geographical regions, without interfering with the local cultures, but only instilling the few fundamental principles of the faith of Muslim law.

As such, when the sources of Muslim law do not express clearly on new situations caused by new social changes and by challenges presented by biomedicine, the doctors of Muslim law (muftis, fuqaha, ulama) use the analogical method (qiyas) and personal interpretation (ijtehad) and issue fatawas, i.e., juridical opinions with which to explain to the faithful the prescriptions contained in the Sources, indicating how to behave in the case in point. Influential fatwas, therefore, sometimes offer support for various medical practices and facilitate the articulation of laws that regulate these practices. To be sure, a fatwa represents at least morally, the rule of conduct to be followed for the faithful of the same juridical school and hence, may be contradicted by the opinions of other jurists.

In addition to fatwas issues by prominent jurists, to provide more adequate answers to the challenges of modernity and specifically to respond to the technological advances in medicine that go beyond the traditional competences of the jurists, Muslims increasingly depend on the opinions provided by meetings, conferences, congresses and academies that bring together jurists and experts from various parts of the Muslim world (Atighetchi 2009).

Regarding individual Muslim countries, while the constitutions contain an article specifying that Shari'a forms one of the sources of the Laws of the state, it is the State that is authorized to issues the law and the various State-appointed muftis are solicited to justify, from the juridical-religious point of view, the political and social programs of the government. However, regarding bioethics and the delicacy of the subjects in question, state legislations generally give great considerable weight to the opinions of the most authoritative jurists residing in the country. That said, the above helps explain how the different countries might take on different positions on bioethical issues and explain why they can each find authority in the classic juridical reflection and be legitimized from the religious point of view.

While a considerable amount of different and even contradictory responses may be seen when there are no clear indications by the Sacred Sources, this should not be seen as a sort of ethical pluralism intrinsic to the Muslim communities (Atighetchi 2009). Ethical relativism is unacceptable according to the Muslim point of view. The truth is already present in the Sacred Sources, which needs to be interpreted correctly by the different jurists, who then must achieve consensus. To be sure, many professionals seek out the opinion of theologians to find answers to the new bioethical issues, but these can be based only on analogies and not on "explicit doctrines, the conclusions of these processes only represent personal interpretations that are potentially different form one another.

While religion affects the ethical behavior of many followers in the Arab countries, it is not the sole determinant of people's practices. Mohamed Arkoun writes: "The Qur'an does not impose definitive solutions to the problems of human existence. It attempts to instigate man to look upon himself and the world…." (Arkoun 1978). Essentially, people must find solutions to problems inherent to human existence together, as there are no standards that prescribe proper behavior in all circumstances and contexts. Thus, it is essential to articulate a set of shared ethical guidelines that are based on human rationality and are multi-denominational and multidisciplinary.

Whether this turns out to be equivalent to Western bioethical principles is not the issue. That said, there have been several commentators who have gone back to the Qur'an to find sources for the principles of "Western" bioethics, which are those of principalism and include the principles of autonomy, beneficence, non-maleficence, and justice (Aksoy and Tenik 2002; Serour 1994). However, the identification of these principles in the Qur'an should not come as a surprise, as they are quite straightforward, as God summons the believer to make a responsible choice according to his faith, to invite to righteousness, do good, to avoid evil, and to apply justice (Qur'an).

If universal principles of bioethics exist, what needs to be recognized is that Western and Islamic scholars might attach different weights and priorities to these principles. Differences that can be partially explained by Western bioethics being rights-based with a strong emphasis on individual rights; whereas Islamic bioethics is based on duties and obligations. As such, variations between Western bioethics and Islam arise in the interpretation and application of these principles, that is, in the attempt to adapt them to local cultures and customs. By way of example, the Western world gives priority to the principle of autonomy, which is explained by its liberal-individualistic political culture; whereas in the Muslim context, a collective interest is considered in addition to that of the individual.

Furthermore, even within the Muslim community, as there is no supreme juridical-religious authority that exists in the religion of Islam (as explained previously), a vast range of positions for several bioethical issues will always exist. Such differences are based on the different interpretations of the Qur'an, although all have the intention of being legitimized by the Sacred Texts. Realizing this state of affairs, one of the goals of this volume is to describe how and in what situations these seemingly universal principles of bioethics are applied differently in an Arab context. To achieve this goal, the authors of the individual chapters represent indigenous scholars from the Arab region who have had direct and personal involvement of the application of these principles in their cultural and social contexts. It is for this reason that makes this collection of essays unique.

References

Aksoy, S., and A. Tenik. 2002. The 'four principles of bioethics' as found in 13th century Muslim scholar Mawlana's teachings. *BMC Medical Ethics* 3: E4. Retrieved from http://www.ncbi.nlm.nih.gov/pubmed/12370082.

An-Na'im, A.A. 1990. Human rights in the Muslim world: Socio-political conditions and scriptural imperatives: A preliminary inquiry. *Harvard Human Rights Journal* 3: 13–52.

Arkoun, M. 1978. *L'Islam hier-demain*. Paris: Buchet/Chastel.

Atighetchi, D. 2009. *Islamic bioethics: Problems and perspectives*. Dordrecht: Springer.

Bernard, C. 1865. *An introduction to the study of experimental medicine*. Macmillan & Co., Ltd. (First English translation, 1927).

Boustany, F.N. 2011. *Bioethics and Monotheistic Religions*, Ethics and law in biomedicine and genetics: An overview of national regulations in the Arab States. Cairo: United Nations Educational, Scientific and Cultural Organization (UNESCO).

Darwish, B. 2014. Arab perspectives. In *Handbook of global bioethics*, ed. H.A.M.J. ten Have and B. Gordijn. Dordrecht: Springer.

Engelhardt, H.T., Jr. 1998. Critical care: Why there is no global bioethics. *The Journal of Medicine and Philosophy* 23 (6): 643–651. https://doi.org/10.1076/jmep.23.6.643.2555.

Free Online Islamic Course. 2016. The sources of Islamic law. Available at: http://free-islamic-course.org/stageone/stageone-module-4/sources-islamic-law.html.

Qur'an. Surah 3. Al-i'Imran, Ayah 104. Available at: http://quran.com/3/104-116.

Serour, G. 1994. Islam and the four principles. In *Principles of health care ethics*, ed. R. Gillon, 75–91. London: Wiley.

Part I

Ethical Issues in Research

What Kind of Research Ethics for the Arab Region?

Henry Silverman

The international guidelines on research ethics rely predominantly on deontological prescriptions that emphasize respect for autonomy, maintaining privacy and confidentiality, and ensuring justice, as well as consequentialistic argumentation that focuses on minimizing harms, maximizing benefits, and providing safeguards to participants prone to be vulnerable. These two main ethical theories represent the dominant ways of evaluating ethical behavior in the West. However, many find arguments from deontology and consequentialism difficult to apply and often inadequate to cover complex situations. Alternatively, the authors of the Belmont Report put forth prima facie principles of respect for persons, beneficence, non-maleficence and justice and when these principles conflict with each other, one uses moral judgement and intuition to balance these principles in an effort to identify a morally correct of action. The use of these principles to guide ethical behavior is known as principlism, as originally developed by Beauchamp and Childress (2012). These principles have been regarded by many as universal and assumed to transcend traditional and cultural boundaries.

Despite claims that principlism offers a framework for problem solving that is neutral between competing religions, cultures, and philosophical theories and hence, can be shared by everyone regardless of their backgrounds (Gillon 1994), it has been criticized on two accounts. First, it is overly reliant on a Western value system that does not overlap fully with value systems of other cultures. It is instructive to note that the initial guidelines regarding research ethics were conceived mainly from a Western bioethics framework without participation from the South, i.e., from the low- and middle-income countries (LMICs). The blanket application of so-called universal principles drawn from a western bioethics may be inappropriate to communities who reject the Enlightenment view of individuals considered in isolation, as opposed to living within a web of relationships (Israel 2015). Rather than endorsing

H. Silverman (✉)
University of Maryland, Baltimore, MD, USA
e-mail: hsilverm@medicine.umaryland.edu

H. Silverman (ed.), *Research Ethics in the Arab Region*, Research Ethics Forum 5,
https://doi.org/10.1007/978-3-319-65266-5_3

an alleged set of universal principles, many contend that ethical standards should incorporate local values and cultural norms (Christakis and Levine 1995).

A second concern with a Western-based bioethics, especially when applied to international settings, is that current concepts of research ethics ignore that "interactions between researchers and research participants are grounded in the broader structural relationships of domination and subordination through research" (Israel 2015). This second challenge to the apparent neutrality of research ethics has come from postcolonial theorists, who recognize that contemporary social relations occur in the aftermath of colonialism. To respond to this postcolonial viewpoint, a more "just" research "ethic" should enable and promote social justice (Cannella and Lincoln 2011; London 2010) as well as the "empowerment" of research participants (Hammersley and Traianou 2014). In contrast, the current research enterprise is focused on a narrower concept of distributive justice that views "research as a commodity to be allocated by market mechanisms" (London 2010) and that the central issue of fairness is a micro-level concern of preventing exploitation within individual transactions, and hence, is mainly focused on the fair distribution of the benefits of research across the involved population (Denzin and Giardina 2007). My aim in this chapter is to further explore these competing viewpoints of a contemporary approach to research ethics and advance the concept that arguing for a distinction between universalism and relativism fails to do the heavy moral lifting needed for a more "inclusive" bioethics that leads to an "emancipatory" bioethics for international collaborative relationships.

Universalism or Relativism?: The Inadequacy of the Principlism Approach

With the increasing prominence of collaborative research activities between Western investigators and those in LMICs, the question has been raised as to whether ethical rules governing the conduct of research are the same wherever research is performed or do they vary according to the cultural setting? (Christakis and Levine 1995; Tangwa 2004).

The tension, as framed by Macklin, asks whether ethical standards for research are universally applicable or are variations permissible relative to cultural norms and other differences (economic or political) among countries? Respect for diversity fuels this form of ethical relativism, which "rejects the notion that a single set of ethical standards for research should prevail in our culturally diverse world". Macklin responds to this tension between universalism and relativism (or pluralism) by stating that "These substantive principles constitute ethical standards, and should be applied universally…Procedural requirements, on the other hand, may vary according to cultural and other differences in multinational research" (Macklin 2008). In other words, ethical standards are higher order universal principles that will generate different codes of conduct in each society (Macklin 1999).

Macklin further opines that a problem with ethical relativism that ignores "ethical standards widely accepted elsewhere, [is that it would allow] virtually any standard a country desired" (Macklin 2008). Similarly, Tangwa states: "At the level of application, the important thing again is to grasp the ethical imperative underlying the guideline and cultural and circumstantial particulars will then do the work of 'shaping and colouring' the guideline without any need for further deliberate effort" (Tangwa 2004).

There is recognition, however, that international documents do not "transplant well" to geography (Israel 2015) and that Western ethical codes can have the "effect of silencing indigenous approaches to ethics" (Tikly and Bond 2013). For example, a researcher from Africa who graduated from a research ethics training program situated in Canada concluded: "While the adoption of Canadian models is tempting because it would be easier, it does not necessarily fit within local contexts, especially when it comes to Islamic bioethics" (De Vries and Rott 2011). Another student pointed out the model of ethical reasoning that is almost universally taught – principlism – is not an easy fit in most developing countries, where the principles may not fit seamlessly with cultural values (De Vries and Rott 2011).

In general, bioethics students from LMICs find several problems with the principlism approach they were learning. For example, students from non-Western cultures frequently identify the principle of autonomy as being most problematic, as they see a disjuncture between their cultural values and the individualism implicit in Western notions of autonomy. A student from a Muslim country noted: "…in [Islam]…justice [is more important] than autonomy…Islam said first your neighborhood…not first yourself" (De Vries and Rott 2011). Indeed, in the West autonomy is conceived in a radically individualist manner, and as such, much emphasis is placed on individual's rights, autonomy, self-determination, and privacy. However, this contrasts with the more relational definitions "of a person found in many non-Western societies that stress the embeddedness of the individual within society and define a person by means of relations to others" (Christakis and Levine 1995). Indeed, critical scholars have rejected the idea that individuals can be considered in isolation, (Israel 2015). Similarly, Chilisa argues that an African research ethics could combine the African concepts of Ma'at (balance and harmony), Ujima (collective work), and Ubuntu (togetherness), which in the context of research would respect "the importance of consensus, interconnectedness and community" (Chilisa and Preece 2005).

These concepts that embrace a "web of relationships" have implications for informed consent, as many from LMICs have found the application of autonomy to be most challenging for the informed consent process. For example, in a study investigating informed consent processes in rural India, 63.2% of potential research participants said they would need to at least consult with other individuals e.g., family, friends, or neighbors in the village. Also, four of seven women said they would not be able to decide for themselves and would abide by decisions taken by others, e.g., husband or mother-in-law (DeCosta et al. 2004).

Macklin maintains, however, that other cultures can "adjust" the concept of autonomy to incorporate more communal ideas of autonomy. She argues that the four principles are sufficiently abstract that they can "float above", and yet account for the peculiarities of culture. However, others believe that rather than "adjust", the focus of the consent process may need to "shift" from the individual to the family or to the community, as it may be necessary to secure the consent of a participant's family or social group in addition to or even instead of the consent of the participant, assuming that proxy consent is obtained in good faith without the potential for exploitation of the participant (Christakis and Levine 1995; De Vries and Rott 2011).

The example that Macklin gives to demonstrate that the principle of autonomy can be incorporated in the value systems of other cultures actually reveals the difficulties of cultures "adjusting" to this principle. Her example describes a previous randomized clinical trial of adjuvant treatment for breast cancer conducted in Vietnam. The investigators were made aware that patients in Vietnam depend on their physicians to choose the appropriate treatment for them and hence, they wanted to withhold any elements of the consent script that would suggest uncertainty by the treating doctor and that treatment would be determined by randomization. The institutional review board (IRB) in the U.S. disagreed and required no alteration to the elements of informed consent. Three months after the trial, the investigators performed a survey involving a small sample of the study participants to determine their understanding of the informed consent. Macklin states that the results of this survey suggest that the women demonstrated an understanding that their treatments were determined by randomization. However, the survey results specifically showed that the participants "were evenly split in answering whether they or the research plan decided treatment", which led the investigators to conclude that "it is unclear whether they understood that their treatment was determined by randomization" (Love and Fost 1997).

This example compels a re-examination of the ethical underpinning of informed consent and the strict application of and the role of autonomy for a valid consent. Does informed consent serve to advance only autonomy or is it better equated with "respect for persons", in which case informed consent may need to accommodate values other than autonomy? (Dickert 2009) Recently, commentators have recommended that other ethical functions, including "promoting concordance with participants' values", are necessary for a valid informed consent (Dickert 2017). This would entail that the informed consent process should respect values that are fundamental in different cultural settings. Accordingly, in the Vietnam study, approving the request for an "altered" consent process would have been justified to respect the cultural values of the Vietnam participants.

Western bioethicists point out, however, that an informed consent process that ensures autonomous authorization provides a protection mechanism for potential participants for research involving more than minimal risk. But limitations in understanding of certain elements of informed consent that interferes with authorization may not preclude participants the ability to control their enrollment choices and additionally, other safeguards can be instituted to provide additional protection. Indeed, in the post-trial survey study, participants in the Vietnam study demonstrated they understood that they had control over their enrollment choices (Mandava et al. 2012; Miller and Wertheimer 2011). Commentators have claimed that autonomous authroization is not always necessary for a valid consent (Miller and Wertheimer 2011).

Furthermore, even in Western contexts, waivers and alternations of consent are permissible when it meets several criteria, which include: (1) subjects are exposed to no more than minimal risk; (2) the waiver or alteration does not adversely affect subject rights and welfare; (3) the research could not practicably be carried out without the waiver or alteration; and (4) subjects will be provided with additional pertinent information after participation, when appropriate.

If autonomous authorization is not necessary in certain research performed in the West, then in contexts where other cultural values conflict with autonomy, one can ask whether traditional in-depth informed consent can be altered, as was requested in the Vietnam study, under an expanded concept of "impracticableness" and a broaden concept of participants' rights? Christakas asks that rather than searching for a single model of transcultural research ethics, there should be discourse between holders of different ethical systems that requires mutual understanding "of the very meaning of what ethical systems are and what their function is" (Christakis 1992).

There is an emerging critique of and distrust for insisting on a universal Western ethic. In India, for example, Chattopadhyay questioned the threat of a 'neocolonial moral imperialism', which would deliver an American or European mantra of universal ethical principles (Chattopadhyay 2011). Similarly, Tangwa states: "Most of these codes have been firmly based in a Western tradition and given their aim of universalizing that paradigm, have invoked deep suspicion in other communities (Tangwa 2004). Indeed, some see the global export of principlism as part of broader international flows of capital, students, and academics, as well as knowledge and ideology (Israel 2015). It is thought that researchers who fail to comply with imported ethical requirements risk losing their funding or having their papers rejected by publishers. DeVries and Rott portrayed some training programs sponsored by international funders (e.g., World Health Organization, Fogarty International Center, UNESCO, and the Welcome Trust) as a one-way flow of western ideas and influence (De Vries and Rott 2015). Recent commentators, however, have documented that non-Western bioethical concepts are also taught in such training programs (Matar et al. 2014; Ndebele et al. 2014).

When international researchers resist the roll out of universal ethical norms, they may be seeking guidelines that display greater cultural sensitivity and incorporation of a broader set of ethical values. For others, opposition to universalistic claims is not simply targeted at insensitivity to other values, but draws on an even greater agenda that calls for a deeper understanding of and engagement with how different societies, cultures, and communities understand ethics and the conduct of ethical research.

A Research Ethics Informed by Post-colonial Theory

In addition to the inclusion of ethical values embraced by other cultures, postcolonial theory provides an additional context for understanding a more inclusive research ethics. In essence, the postcolonial condition should serve as a basis for developing an emancipatory research ethics driven by a social justice imperative rather than one based on "narrow" concept of distributive justice.

As pointed out by King et al., justice is the least well understood and most neglected of the ethical principles presented in the Belmont Report (King et al. 1999). In the Belmont Report, the principle of justice was narrowly focused on fair selection of subjects and the fair distribution of the benefits of research across a population (King 2005). Seemingly, this idea of justice mandates that there should be a fair balance between what each side gains from the research relationship (Hammersley and Traianou 2014), but without a normative account of what is fair, the concern remains that the researcher gains much more than those who are researched. Specifically, researchers are portrayed as extracting data and information for free in order to generate research products, which even if these do not produce immediate financial return, nevertheless potentially provide benefits in terms of reputation and promotion prospects. In effect, the charge is that the relationship between researcher and researched has sometimes been or perhaps intrinsically exploitative.

This focus on distributive justice that embraces exploitation as the fundamental concern of fairness in international research has led commentators to consider that it is the amount of benefits rather than the kind of benefit that matters the most in transactions between countries in the North and South. As such, research is regarded "as a commodity to be allocated by market mechanisms" (London 2010) and the measure of fairness depends on whether researchers and sponsors on one hand, and the host communities on the other hand, have received sufficient economic benefits for themselves.

This utilitarian market driven approach is particularly evident in much of the research that is conducted by sponsors and some aid agencies. That is, the dominant principle or ethic is 'value for money' and economic growth, which becomes the main criterion through which development and progress are evaluated. Favored methodologies reflect these concerns and include, for example, forms of econometric and cost benefit analysis and randomized control trials (Israel 2015). Such an emphasis has led to focusing solely on economic growth (e.g., the predominant interests of randomized clinical trials) rather than on the development of capabilities that individuals and groups require to realize their valued functionings, something that is more highly valued due to the effects of colonialism. The concern with 'value for money' has the effect of privileging some kinds of research questions and problems while silencing others, for example, social justice issues (Santos 2012). Indeed, the narrow focus of the principle of justice in the Belmont report fails to take into account social justice, "including historical patterns of oppression and domination" (Friesen et al. 2017). A conception of justice informed by post-colonial approaches has in recent years appeared as a stronger more active principle, one that is related to past, present, and future distributions of power.

Crucially, "colonized and formerly colonized groups continue to struggle against it effects" and trying to respond to the "emergence of a new imperialism", by which is meant the economic, political, military and cultural hegemony of the U.S. and its Western allies within contemporary globalization.

Essentially, postcolonial theorists have recognized that contemporary social relations, including the research endeavor, occur in the presence or the aftermath of colonialism. Postcolonial theory makes a distinctive contribution to the understanding of research ethics by using the postcolonial "condition" as a basis for deconstructing dominant approaches to research ethics (Israel 2015). Cannella and

Lincoln calls for a new ethical relation between North and South that would "address contemporary political and power orientations by recognizing that the investigator and investigated (whether people, institutions or systems) are subjects of the presence or aftermath of colonialism" (Cannella and Lincoln 2011).

As such, current debates about fairness in research have focused on whether the knowledge generating activities will serve as a means of expanding the capacity of the health related social structures in a community to meet the health needs of community members and improve the health of burdened populations (London 2010). As a consequence of this shift in focus between competing concepts of justice is that the empowerment of research participants is an ethical imperative (Hammersley and Traianou 2014) and that to "tackle the question of how to do research fairly in an unjust world, we need to move beyond the narrow rubric of exploitation…." (London 2010). Consideration of the post-colonial condition provides a context for identifying issues and questions for research and understanding ongoing inequalities in the research process.

In addition to issues revolving around the subject matter of justice in post-colonial conditions, attention is required on procedural justice, that is, the research process itself. Specifically, people whose lives are being investigated must participate on at least equal terms in the development and conduct of research. Typically, research participants have been viewed principally as informants rather than as active participants in the research process and in this sense, researchers were viewed as being predatory by co-opting informants to their purposes (Cannella and Lincoln 2007). As such, doing research "on" people rather than "involving" them in the research process is viewed as itself unjust, because it involves a differential distribution of rights or power. Second, the argument that doing research on certain types of people without involving them in the research as partners is unjust, because it is believed that the wider context within which the research function change, marginalizes or oppresses those people.

A new way forward would embrace a "countercolonial solidarity" that revolves around the politics of partnership in a context where research increasingly takes place in cross national teams (Cannella and Lincoln 2011). It would involve engaging with the complexities of power relationships between researchers and researched in post-colonial settings. Such an emancipatory intention is to bring to the forefront the voices and experience of those who have been historically marginalized by the colonial encounter. "Giving an increasing say to other communities, peoples and cultures and incorporating their views in international regulatory documents…is one way of helping to complete the process of decolonization in a world increasingly becoming a global village." (Tangwa 2004).

Here the implication is that a participatory approach is required in order to achieve this goal and the primary methodology ought to include a dialogical approach between the interested parties (Tikly and Bond 2013). It would seek to identify key ethical questions at each stage of the research process. Who defines the research questions and in whose interests? How are the roles and responsibilities defined within cross cultural teams? What are the theoretical and methodological assumptions guiding the research? How can the research be conducted ethically and in the best interests of the researched? Who benefits from the research findings? To what extent can the research contribute to the development of an ecology of knowledge and to an epistemology of the South that can act in the interests of the historically marginalized? (Tikly and Bond 2013).

There is recent evidence that such a dialogical approach has taken place insofar that community partnership is being recognized as an important ethical principle in research. For example, in the framework developed by Emanuel and colleagues, collaborative partnership is one of the eight ethical requirements of international research (Emanuel et al. 2004). Furthermore, the revised CIOMS has a new guideline on community engagement that recommends a proactive and sustained engagement with the communities from which individuals will be invited to participate that shows respect for them and for the traditions and norms that they share (Council for International Organizations of Medical Sciences (CIOMS) and World Health Organization (WHO) 2016). The idea is to construct a critical research ethics agenda in which "societal structures, institutions and oppressions become the subject… of research (rather than human beings) [with a view to] avoid further…subjectification of an or the Other" (Cannella and Lincoln 2011).

References

Beauchamp, T., and J. Childress. 2012. *Principles of biomedical ethics*. Oxford: Oxford University Press.

Cannella, G., and Y. Lincoln. 2011. Ethics, research regulations and critical social science. In *The Sage handbook of qualitative research*, ed. N. Denzin and Y. Lincoln, 4th ed., 81–89. Thousand Oaks: Sage.

Cannella, Gaile, and S., Yvonna Lincoln. 2007. Predatory vs. Dialogic ethics constructing an Illusion or ethical practice as the core of research methods. *Qualitative Inquiry* 13: 315–335. https://doi.org/10.1177/1077800406297648.

Chattopadhyay, S. 2011. Facing up to the hard problems: Western bioethics in the eastern land of India. In *Bioethics around the globe*, ed. C. Myser, 19–38. Oxford: Oxford University Press.

Chilisa, B., and J. Preece. 2005. *Research methods for adult educators in Africa*. Cape Town: Pearson/UNESCO.

Christakis, N.A. 1992. Ethics are local: Engaging cross-cultural variation in the ethics for clinical research. *Social Science & Medicine* 35 (9): 1079–1091.

Christakis, N., and R.J. Levine. 1995. Multinational research. In *Encyclopedia of bioethics,* Revised ed. ed. W. T. Reich. New York: Schuster Macmillan.

Council for International Organizations of Medical Sciences (CIOMS), & World Health Organization (WHO). 2016. *International ethical guidelines for health-related research involving humans* Vol. Retrieved from: http://www.cioms.ch/index.php/12-newsflash/400-cioms-inernational-ethical-guidelines

De Vries, R., and L. Rott. 2011. Bioethics as missionary work. The export of western ethics to developing countries. In *Bioethics around the globe*, ed. C. Myser. Oxford: Oxford University Press.

De Vries, R., and L. Rott. 2015. Bioethics as missionary work. The Export of Western Ethics to Developing Countries *Bioethics Around the World.*

DeCosta, A., N. D'Souza, S. Krishnan, M.S. Chhabra, I. Shihaam, and K. Goswami. 2004. Community based trials and informed consent in rural north India. *Journal of Medical Ethics* 30 (3): 318–323.

Denzin, N., and M.D. Giardina. 2007. Introduction: Ethical futures in qualitative research. In *Ethical futures in qualitative research: Decolonizing the politics of knowledge*, ed. N. Denzin and M. Giardina, 9–44. Walnut Creek: Left Coast Press.

Dickert, N.W. 2009. Re-examining respect for human research participants. *Kennedy Institute of Ethics Journal* 19 (4): 311–338.

Dickert, N. 2017. Re-framing consent for clinical research: A function-based approach. *American Journal of Bioethics*. In Press.

Emanuel, E.J., D. Wendler, J. Killen, and C. Grady. 2004. What makes clinical research in developing countries ethical? The benchmarks of ethical research. *The Journal of Infectious Diseases* 189 (5): 930–937. https://doi.org/10.1086/381709.

Friesen, P., L. Kearns, B. Redman, and A.L. Caplan. 2017. Rethinking the Belmont report? *The American Journal of Bioethics* 17 (7): 15–21. https://doi.org/10.1080/15265161.2017.1329482.

Gillon, R. 1994. Medical ethics: Four principles plus attention to scope. *British Medical Journal* 309: 184–188.

Hammersley, M., and A. Traianou. 2014. An alternative ethics? Justice and care as guiding principles for qualitative research. *Sociological Research Online* 19 (3): 1–14. Retrieved from: http://www.socresonline.org.uk/19/13/24.html.

Israel, M. 2015. *Research ethics and integrity for social scientists: Beyond regulatory compliance*. 2nd ed. London: Sage.

King, A. 2005. Justice beyond Belmont. In *Belmont revisited: Ethical principles for research with human subjects*, ed. J.F. Childress, E.M. Meslin, and H.T. Shapiro, 136–147. Washington, DC: Georgetown University Press.

King, N., G. Henderson, and J. Stein. 1999. *Beyond regulations: Ethics in human subjects research*. Chapel Hill: University of North Carolina Press.

London, A.J. 2010. Justice in the application of science: Beyond fair benefits. *The American Journal of Bioethics* 10 (6): 54–56. https://doi.org/10.1080/15265161.2010.483184.

Love, R.R., and N.C. Fost. 1997. Ethical and regulatory challenges in a randomized control trial of adjuvant treatment for breast cancer in Vietnam. *Journal of Investigative Medicine* 45 (8): 423–431.

Macklin, R. 1999. *Against relativism: Cultural diversity and the search for ethical universals in medicine*. New York: Oxford University Press.

———. 2008. Appropriate ethical standards. In *The oxford textbook of clinical research ethics*, ed. E.J. Emanuel, C. Grady, R.A. Crouch, R.K. Lie, F.G. Miller, and D. Wendler. New York: Oxford University Press.

Mandava, A., C. Pace, B. Campbell, E. Emanuel, and C. Grady. 2012. The quality of informed consent: Mapping the landscape. A review of empirical data from developing and developed countries. *Journal of Medical Ethics* 38 (6): 356–365. https://doi.org/10.1136/medethics-2011-100178.

Miller, F.G., and A. Wertheimer. 2011. The fair transaction model of informed consent: An alternative to autonomous authorization. *Kennedy Institute of Ethics Journal* 21: 201–2018.

Matar, A., S. Garner, J. Millum, B. Sina, and H. Silverman. 2014. Curricular aspects of the Fogarty bioethics international training programs. *Journal of Empirical Research on Human Research Ethics* 9 (2): 12–23. https://doi.org/10.1525/jer.2014.9.2.12.

Ndebele, P., D. Wassenaar, S. Benatar, T. Fleischer, M. Kruger, C. Adebamowo, et al. 2014. Research ethics capacity building in Sub-Saharan Africa: A review of NIH Fogarty-funded programs 2000-2012. *Journal of Empirical Research on Human Research Ethics* 9 (2): 24–40. https://doi.org/10.1525/jer.2014.9.2.24.

Santos, B. 2012. The public sphere and epistemologies of the south. *African Development* 37 (1): 43–68.

Silverman, H., and S. Osman. 2017. Applicability of Dickert's function-based approach to informed consent in international settings. *The American Journal of Bioethics* 17 (12): 25–27. https://doi.org/10.1080/15265161.2017.1388873.

Tangwa, G.B. 2004. Between universalism and relativism: A conceptual exploration of problems in formulating and applying international biomedical ethical guidelines. *Journal of Medical Ethics* 30 (1): 63–67.

Tikly, L., and T. Bond. 2013. Towards a postcolonial research ethics in comparative and international education. *Compare: A Journal of Comparative and International Education* 43 (4): 422–442.

U.S. Department of Health and Human Services. Code of federal regulations. 45 CFR 46.116(d). *Protection of human subjects*. Available at: https://www.law.cornell.edu/cfr/text/45/46.116.

Exploitation and the Matter of History

Robert Wachbroit

Introduction

Exploitation is one of the most-discussed topics in the ethics of clinical research. This is not due to any particular scandal or crisis – no one has claimed that there has lately been a significant rise in the amount or range of exploitation in clinical research. The special attention on exploitation comes from an appreciation that, within the broad field of biomedical ethics, exploitation is a distinct concern of research ethics. In contrast, many of the other ethical concerns that inform the regulations of human subject research – the importance of valid consent, the requirement of a favorable risk-benefit ratio, the responsibility to protect privacy, etc. – also inform the regulations and policies of clinical care and treatment. Despite their different aims and procedures, health research and clinical care must attend to the requirements of consent, reasonable risk, privacy, etc., in order to be ethical. Consequently, ethical analyses and policies for one context often extend to the other.[1] This has not been the case with the issue of exploitation since it is not regarded as a pressing matter in clinical care.[2] In contrast, it is a pressing matter in health

[1] Nevertheless, the ethics requirements are not entirely identical. For example, the demand for valid consent is typically more rigorous and detailed in health research than in clinical care. See also, Litton, P. and Miller, F. G. (2005), A Normative Justification for Distinguishing the Ethics of Clinical Research from the Ethics of Medical Care. *The Journal of Law, Medicine & Ethics*, 33: 566–574.

[2] This is not to deny that exploitation can occur in clinical care. The point here is that as a matter of fact far more has been written about exploitation in health research than about exploitation in clinical care.

R. Wachbroit (✉)
Department of Epidemiology and Public Health, University of Maryland,
Baltimore, MD, USA
e-mail: rwachbroit@som.umaryland.edu

H. Silverman (ed.), *Research Ethics in the Arab Region*, Research Ethics Forum 5,
https://doi.org/10.1007/978-3-319-65266-5_4

research and has shaped how importantly different research ethics is from clinical ethics.[3]

Despite the serious attention that has been given to understanding exploitation in health research, no consensus has emerged regarding its meaning – what constitutes exploitation in research – or its moral force – how should cases of exploitation be addressed or remedied.[4] Part of the explanation for this, as I will try to show below, rests on what commentators take as a paradigm of exploitation. For many, that paradigm is the sweatshop. While this picture of exploitation certainly captures many cases we would recognize as exploitation, the picture is different from what others might have considered the paradigm of exploitation many years ago –the colonialist. The salient differences between these paradigms are that, according to the sweatshop paradigm, (1) history is not relevant to identifying exploitation (in the sweatshop and elsewhere), and (2) exploitation is straightforwardly remedied (in the sweatshop and elsewhere) by simply increasing the employees' wages and perhaps improving their working conditions. The colonialist paradigm is more complicated.[5] Not only does it depend upon history, a simple redistribution of wealth might not be considered an adequate or appropriate remedy. These differences can affect our understanding and response to cases of exploitation in health research.

Defining the Concept

We should begin by noting that the concept of exploitation can be used simply as a description with no moral assessment implied. Consider cases where A takes advantage of B. We might say that the boxer exploited his opponent's fatigue in order to win the match by taking advantage of his opponent's fatigue. But simply taking advantage of someone is not enough to constitute exploitation. We wouldn't say that shopping online to take advantage of lower prices means that the shopper is exploiting the online retailer. Consequently, in order to give a definition of exploitation, we need to carefully identify what taking advantage means in the case of exploitation. Furthermore, when exploitation is understood as a moral judgment, we need to be explicit in the moral complaint being registered.

Much of the modern discussion of exploitation has been framed and advanced by the incisive writings of the late Alan Wertheimer.[6] He gives a succinct definition of exploitation:

> A exploits B means that A takes unfair advantage of B.

[3] See, for example, Hawkins, J. and Emanuel, E. (2008), *Exploitation and Developing Countries*, Oxford University Press, p 12.

[4] Many are neatly summarized in Wertheimer (2011), *Rethinking the Ethics of Clinical Research*, Oxford University Press, Chap. 5, and in https://plato.stanford.edu/entries/exploitation/

[5] For example, see: Cannella G, & Lincoln Y. (2011). Ethics, research regulations and critical social science. In Denzin N & Lincoln Y (Eds.), *The Sage Handbook of Qualitative Research* (4th ed., pp. 81–89). Thousand Oaks, CA: Sage.

[6] His last and most relevant writing on the matter is Wertheimer (2011), Chap. 5.

This definition, as Wertheimer ably shows, fits many cases we recognize to be ones of exploitation. Despite the lack of consensus, I will refer to it as "the common definition." A paradigm example is the sweatshop:

> *Sweatshop*. B is a poor framer who can no longer make an adequate living from his farm. A owns a nearby factory and offers employment. B works at the factory long hours but receives little more than subsistence wages. As a result, A reaps enormous profits.

Wertheimer's analysis contains a frank admission and an uncomfortable claim. He acknowledges that he has no satisfactory account of what an unfair transaction is. A simply receiving an unequal or even an excessive amount of benefit compared to B need not amount to unfairness.[7] We are left therefore, as some have said about pornography,[8] that, while we cannot precisely define an unfair transaction, we know it when we see it. The issue is that we have no normative baseline to draw upon. This might not raise as much concern as his further claim about the moral significance of exploitation.

In some cases exploitation results in the exploited being harmed. In some cases the exploited have been forced into their exploitation. In either case the moral assessment is clear. It is *prima facie* wrong to harm someone. This would be the situation if *Sweatshop* was changed so that B was receiving less than subsistence wages and was therefore suffering malnutrition. It is also *prima facie* wrong to coerce people and so violate their right of self-determination. This would be the situation if *Sweatshop* was changed so that B was a slave. Nevertheless, these varieties of exploitation are not exhaustive. Exploitation can occur even though both A and B are benefiting and B has validly consented to the situation or transaction. Indeed, that is assumed in *Sweatshop*.[9] How are we to assess these cases of mutually advantageous consensual exploitation (MACE). According to Wertheimer, although engaging in such arrangements is unfair, they should nevertheless be permitted – not only should they not be interfered with when they occur, they should not even be prevented. The moral significance of MACE barely registers. If B's rights have not been violated and if B stands to benefit from the situation, its unfairness counts for little and so we should not intervene. This is because it is better to benefit from an unfair situation than not to benefit at all. It would seem that, when it comes to

[7] See Wertheimer (2011) p 208ff. The surgeon who grossly overcharges his patient for an emergency, life-saving surgery could be guilty of exploitation even though the patient is getting greater value from the transaction – the value of an identifiable (non-statistical) life saved is usually thought to be much greater than the value of the money from even an overcharged fee.

[8] Justice Potter Stewart's remark in Jacobellis v. Ohio, 378 US 184 – Supreme Court 1964.

[9] Some might argue that B could not give valid consent because he had little choice, and so no viable alternative, given his economic situation. Nevertheless, Wertheimer would argue that making such hard choices is not the result of coercion, and so does not undermine valid consent, as long as B's rights were not violated. "We do *not* say that a patient's consent to surgery is involuntary, coerced, or invalid just because her only alternative is to die ..." See Wertheimer (2011) p 232.

exploitation, concerns about fairness or distributive justice should have no effect on public policy as it affects clinical research.[10]

Some scholars have offered different analyses of exploitation and its significance. Exploitation involves, to mention a few, using B as a mere means or it consists in failing to respect B as a person or it results in gross inequalities between A and B. A good deal has already been written adjudicating among these different proposals and whether they improve upon Wertheimer's account.[11] I don't wish to enter that specific fray. Instead, I would like to begin with a new definition, one that is more general and so might accommodate these different analyses and yet in some ways be more specific.

> A exploits B means that A wrongly benefits from B's vulnerability.

First of all, I've replaced the idea of taking advantage with the more explicit idea of benefiting from a vulnerability. To take advantage of someone in the case of exploitation is surely more than simply A benefits more than B in a transaction. The outcome of most paid employment is that the employer's profits are more than the wages of the employee, but most people would not regard merely being paid to do a job as exploitation. Of course, some Marxists would disagree.[12] In the case of *Sweatshop* the exploitation arises out of B's economic desperation. It is because of this vulnerability that B accepts A's offer of subsistence wages, resulting in A taking advantage of B.

The importance of the connection between exploitation and vulnerability can be underscored by considering challenge studies, such as this fictitious example:

> *Frostbite*. Researchers are conducting a study of a drug designed to prevent the damage from severe frostbite. The researchers want to work in Egypt because it is far less expensive to run a study there than in any Western country, and in past studies, they have found it easy to recruit and retain subjects in rural areas. Half of the participants will be given this drug, the other half not. All will be exposed to conditions that would lead to frostbite and all will be treated for any severe damage from frostbite that does occur. The researchers have adopted culturally appropriate informed-consent procedures and will offer subjects compensation for any injury that might occur as well as payment that is generous but not extravagant by local standards.[13]

[10] Wertheimer calls this the "Permitted Exploitation Principle" (PEP). He acknowledges that while he believes that the theoretical arguments against it are not compelling, its validity does depend upon PEP not in fact encouraging exploitation. Cf. p. 242.

[11] See Wertheimer (2011) and https://plato.stanford.edu/entries/exploitation/.

[12] To greatly simply the thought of some Marxists, if workers are creating more value than they need for their own consumption – i.e., generating a profit for their employer – they are being exploited. Cf. Roemer, J. (1988), *Free to Lose*, Harvard University Press.

[13] The idea of this case is due to David Wasserman who developed it for a course on research ethics we co-taught years ago.

Whatever complaint we might have about *Frostbite*, it is not a case of exploitation. The research team is not benefiting from the participants' vulnerabilities and so they are not guilty of exploitation.[14]

The second change is to replace "unfair" with "wrongly benefits." This might seem to be a step backwards because it is less specific. This change is warranted because, as we will see, claiming that exploitation is just a matter of unfairness might seem to prejudge matters too quickly based on an examination of simple transactions. Hence, the more general term "wrongly."

Some comments and clarifications of this definition are in order. First, it should be acknowledged that exploitation can occur even if, as in the case of *Sweatshop*, A fails to make a profit because the factory's product is not selling well. As long as A had a reasonable expectation that his enterprise, if successful, will wrongly benefit from B's vulnerability, then it amounts to exploitation. Unsuccessful outcomes do not make exploitation disappear or render it insignificant. I will forgo trying to modify and so complicate and muddy the definition in order to incorporate this acknowledgement. For our purposes, we will retain the succinct definition with the understanding that exploitation can occur even when, despite reasonable expectations, the exploiter fails to benefit.

I should also note the importance of the phrase, "wrongly benefit," in the definition. Simply benefitting from another's vulnerability is not necessarily exploitation. The clear example of this is clinical care. Clinicians are typically paid or otherwise receive a benefit for administering care and treating people's diseases and injuries. No one regards this profiting from other's vulnerabilities as wrongly benefiting – i.e., as exploitation.

One of the advantages of this definition is that it covers cases we would recognize as exploitation but do not fit the common definition. Consider the following:

> A sells candy to children. He sells it at the standard price and there are others who sell candy in the neighborhood. C is a dentist who among other things treats cavities in children. He charges the standard fee and there are other dentists in the neighborhood.

At this point we would regard A and C as perfectly ordinary; we would not likely raise any moral objections to what they were doing. But suppose that A and C are the same person. We would then regard him as acting unethically. Surely one of our objections would be that he is exploiting the children.[15] What, we may ask if we were following the common definition, is the unfair transaction? By design there is nothing unfair in the price in which his selling the candy and there is nothing unfair in the price he is charging for treating cavities. Nevertheless, he is wrongly benefiting

[14] One might object that this is a case of exploitation if the participants were economically desperate and so vulnerable. But that would be a different case since that vulnerability is not assumed in *Frostbite*. This might be clearer by changing the location of the study. For example, challenge studies done in US examining malaria treatment are not necessarily exploitative even though malaria is not a health concern in the US.

[15] We might also say that he is violating his professional responsibility as a dentist, but, as we will see, that cannot be the entire moral complaint.

from the children's vulnerabilities, which is what we mean by saying that he is exploiting them.

To summarize, the proposed definition of exploitation has two clear advantages over the common one: (1) it clearly displays the connection between exploitation and vulnerability, and (2) it covers all the standard examples of exploitation as well as ones such as *Candy-Selling Dentist*.

We can now see that the moral assessment of exploitation has two issues to examine. First of all there is the obvious objection arising from *wrongly* benefiting. As I mentioned earlier, this can easily include unfair transactions. The common definition however presents this as the only moral objection as far as exploitation is concerned. It invites the conclusion that we can effectively eliminate exploitation by appropriately changing the distribution of benefits between the exploiter and exploited. Indeed, that would be a correct conclusion to draw from *Sweatshop*. If we appropriately raised the workers' wages (and perhaps improve the working conditions), the workers might still be sweating but they would not be exploited. That sort of response is not available for *Candy-Selling Dentist*. Changing the dentist's professional fees would not eliminate the exploitation.[16] By insisting that the exploiter wrongly benefits and not simply unfairly benefits, we do not confine ourselves to a single type of assessment.

The other objection to exploitation attends to the circumstances of the vulnerability itself. A might be responsible for or complicit with regard to the vulnerability of B that A is benefiting from. It is important to distinguish clearly the different possible moral objections. Creating someone's vulnerability or making someone vulnerable can certainly amount to harming that person and so in many cases can be understood as a moral wrong.[17] Nonetheless, in some cases, benefiting from that moral wrong – benefiting from a vulnerability one created in another – can be an additional, separate wrong. Thus some people might have second thoughts about *Candy-Selling Dentist* and so reconsider the claim that the candy-seller's action on its own is blameless. Some might object that he is harming the children or at least those who subsequently need to see a dentist. But even if we grant that the candy-selling is wrong, the candy-selling dentist benefiting from his practice of treating the children's subsequent cavities is an *additional* wrong. It is the wrong of exploitation.[18]

This last point illustrates an interesting logical feature of exploitation that characterizes some cases of exploitation. Suppose, and let me use different names for

[16] What would a fair benefit be for the candy-selling dentist or for the children? If we allow any benefit to the dentist, including training and "loss leader" advertising, we still have exploitation. Nor would giving the children additional benefits address the exploitation.

[17] The boxer causing his opponent's fatigue and so harm would arguably not be considered a moral wrong because of the contestants prior understanding and agreement.

[18] The general question is: When do the beneficial consequences of a wrong, beneficial to the perpetrator, constitute an additional wrong? In some cases they do not. For example, consider the robber who successfully invests his stolen money. His return on these investments is not regarded as an additional or further wrong. But if the robber used the stolen money to successfully bribe people investigating the robbery, that would be an additional wrong, distinct from the robbery.

variables to avoid a possible confusion, that X exploits Y. Suppose a different person Z were to treat Y in the same manner as X has been treating Y. Would Z necessarily be exploiting Y? In the case of *Sweatshop* the answer is surely yes. If someone else were running the factory but still paying the workers subsistence wages, that would be a morally irrelevant change. Z would be just as morally liable as X. It would still be a case of exploitation. The logical feature operates differently in *Candy-Selling Dentist*. As we have already in effect noted, if a dentist other than the candy-selling one were to treat these same children in the same way – i.e., professionally treating the cavities – he would not be acting wrongly or exploiting the children even though he would be benefiting from his dental practice to the same amount as the candy-selling dentist would be benefiting from his dental practice. The general conclusion is that history can matter. Exploitation might not simply depend upon the details of the *current* transaction.

One might object to my argument by claiming that *Candy-Selling Dentist* is a peculiar case. Let me respond by showing how easily other cases can be generated. Indeed, let me present a simple modification of *Sweatshop*:

> *Sweatshop 2*. B is a poor farmer who can no longer make an adequate living from his farm. **B's farm was adequate until A's factory moved in and diverted many of the resources, especially water.** A owns a nearby factory and offers employment. B works at the factory (long hours but receives little more than subsistence wages). As a result, A reaps (enormous) profits.

We cannot address *Sweatshop 2* as we might have addressed *Sweatshop*. There is now a history involved. We are invited to assume that the workers in *Sweatshop 2* have validly consented to their employment and derive some benefit. Should we conclude, as Wertheimer has argued, that since the workers are not now being harmed nor having their rights violated, we should neither stop nor prevent this exploitation? Let me sharpen this question by considering a further modification:

> *Sweatshop 3*. B is a poor farmer who can no longer make an adequate living from his farm. **B's farm was adequate until A's factory moved in and diverted many of the resources, especially water.** A owns a nearby factory and offers employment. B works at the factory **and receives proper wages**. As a result, A profits.

Even if A raised wages to the proper amount for that area and improved working condition, A would still be guilty of exploiting B in the same way that the candy-selling dentist is guilty of exploiting the children.

What I hope we can now see is that the common definition takes as its exemplar that of the opportunistic capitalist. As far as that definition is concerned, everything depends upon the current transaction and the distribution of benefits. In contrast, the definition defended in this paper could be said to take as its exemplar that of the colonialist expropriating land, resources, and people. Indeed, for some the paradigm of exploitation is colonialism. This contrast in definitions is particularly striking when we consider the issue of exploitation as it might arise in clinical research conducted in less developed countries. Is the researcher to be compared – favorably or unfavorably, as we will see – to the opportunistic capitalist or to the colonialist?

The Colonialist Paradigm: The Importance of History

My using the word "colonialist" is meant to be suggestive only and not an attempt to present a theory or analysis of that complex phenomenon. Colonialism included the low, repellant goals of thief, plunder, rape, and enslavement, and sometimes it was driven by the allegedly high goals of "saving souls" or extending the fruits of civilization, albeit conducted with hard paternalism. My point here in alluding to colonialism is that the response or remedy for any particular case of colonialism is a matter of ongoing debate and controversy. I do not want to suggest that the exploitation arising from colonialism is the most salient or egregious wrong of colonialism. We can however learn something by considering the challenge of addressing exploitation from colonialism.

Simply ending the colonial activity – the occupying power moving out and ceding authority – does not necessarily end the exploitation. Although no longer present or in charge, the colonialist could continue to wrongly benefit from the vulnerabilities of the formerly colonized, vulnerabilities which the colonialist might well have created or exacerbated. For example, the colony might still depend upon the "Mother Country" for trade or basic needs. Indeed, the benefits might not be so much economic but rather matters of culture, status, self-image, and dignity. The former colony might retain what the colonialists have left behind, including language, administrative and education institutions, measures of achievement, or conceptions of well-being and self-respect. Even if such legacies are an improvement over the colony's earlier way of life, this progress can carry a sting: the colonized didn't, and perhaps couldn't, discover or develop these improvements by themselves but had to be taught them like children. The colonialists, whatever their other faults, are thereby acknowledged to be a superior and civilizing force. So when a member of a former colony achieves distinction in a field introduced by the colonialists, such as science, that accomplishment can add to the glory of the Mother Country's "civilizing mission."

None of this is to deny that some of the colonialist's legacy can be real improvements and significant benefits. And so it underscores the problem of responding to or remedying exploitation. Because of a history between the exploiter and the exploited, a mere redistribution of benefits arising from the current transaction might be inadequate and not be to the point. We need to respond to the history.

Exploitation in Clinical Research

In contrast to the aim of clinical work, which is the care and treatment of the patient, the aim of clinical research is knowledge and not the well-being of the human subject. To be sure, researchers – or more accurately stated, the research team, which includes not only the investigators but also the support staff, sponsors, and supporting institutions – are not indifferent to the well-being of the people who participate in their studies. They do take care, but only to a certain extent. Researchers will intentionally place their participants at risk, not for the benefit of these participants but in order to obtain knowledge. Because researchers will therefore often use people and their vulnerabilities in order to generate knowledge, exploitation is a legitimate worry, especially when the research is conducted on people in a low- to middle-income country (LMIC).

There are two types of cases that are sometimes presented as raising a concern about exploitation. In the first type of case the research team wants to perform an experiment that would be unethical to do in the US or any other developed country because of its wealth and health care system but might be permitted in a LMIC because of its poverty and health care system. For example:

> *The S2 Trial.* Researchers want to determine whether S2 is a better drug than S1, which is already used for treating a life-threatening disease in the US. They wish to conduct a trial with placebo controls so that the results would be clearer and come quicker. They cannot conduct the clinical trial in the US – it would be rejected by any US IRB – because they would be interfering with participants getting the standard treatment of S1. They decide to conduct the experiment in a LMIC in which people do not standardly get treated with S1. The researchers cannot be accused of interfering with the participants getting treated with S1 since such treatment is not part of the standard of care in the LMIC.[19]

In the second type of case the research team wants to perform an experiment in a LMIC because doing so would be cheaper, but, if the experiment is successful, the resulting drugs would be marketed in developed countries and not in the LMIC because of its cost.

> *The Modified S2 Trial.* Researchers want to determine whether S2 is a better drug than S1, which is already used for treating a life-threatening disease in the US. They wish to conduct a trial with active controls (i.e., S1). Although they can conduct the clinical trial in the US, it would be much cheaper to do so in a LMIC even though S1 treatment is not the standard of care in the LMIC. Nevertheless, if the experiment is successful and S2 is shown to be superior to S1, S2 will be available in the US and other developed countries but will not be available in the LMIC because of its cost.

The question of exploitation in either case is: Are the researchers wrongly benefiting from the LMIC participant's vulnerabilities – e.g., poverty, lack of standard access to S1, and the life-threatening disease being studied?

In *The S2 Trial* researchers are letting participants in the placebo die from their disease, which would be their normal fate given local conditions, in order to obtain further knowledge even though the researchers know how to rescue them. Since this is an experiment, the fate of those in the treatment arm could be better or worse than those in the placebo arm. The charge of exploitation arises from the claim that the research team wrongly benefits from the deaths in the placebo group – the research

---

[19] This is an abbreviated and schematic rendering of the Surfaxin trial. See, for example, Hawkins and Emanuel (2008), Chap. 2.

team already has the ability to prevent those deaths but do not exercise their ability because they want to gain some knowledge.

Claiming that *The Modified S2 Trial* is exploitative is more difficult to sustain. Presumably the experiment would not be exploitative if exactly the same one were carried out in the US. The difference is that US participants are being placed at risk for the benefit of US health care whereas LMIC participants are being placed at risk but not for the benefit of the LMIC health care. To be sure, the trial conducted in an LMIC would generate some benefits. The LMIC participants in the active control arm would be receiving life-saving treatment they would otherwise not get and the LMIC participants in the treatment arm might benefit as well. In either case, the participants would at least have their health monitored, which might lead to some needed health care, and the presence of the research team might contribute modestly to the economy of the LMIC. Such benefits are however small compared to the benefits the US would receive if the trial were successful. If we focus our attention to the common definition, we might hold that this disparity in benefits is unfair and so conducting the modified S2 trial in the LMIC is a case of exploitation.

This conclusion would need further argument because an unequal distribution of benefits is not the same thing as an unfair distribution of benefits, much less taking unfair advantage, which the common definition demands. If the workers in a factory are receiving a proper wage, we don't regard it as exploitation just because the owner of the factory is making more money. One might object that that is not a good comparison – unequal health benefits can lead to unfairness in a way that unequal economic benefits do not. As a response, consider a case where S2 would not be available even if the trial were successful because S2 does not address a health concern of the LMIC. This is the situation in *Frostbite*, which we noted is not a case of exploitation.

I don't want to suggest that there can be no moral objection to *The Modified S2 Trial*. If S2 did not address a health concern in the LMIC, one might still object, for example, that needed resources were being diverted to something that is not a priority for the LMIC. But such concerns would also have to take into account the benefits for the LMIC that might arise, including providing locals with training and experience in clinical research which could be later directed at the LMIC's priorities.

If we focus on the common definition, it might well seem that the charge of exploitation in clinical research turns on current transactions; that history does not come into the analysis. In particular, considerations about the colonialist paradigm do not seem relevant. The research team, it will be emphasized, did not caused the health vulnerabilities of the potential participants from the LMIC. These vulnerabilities were already in place before specific research projects were proposed.

Some writers have challenged this picture by examining the behavior of pharmaceutical companies who enhance their profits by pricing drugs so that they are not affordable in LMICs. The resulting lack of suitable drugs can lead to a poor health status – hence, vulnerabilities – in these countries.[20] The challenge is filling out and establishing the suggested complex causal connections. Furthermore, not every new drug is relevant to a LMIC's health priorities. But even putting that matter aside, having an adequate supply of needed drugs means little without the appropriate local expertise in diagnosing, distributing, and administering the medication. Perhaps this picture places too much emphasis on the availability of drugs. As every public health practitioner knows, a lot more goes into a population's health status than the availability of certain drugs. Why should individual researchers and their teams, pursuing a well-defined but limited investigation, be under an obligation to respond to these concerns?

I want to present a different set of issues that better fit the colonialist paradigm of exploitation and so call for the revised definition. As just mentioned, the health status of any country or region depends in part upon the availability of local expertise – including physicians, nurses, researchers, and their supporting institutions. The availability of this expertise is threatened by what has been gruesomely called, "brain drain." As locals have become trained and skilled in the diagnosis and treatment of various diseases, the better and more promising professionals will often be recruited by US and European universities, institutes, and hospitals. The result is that locals will have poorer health in part because they have fewer well-trained professionals in their country, the better ones having left the LMIC in order to pursue their careers.

This recruitment of local expertise who are capable and promising, this draining of local talent, takes place in a several ways. Local experts will learn in their training and work of opportunities abroad. Visiting professionals can identify ambitious and talented people and encourage them to pursue careers elsewhere. And frequently, the establishment of an international research project can have the unintended consequence of brain drain.

Clinical research does not typically helicopter into a LMIC fully formed. Depending upon the details of the project, it will need cooperation and assistance on the ground, usually employing local expertise for help in such things as recruiting participants, gathering and analyzing data, monitoring and responding to adverse events, giving presentations, and preparing publications. This experience and training will often present opportunities for these locals to go to developed countries to follow their interests, pursue their ambitions, and advance their careers. And who can blame them since the prospects in their own country might be severely limited? Some will no doubt return to their home country to help address local health needs and priorities. But many will not and the result will be a decrease in the potential expertise available to develop and administer local health care. It's not too far off to see this recruiting of talent as comparable to the expropriation of a local resource.

[20] Cf. Thomas Pogge, "Testing Our Drugs on the Poor Abroad," in Hawkins and Emanuel (2008). It is important to acknowledge that the cost of a drug might not be the only or the even primary problem for its inadequate use in a LMIC. Even when the country has the drug, challenges can exist in distributing the drug (roads and distribution networks are deficient) or from the lack of local experts who can correctly identify health needs and administer the drug.

Suppose a research team has been complicit in an LMIC's brain drain. As I have already mentioned, this could occur in a variety of ways, including past recruitment efforts of local talent by the sponsor or the supporting institution – usually a university or hospital. With that history we should worry about that team conducting clinical research in that LMIC. Is the research examining a medical condition that has been caused or aggravated by the loss of local expertise in health care? If so, then the research would be guilty of exploitation in the same way that the factory owner A is guilty of exploitation in *Sweatshop 2* or *Sweatshop 3*. It is not at all clear how you could judge these cases as exploitation if you stick simply with the common definition. Questions about the distribution of benefits between the research team and the potential participants are not what matters. That is why a new definition of exploitation is offered.

Let me make clear that I am not claiming that all cases of exploitation in clinical research arise from a brain drain. Many cases such as *The S2 Trial* might be solely about current transactions and so would be nicely captured by the common definition. But once we take history into account, as the new definition invites us to do, we can begin to see research teams conducting studies in the LMICs in a different light. Is the research team – in the broad sense including investigators, sponsors, and supporting institutions – complicit in the participants' vulnerability? Is the research team benefiting from this vulnerability? Are they guilty of exploitation?

Responding to Exploitation in Clinical Research

I mentioned earlier that even though most people morally object to exploitation, several thoughtful commentators have argued that mutually advantageous consensual exploitation (MACE) should not only be tolerated it should not even be prevented. As far as the current transaction is concerned, the exploited have consented and they are benefiting. These matters trump any concern about the unfairness of the transaction. The wrongness of MACE is a modest stain that we should not interfere with. If, however, we look beyond the current transaction and bring history into account, as the new definition of exploitation invites, our assessment and response to exploitation becomes more complex and nuanced. But even on the common definition, the assessment of exploitation in clinical research is significantly incomplete.

Discussions of exploitation in clinical research typically view only two groups as possible beneficiaries in clinical research – the research team on the one hand and the participants and perhaps their community on the other. This treats clinical research too much like a commercial transaction or a contract governing an exchange of goods between two parties. We need to be reminded in these discussions that there is a third beneficiary – our body of scientific knowledge. The person coming from a developed country to build a factory in a LMIC is aiming to benefit himself. The factory might also benefit the workers in the factory and perhaps some others in the LMIC. In clinical research the aim is to generate generalizable knowledge, specifically to add to *our*[21] understanding and abilities regarding the diagnosis and treatment of disease. It is so significant an undertaking that we believe that, under suitable restrictions and oversight, we are justified in exposing participants to some risk even when they will not benefit from this exposure at all. The importance of this aim complicates any policy or response regarding exploitation in clinical research.

Let me affirm and repeat the consensus view that efforts to achieve the aim of research do not overrule ethical considerations. The requirement of valid consent from the participants, for example, does constrain the conduct of research. Nevertheless, ethical codes and guidelines have undergone revisions in order to strike a proper balance between achieving the aims of research and the ethical requirement of protecting the rights and welfare of participants. For example, the Nuremberg Code asserted that no experiment could proceed without the clear and explicit consent of the participant.[22] It soon became apparent, however, that we could not experimentally evaluate important areas of medical knowledge regarding diagnosing and treating head trauma patients, children, and people with cognitive disorders because clear and explicit consent was usually not feasible. Rather than forgo such research, additional guidelines and requirements were developed to protect participants so that such research could ethically proceed.

We therefore have three possible responses to a case of exploitative clinical research: we could stop the research, eliminate the exploitation, or establish requirements that specifically protect participants who are being exploited.

Stopping the research is the least attractive option. This is not because of those cases where the participants might derive some benefit. If the research proposal is warranted scientifically – the study would make a justified contribution to our biomedical knowledge – then stopping the research means blocking a reliable method for generating knowledge that would enhance our understanding and ability to diagnose and treat disease. Nevertheless, this option must be taken if the research cannot be made ethical. Conducting that research would not only be wrong in itself, but also knowingly pursuing unethical research undermines public confidence and support for the general research enterprise and its supporting institutions. The success and trust in medical research is due in part to the belief that researchers are governed by ethical regulations – just because something can be effectively tested in a particular way does not mean that it will. Because stopping research can have such significant consequences, it should not be considered unless the other two options are not available.

Eliminating the alleged exploitation in the research would be a more straightforward response. If we confined ourselves to the common definition of exploitation, we should be able to effectively address exploitation by changing the distribution of benefits. If the potentially exploited receive sufficient benefits, they can no longer claim to be exploited. There are two immediate problems with this response: While

[21] It is important to note that this first person plural does not refer to just the people in developed countries.

[22] The Nuremberg Code (1947) In: Mitscherlich A, Mielke F. *Doctors of infamy: the story of the Nazi medical crimes*. New York: Schuman, 1949: xxiii–xxv.

increasing benefits might be a straightforward response for a commercial transaction such as *Sweatshop*, it is not clear what an increase in benefits for participants means in clinical research. Since it is *research*, there is no guarantee that the participants receiving the experimental treatment will get any benefit at all. Indeed, they might be harmed. If the research team could guarantee a therapeutic benefit, it would not be research. Consequently, the only other possibility would be to give participants benefits that are not part of the clinical trial – e.g., money or free medical exams. But IRBs or RECs generally view such "indirect benefits" with suspicion. Do they generate an "undue inducement" that entices people to accept participation in a trial they would otherwise reject? It might seem that we have traded one ethical problem for another.[23]

The other problem is that increasing benefits from the transaction might not address the charge of exploitation at all. That is one of the insights of the proposed alternative definition of exploitation. If the research team bore some responsibility for the participants' vulnerability, paying the participants off would be no better than the candy-selling dentist offering discounts for his dental service.

Looking at the preferred definition, perhaps we could eliminate the exploitation by selecting different participants or by addressing the concern over "wrongly benefiting." Either response could face considerable practical obstacles. Simply selecting different participants might just change who is being exploited and not the charge of exploitation. And so it might require redesigning the trial – e.g., changing it from placebo controls to active controls if we are examining a Phase III study. But such redesigns, even if possible, can easily increase the cost and burden of the research project to the point where its priority for the members of the research team drops. There are always many interesting research questions to investigate. There is no guarantee that the project would continue to be pursued should it become more expensive and burdensome.

What about the third option? Are there special protections that could allow the research to proceed as designed but address the complaint about exploitation? Since we do acknowledge the possibility of MACE, special considerations regarding obtaining consent or ensuring that the trial has only reasonable risks do not seem to be to the point. I would like to end this paper with a suggestion that requires a good deal more discussion than I can give here.

Consider *Sweatshop 3*. The salaries are already adequate, the workers have consented to work. The charge of exploitation arises not from the current transaction but from a history of transactions that at a minimum have undermined the dignity of the workers. Increasing their benefits will not address that concern, but inviting them to have greater control in the sweatshop – perhaps even assuming a partnership with A – would be a move in the right direction. Arguably, it could begin to repair their dignity.

---

[23] One might wonder why "undue inducement" is a concern regarding participating in a clinical trial but not so much a concern regarding working in a factory. For a discussion of some of these difference, see Wachbroit (2013), "Human Subjects, Research Use of," in *The International Encyclopedia of Ethics*. Edited by Hugh LaFollette, Blackwell Publishing Ltd.

A comparable effort in the case of clinical trials in LMICs would be to arrange for local experts to be partners in the study. They would not be merely hired staff to assist the investigators helicoptered in from the developed country. They would be the investigators themselves, appropriately trained to oversee the project and deal with the challenges that arise. Two welcome consequences can be expected. Not only would we get the benefits of new knowledge from the clinical trial, but we would also have enhanced the capacity of the local experts to deal with the health issues their country faces. Of course I do not want to dismiss the practical challenges that such a move presents. We need to have an informed discussion of this proposal. Nevertheless, I believe it is a more promising response, particularly in the case of MACE, than simply proclaiming that we should not interfere to stop or prevent exploitation as long as it does not currently violate rights or harm participants. History does matter.

Research Involving Persons Likely to be Vulnerable

Nahed M. Ali

Introduction

The Master's candidate was invited to a meeting of the Research Ethics Committee (REC) to discuss the changes being required by the members who reviewed her proposal. The Master's candidate displayed obvious annoyance and anger on her facial expression. Shortly after the meeting started, she stated:

> I did not expect all these changes! My thesis highlights a very simple idea. It is about the prevalence of domestic violence among pregnant women attending the primary health care units in our Governorate. There is no risk in such a type of research, as no procedures are being done that can be considered invasive. Participants will answer some questions about whether they were exposed to domestic violence, by whom and the impact of the incident on them and their pregnancies.
>
> The primary reviewer remarked to the Master's candidate: "I will discuss all these points with you and I think we need to plan a workshop about research involving vulnerable populations.

The above conversation actually took place in one of the universities in the Arab region. It reflects inadequate knowledge and appreciation among researchers regarding the involvement of vulnerable groups in research as well as a lack of appreciation of the risks in research involving such individuals. Furthermore, as shown in Table 1, the current regulations in the countries in the Arab region inadequately discuss who might be vulnerable in research (Alahmad et al. 2012) and only three mention the need for additional safeguards, although specification of such safeguards are not mentioned (Silverman 2011). Such deficiencies are worrisome, as the majority of research ethics abuses in the past several decades have involved vulnerable groups.

N.M. Ali (✉)
Faculty of Medicine, Suez Canal University, Ismailia, Egypt
e-mail: Ali.nahed@med.suez.edu.eg

H. Silverman (ed.), *Research Ethics in the Arab Region*, Research Ethics Forum 5,
https://doi.org/10.1007/978-3-319-65266-5_5

Table 1 Vulnerability in research ethics regulations in the Arab Region

Country	Guidelines/law	Authorized body	Year	Mention of vulnerability
Bahrain	Health research structure and procedures	Ministry of Health	2009	No mention
Egypt	Profession Ethics Regulations	Resolution of the Minister of Health & Population No. 238	2003	Article 56: Surrogate consent in case of minors/incapacitated person. Research should pertain to his sick condition
Jordan	Law of clinical studies	A royal decree	2011	No mention
Saudi Arabia	The law of ethics of research on living creatures	Royal decree No. M/59	2011	Article 24–26: Scientific research involving prisoners, minors, incompetent persons, pregnant women and fetuses. Definition of vulnerability and classification of vulnerable groups
	Clinical trials requirements guidelines	Saudi Food & Drug Authority	2013	
Kuwait	Ethical guidelines for biomedical research	Kuwait Institute for Medical Specializations (KIMS), Ministry of Health	2001	Additional safeguards should be provided if vulnerable populations are studied. The guidelines do not clarify these safeguards
Lebanon	Law of medical ethics (modification)	Parliament	2012	Surrogate consent in case of minors/incapacitated persons
Qatar	Policies, regulations and guidelines for research involving humans	Supreme Council of Health	2009	Additional protections for research involving pregnant women, human fetuses, neonates, prisoners and children. The guidelines do not clarify these safeguards
Sudan	National guidelines for ethical conduct of research involving human subjects	Ministry of Health	2008	Ethical justification for involving vulnerable groups. Additional safeguards for involving children and pregnant women in research. The guidelines do not clarify these safeguards
United Arab Emirates	Guidance for conducting clinical trials based on drugs/medical products and good clinical practice	Ministry of Health-Drug Control Department (DOD)	2006	Surrogate consent in case of minors/incapacitated person

Definition of Vulnerability

The term 'vulnerability" is used frequently in the context of health research and guidelines offer various definitions. For example, the Belmont Report defines vulnerability explicitly on individuals' "dependent status and their frequently compromised capacity for free consent" (National Commission for the Protection of Human Subjects of Biomedical and Behavioral Research 1979). The ICH Tripartite guidelines offer the following definition: "Individuals whose willingness to volunteer in a clinical trial may be unduly influenced by the expectation, whether justified or not, of benefits associated with participation, or of a retaliatory response from senior members of a hierarchy in case of refusal to participate" (International Conference on Harmonization (ICH) 1996). Finally, the Council for International Organizations of Medical Science (CIOMS) states that "persons are vulnerable because they are relatively (or absolutely) incapable of protecting their own interests. This may occur when persons have relative or absolute impairments in decisional capacity, education, resources, strength, or other attributes needed to protect their own interests. In other cases, persons can also be vulnerable because some feature of the circumstances (temporary or permanent) in which they live makes it less likely that others will be vigilant about, or sensitive to, their interests. This may happen when people are marginalized, stigmatized, or face social exclusion or prejudice that increases the likelihood that others place their interests at risk, whether intentionally or unintentionally (Council for International Organizations of Medical Sciences (CIOMS) and World Health Organization (WHO) 2016).

Categories of Vulnerable Participants

In an attempt to add specification to these definitions, guidelines frequently provide long lists of groups who might be considered vulnerable (Hurst 2008). Herein are some examples of vulnerable groups (Lott 2005).

- **Children/minors:** Children are always considered as a vulnerable group mainly due to their evolving decision making capacity. Accordingly, many countries have laws/guidelines or common practices regarding the age of adulthood, which is most commonly taken to be the age of 18 years old. RECs must be familiar with their relevant national regulations regarding such thresholds. That said, in some types of research, adolescents might be considered to have decision making capacity below the stated age of adulthood if there is a common practice regarding the concept of an 'age of maturity' or "emancipated minor'.
- **Elderly persons:** Some elderly persons of advanced age might be considered vulnerable, for example, if they are institutionalized or have developed a certain degree of dementia. These attributes will affect their ability to provide voluntary consent when being recruited in research.

- **Subordinate members of hierarchical groups:** Individuals in a subordinate role "may be unduly influenced, whether justified or not, by the expectation of preferential treatment if they agree to participate in the study or by fear of disapproval or retaliation if they refuse" (Council for International Organizations of Medical Sciences (CIOMS) and World Health Organization (WHO) 2016). Examples of such groups are patients, students, employees, policeman, prisoners, members of the armed forces and workers in settings where research is conducted.
- **Mentally ill:** some mentally ill individuals are not capable of giving a valid informed consent, although just the mere presence of a mental illness does not necessarily confer vulnerability, e.g., a person with mild schizophrenia.
- **Terminally ill:** the vulnerability of such persons may exist if the patient looks to research as a last effort for treatment. This is considered a specific type of a medical vulnerability, i.e., a situation where a patient has a serious health-related condition for which there are no existing satisfactory treatments. Also, the consent process for terminally ill patients may be affected by deficit decision making capacity loss and possible influence from their family members who are fearful of losing a loved one.
- **Pregnant women**: due to their pregnant state, women may be more prone to health risks (e.g., diabetes and hypertension) and their fetuses might be more prone to developmental abnormalities.
- **Prisoners**: prisoners are involuntarily confined or detained in a penal system institution and have been deprived of freedoms normally enjoyed by other individuals. Their subordinate setting makes it less likely they can make a voluntary decision under a real or perceived threat of ensuing harm (coercion). Also, prisoners may be unduly influenced by potential gains offered by research participation, such as reduced prison time or other incentives (more or better food, increased access to entertainment or exercise facilities, increased 'free' time, etc.).

Vulnerable Groups Relevant to the Arab Region

- **Refugees:** Refugees are persons who have been displaced from their permanent homes or residences and now live elsewhere – within foreign boundaries – as non-citizens (Leaning 2001). Several factors contribute to the vulnerability of refugees, including the lack of political and civil rights, the lack of basic human needs, low levels of literacy, and fear that their immigrant status will not be approved by the higher authorities in their temporary countries. Recruiting refugees into research is not unethical as long as the research is responsive to their health care needs (Block et al. 2013).

- The Office of the United Nations High Commissioner for Refugees (UNHCR), also known as the UN Refugee Agency (Office of the United Nations High Commissioner for Refugees (UNHCR) 2016), mentioned that the number of refugees in the Middle East is likely to increase, which can be attributed to many factors, such as:
  - Continued unstable political situation,
  - Continued military confrontation,
  - The ongoing destruction of infrastructure, which presents a major obstacle for people to return to their homes and
  - High levels of insecurity and violence
  - The UNHCR added that Lebanon and Jordan are considerably affected by the security situation in the neighboring Syrian Arab Republic (Syria) and the influx of Syrians into the country, as well as by the conflicts in Iraq and Gaza.
- **Internally displaced persons (IDPs):** IDPs are defined as individuals who have been forced to leave their homes or places of habitual residence as a result of or to avoid the effects of armed conflict, situations of generalized violence, violations of human rights or natural or human-made disasters – and who have not crossed an internationally recognized state border (United Nations 2014).
- In reference to the last two groups, Table 2 shows that there are millions of refugees and IDPs in several Arab countries affected by political instability.
- **Poverty:** Although poverty is not, in it of itself, a cause of vulnerability, factors associated with poverty accounts for their vulnerability (Grady 2009). For example, poverty is usually related to illiteracy/low level of education and little familiarity with research and poor understanding to the study risks, all of which makes the informed consent process questionable (Grady 2009).

Individuals living in poverty frequently lack health insurance or have limited health care options from public assistance programs rendering them more likely to enroll in research, especially clinical trials, as an alternative means of gaining access to needed medicines. This desperation for medical care fueled by an inducement that might be considered "undue" is amplified by the lack of insight and understanding of what constitutes research (Schuman 2012).

Table 2 Number of refugees, internally displaced persons (IDPs), and others of concern to UNHCR in several Arab countries affected by political instability as at December 2015

Country	Total of refugees and people in refugee-like situations	IDPs	Others of concern to UNHCR
Iraq	264,107	4,403,287	3,599
Libya	6,085	434,869	8
Sudan	628,770	3,218,234	19
Syria	4,872,580	6,563,462	8,247
Yemen	15,896	2,532,032	13

5.2 million Palestinian refugees registered by UNRWA
Source: The UN Refugees Agency. Global forced displacement trends in 2015. Retrieved from http://www.unhcr.org/statistics/unhcrstats/576408cd7/unhcr-global-trends-2015.html

Similar to the Development Index, poverty can also be described in multidimensional factors. The Multidimensional Poverty Index (MPI) identifies deprivations across the three dimensions: health, education and standard of living. Table 3 illustrates the population who are multi-dimensionally poor (suffering acute deprivations in 33% or more of weighted indicators) in several Arab countries.

- **Illiteracy and Unemployment:** Illiteracy and unemployment are highly prevalent in several countries in the Arab region and represent factors that can account for vulnerability (Table 4). The UN Human Development Reports use the adult literacy and unemployment rates as indicators for development in resource limited countries (United Nations 2014). The report defined the Adult Literacy Rate as the percentage of the population ages 15 and older who can, with understanding, both read and write a short simple statement on their everyday life. The unemployment rate is the percentage of the labor force population ages 15 and older who are not in paid employment or self-employed, but is available for work and has taken steps to seek paid employment or self-employment. Table 4 shows that both the illiteracy rate and unemployment rates are high in several countries in the Arab Region compared to the international rate.
- **Homeless People:** While quantifying homelessness is not easy, the UN Human Development Report defines homeless as people who lack a shelter for living quarters as a result of natural disasters or who carry their few possessions with them. They sleep in the streets, in doorways or on piers, or in any other space on a more or less random basis. Their numbers are expressed as a percentage of the total population. In 2009, the percentage of homeless in Egypt was 0.1% (76,780

Table 3 Population in multidimensional poverty in some Arab countries

Country	Year	Intensity of deprivation of multidimensional poverty (% of intensity of deprivation)	Population near multidimensional poverty (%)	Population in severe multidimensional poverty (%)	Population below national income poverty line (%)
Egypt	2008	40.3	8.6	1.5	25.2
Iraq	2011	39.4	7.4	2.5	22.9
Jordan	2009	36.8	4.1	0.1	13.3
Palestine	2006/2007	36.9	7.4	0.1	21.9
Yemen	2006	50.9	16.7	18.4	34.8

Source: United Nation Development Programme- UN human development report 2014. http://hdr.undp.org/en/content/human-development-report-2014

Intensity of deprivation of multidimensional poverty: Average percentage of deprivation experienced by people in multidimensional poverty

Population near multidimensional poverty: Percentage of the population at risk of suffering multiple deprivations (those with a deprivation score of 20–33%)

Population in severe poverty: Percentage of the population in severe multidimensional poverty (those with a deprivation score of 50% or more)

Table 4 Poverty, illiteracy, and unemployment variables in several Arab countries

Country	% of individuals living below National Poverty Line (below $ 1.25 a day)[a]	% of adult illiteracy rate (2005–2012)[b]	% of Unemployment rate (2004–2013)[b]
World	14.5 (2011)	18.8	7.5
Egypt	25.2 (2011)	25.2	9.0
Iraq	18.9 (2012)	21.5	8.0
Jordan	14.4 (2010)	4.5	12.2
Sudan	46.5 (2009)	28.1	19.8
Syria	35.2 (2007)	15.9	8.6
Yemen	34.8 (2005)	34.7	16.2

[a]Source: http://povertydata.worldbank.org/poverty/region/MNA, 2015
[b]Source: United Nation Development Programme- UN human development report 2014. http://hdr.undp.org/en/content/human-development-report-2014

persons) of the total population (76.78 million), while it is 1.3% in Sudan (453,050) of the total population (34.85 million).

- Persons prone to discrimination and stigmatization: Persons belonging to certain types of marginalized groups in the Arab region might suffer from further discrimination and stigmatization due to privacy violations or if their sensitive information becomes disseminated from breaches of confidentiality. Such groups include:
  - Racial, ethnic, and religious minorities
  - Members of political parties not in power
  - Sex workers
  - Lesbians, Gay, Bisexual, and Transgender (LGBT)
  - Substance abusers
  - Individuals charged with criminal activity

Although at first glance having lists of groups who might be vulnerable can be useful, these lists are long and can appear to suggest that almost every potential research participant is prone to being vulnerable. Furthermore, defining vulnerability in terms of groups has been controversial, as other factors that are relevant to the research setting itself might be more important than inclusion of a particular sociodemographic group in order to determine whether an individual is vulnerable (Grady 2009).

As such, a useful definition of vulnerability would combine an internal and an external element, as proposed by Schroeder and Gefenas: "To be vulnerable means to face a significant probability of incurring an identifiable harm while substantially lacking ability and/or means to protect oneself" (Schroeder and Gefenas 2009). The external element of vulnerability refers to the existence of potential harms, whereas the internal element refers to characteristics that make a person unable to protect themselves from the harm. An inability to protect oneself includes intrinsic characteristics ('lacking ability'), such as the ability to provide a valid informed consent, as well contingent elements ('means'), such as political, social or economic circumstances that would make them easily victimized. For example, vulnerable individuals might have unequal power relationships with others or possess substandard mental faculties.

Safeguards for Persons Prone to Being Vulnerable

The potential for harms as well as an inability to protect oneself are both required for vulnerability to be present. These two elements need to be present in order for there to be a special claim for protection, which then requires the institution of safeguards in the research activity that can lessen the incidence of such harms (Hurst 2008).

The identification of the potential harms emanating from the characteristics of the research and the research environment helps to specify the particular safeguards needed to protect individuals from the identified harms (Levine et al. 2004; Schroeder and Gefenas 2009).

Identifiable harms in research include the following:

1. Unfavorable risk/benefit ratio
2. Breach of confidentiality or invasion of privacy
3. Invalid consent
4. Lack of or unfair access to the benefits of research.

An unfavorable risk/benefit ratio can impact directly on subjects' welfare; a breach of confidentiality or a violation of privacy can lead to social risks (e.g., stigma or denied access to health insurance or employability); invalid consent due to deficit decision making capacity can lead to unwanted harms insofar as one does not realize to what they provided consent; invalid consent can also presents dignity harms, as one's autonomy has been denied; and lack of or unfair access to the benefits of research represents a justice issue that amounts to exploitation.

To prevent such harms to potential subjects, special protections must be provided that would need to be tailored to the type of harm to be avoided and the source of the specific vulnerability.

Examples of application of this approach are as follows:

1. **Unfavorable balance of risks and benefits:**

   Investigators and members of RECs should scrutinize the risk/benefit ratio in order to identify potential subjects who are more likely to suffer harms (e.g., individuals who have more co-morbidities). Potential safeguards include:
   - Exclusion of participants at higher risk
   - Risk ceiling of the research set at no more than minimal risk

2. **Potential breaches inconfidentiality or invasion of privacy**
Potential safeguards include:
   - Anonymization of data to prevent identification
   - Data security methods to prevent unauthorized access to sensitive data
   - Specific attention to the enrollment setting to enhance privacy

3. **Invalid consent:**
Potential safeguards include:
   - Assessing the understanding of the potential subjects
   - Requirement for surrogate consent
   - Requirement of an independent monitor to assess the consent process
   - Scrutiny of the incentives to prevent undue inducement.

4. **Prevention of Exploitation (unfair distribution of the benefits)**
Potential safeguards include:

   - Assurances that the research is directly relevant to the needs and the health concerns of the persons who might be vulnerable. As such, "the sponsor, researchers, and relevant public health authority must ensure that the research is responsive to the health needs or priorities of the communities or populations where the research will be conducted" (Council for International Organizations of Medical Sciences (CIOMS) and World Health Organization (WHO) 2016). Hence, the goal of the research is to obtain knowledge that will lead to improved diagnosis, prevention or treatment of diseases or other health problems that are unique to the vulnerable groups.
   - Even if the research is relevant to the health needs of the potential subjects, the requirement of reasonable availability of any developed product related to the research also aims to minimize exploitation.
   - The research cannot be done involving a less vulnerable group. For example, children should not be enrolled in a clinical investigation unless absolutely necessary to answer an important scientific question about the health and welfare of children.
   - Appointment of an advocate for an institutionalized group (e.g., prisoner advocate) to serve on the REC.

Conclusion

Conducting health research involving persons prone to being vulnerable represents an ethical challenge in the Arab region for several reasons. First, national regulations in research ethics are lacking in many of the countries in the region. Second, the existing regulations do not fully address protections for vulnerable groups.

Third, the current political climate in many countries and the existence of violent conflict settings can render certain groups more vulnerable than others, such as refugees, internally displaced persons, and ethnic and political minorities. Fourth, widespread discriminatory practices can lead to enhanced harms to members of certain groups, e.g., homosexuals, sex workers, and those with HIV or HCV. Finally, educationally and economically deprived groups are more prevalent in certain countries in the Arab region.

The implementation of required safeguards for protecting the vulnerable groups is extremely needed in the Arab region. This goal could be achieved through development of national regulations and capacity building of RECs so that adequate safeguards can be included for persons prone to being vulnerable. Also, enhanced awareness regarding the concept of vulnerability is needed among policy makers, members of RECs, researchers, and community members. Finally, efforts should made to enhance the resilence of persons prone to be vulnerable as well as empower them so that they can adequately protect themselves.

References

Alahmad, G., M. Al-Jumah, and K. Dierickx. 2012. Review of national research ethics regulations and guidelines in Middle Eastern Arab countries. *BMC Medical Ethics* 13: 34. https://doi.org/10.1186/1472-6939-13-34.

Block, K., E. Riggs, and N. Haslam. 2013. *Values and vulnerabilities: The ethics of research with refugees and asylum seekers*. Australia: Australian Academic Press.

Council for International Organizations of Medical Sciences (CIOMS), World Health Organization (WHO). 2016. International ethical guidelines for health-related research involving humans vol. Retrieved from: http://www.cioms.ch/index.php/12-newsflash/400-cioms-inernational-ethical-guidelines.

Grady, C. 2009. Vulnerability in research: individuals with limited financial and/or social resources. *The Journal of Law, Medicine & Ethics* 37 (1): 19–27. https://doi.org/10.1111/j.1748-720X.2009.00347.x.

Human Development Report 2014. Sustaining Human Progress: Reducing vulnerabilities and building resilience. Available at: http://hdr.undp.org/en/content/human-development-report-2014.

Hurst, S.A. 2008. Vulnerability in research and health care; describing the elephant in the room? *Bioethics* 22 (4): 191–202. https://doi.org/10.1111/j.1467-8519.2008.00631.x.

International Conference on Harmonization (ICH). 1996. Good clinical practice: Available at: http://www.ich.org/products/guidelines/efficacy/article/efficacy-guidelines.html.

Leaning, J. 2001. Ethics of research in refugee populations. *Lancet* 357 (9266): 1432–1433. https://doi.org/10.1016/S0140-6736(00)04572-4.

Levine, C., R. Faden, C. Grady, D. Hammerschmidt, L. Eckenwiler, J. Sugarman, and Consortium to Examine Clinical Research, E. 2004. The limitations of "vulnerability" as a protection for human research participants. *The American Journal of Bioethics* 4 (3): 44–49. https://doi.org/10.1080/15265160490497083.

Lott, J.P. 2005. Module three: Vulnerable/special participant populations. *Developing World Bioethics* 5: 30–54. Available at: http://www.udo-schuklenk.org/files/module33.pdf.

National Commission for the Protection of Human Subjects of Biomedical and Behavioral Research. 1979. *The Belmont report*. Washington, DC: Department of Health and Human Services. Available at: http://www.hhs.gov/ohrp/humansubjects/guidance/belmont.html.

Office of the United Nations High Commissioner for Refugees (UNHCR). 2016. Available at: http://www.unhcr.org/pages/49c3646c2.html.

Schroeder, D., and E. Gefenas. 2009. Vulnerability: Too vague and too broad? *Cambridge Quarterly of Healthcare Ethics* 18 (2): 113–121. https://doi.org/10.1017/S0963180109090203.

Schuman, J. 2012. Beyond Nuremberg: A critique of informed consent in third world human subject research. *Journal of Law and Health* 25: 123–153.

Silverman, H. 2011. Protecting vulnerable research subjects in critical care trials: Enhancing the informed consent process and recommendations for safeguards. *Annals of Intensive Care* 1 (1): 8. https://doi.org/10.1186/2110-5820-1-8.

Ethical Issues Involving Informed Consent in the Arab Region

Shahd Osman

Introduction

Informed consent is a fundamental requirement for ethical conduct in research involving human participants. The focus on informed consent was a primary subject of the first international code of research ethics developed after World War II. During the war, Nazi physicians committed atrocious acts in the name of human experimentation. After the war, they were prosecuted for war crimes by the Nuremberg Tribunal in Germany 1947. From that trial, the Nuremberg code, which includes ten statements to protect human subjects from exploitation by research, was developed (Nuremberg Code 1949).

The first principal of the Nuremberg Code and cornerstone of this code, is as follows:

> The voluntary consent of the human subject is absolutely essential. This means that the person involved should have legal capacity to give consent; should be so situated as to be able to exercise free power of choice, without the intervention of any element of force, fraud, deceit, duress, over-reaching, or other ulterior form of constraint or coercion; and should have sufficient knowledge and comprehension of the elements of the subject matter involved, as to enable him to make an understanding and enlightened decision. (Nuremberg Code 1949)

The principal of informed consent is included in all research ethics guidelines that emerged after the Nuremberg Code. In 1964, the World Medical Association issued the Declaration of Helsinki, which was geared towards ethics of research involving patients and was last updated in 2013 (World Medical Association 2013). Since important research needs to be performed involving individuals unable to provide consent, e.g., mentally ill and children, the Declaration recommended that

S. Osman (✉)
Public Health Institute, Federal Ministry of Health, Khartoum, Sudan
e-mail: Osman.shahd@gmail.com

H. Silverman (ed.), *Research Ethics in the Arab Region*, Research Ethics Forum 5,
https://doi.org/10.1007/978-3-319-65266-5_6

such individuals can participate in research with surrogate consent. The Belmont report of 1979 covered the issue of informed consent under the principal of "respect for persons", which entails that individuals need to provide their autonomous consent and those who cannot give such consent require protection afforded by surrogate consent (National Commission for the Protection of Human Subjects of Biomedical and Behavioral Research 1979). Based on the western philosophy of liberal individualism, persons are autonomous when they are able to practice self-governance, which means they would not allow the influence of others when making their own decisions (Schuman 2012).

For more clarity regarding informed consent, the Belmont Report described acts that interfere with the voluntariness of research subjects. This included coercion, where the subject may feel endangered by some sort of threat if they do not participate in the research study, and undue inducement, which comprise of inappropriate incentives to participate in a study that might interfere with understanding, particular of the risks and benefits (Ryan et al. 1979).

The CIOMS guidelines was developed to address international research and mentioned further details regarding informed consent compared to the previously mentioned guidelines (Council for International Organizations of Medical Sciences (CIOMS) 2002). In the last update of the CIOMS guidelines in 2016 informed consent is discussed in guideline 9, which covers the three main aspects of an informed consent for individuals that are capable of providing an informed consent; Guideline 10 covers waivers and modifications of informed consent, it emphasizes that competent individuals should provide their consent for research but explains when permission from legal guardians and waiver of consent can be appropriate. Guidelines 16, 17 and 18 focus on specific groups of vulnerable populations describing them as 1- adults incapable of giving informed consent, 2- children and adolescents, and 3- women as research participants; each chapter describes considerations to be taken during the consent process, the importance of an assent and the likelihood of the need of authorization from gatekeepers in cultures where women typically need a permission to participate in research. The guidelines also include an appendix which presents an extensive list of 26 "essential information for the research subjects" that ought to be disclosed for a consent to be informed (Council for International Organizations of Medical Sciences (CIOMS), 2016). Similar "basic" elements of informed consent are summarized in the US Code of Federal Regulations and include the following eight elements (U.S. Department of Health and Human Services 1991):

- A statement that the study involves research, an explanation of the purposes of the research and the expected duration of the subject's participation, a description of the procedures to be followed, and identification of any procedures which are experimental.
- A description of any reasonably foreseeable risks or discomforts.
- A description of any benefits to the subject or to others which may reasonably be expected from the research.
- A disclosure of appropriate alternative procedures or courses of treatment, if any, that might be advantageous to the subject.

- A statement describing the extent, if any, to which confidentiality of records identifying the subject will be maintained.
- For research involving more than minimal risk, an explanation as to whether compensation in case the case of research injury is available.
- A description of whom the subject can contact for questions about the research, research injury and questions about their rights as research subjects, with the contact details provided.
- An explanation that the research is voluntary and the subject may agree to participate or withdraw at any time without penalty or loss of benefits to which the subject is otherwise entitled.

In general, the validity of an informed consent depends on the following: (1) the extent with which researchers have disclosed the information that participants need in order to make an autonomous decision; (2) the extent to which potential participants understand the factual information and appreciate the disclosed information in the light of their situation; (3) the cognitive ability to assess the information; (4) the ability to commit to making a decision; and (5) the extent to which the decision is voluntary (i.e., free from manipulation, coercion and undue inducement).

Issues Regarding Informed Consent in the Arab Region

The guidelines for research ethics in general and for informed consent, specifically, as discussed above, were developed by western countries. Other countries, including those in the Arab region, adopted the basic principles underlying these guidelines. However, applying these principles is challenging to researchers conducting their studies in different contextual environments where the social, economic, and cultural settings may differ from that in western countries. The following sections will elaborate on the challenges investigators in the Arab region face when obtaining informed consent based on western principles.

Social Structure and the Principal of Autonomy

The fabric of Arab societies is different than that found in western societies. Though there is diversity even within the Arab region, there are still some dominant characteristics that contribute to a common social structure. For instance, the majority of people in the region follow Islam as a religion, which has a noticeable effect on behaviors and social opinions. The majority of citizens are Arabs with a culture that considers the family as the building unit of the society, which contrasts with the dominance of the individual in western societies. Overall Arabic traditions and norms prevail and are followed by most of the existing communities (Alahmad et al. 2015).

Informed consent has stemmed basically from the principle autonomy, which reflects a liberalism that emphasizes a concept of individual rights. The lure that is related to the sense of freedom in this principal drives researchers to embrace a notion that might actually be overlooking the social structure and context they are trying to study (Schuman 2012). As such, in societies in the Arab region, the social network is very strong, people commonly live in nuclear and extended families; children (whether males or females) remain living with their parents until they marry and afterwards, and family members remain close both physically and socially. There is a great deal of respect to elders and often within the household there are power positions dominated by the male head (parent). As children mature they assume the dominant position and maintain responsibility for their aging parents. In view of this context, individualism is disregarded in such societies and personal choices usually reflect the common good of the family unit. In tribal areas, the family network extends to larger societal networks where group leaders also possess power positions on a community.

Based on the above, if scholars from Western countries or even scholars from the Arab region try to advocate for a universal informed consent procedure based on the western model of autonomy, they will find themselves ignoring contextual issues that can affect the consent process. For example, when taking an informed consent, researchers might find themselves obliged to take permission from multiple sources before obtaining individual consent from participants themselves (Abdel-Messih et al. 2008a; Nakkash et al. 2009). With regards to gender, Killawi and colleagues noticed in their study done in Qatar (which examines the procedures by which informed consent is obtained) that more women of Arabic backgrounds felt a need to discuss with their husbands or family members before providing consent to participate in the research study. This observation might reflect the power position of males in those societies whereby women are expected to be submissive to the male figure (Killawi et al. 2014).

Several studies in African and Middle-Eastern contexts advocate for a stepwise approach of consent that will take permission from gatekeepers followed by a discussion with the potential participants that then permits them enough time to discuss with friends and family before making a decision to participate (Abdel-Messih et al. 2008b; Alaei et al. 2013; Tindana et al. 2006). The strategies used for each study will probably need to be context specific. However, the key issue that can help guide researchers seeking consent is understanding and acknowledging that they need to prioritize the values of the participants (collectivism) rather than those from western thought (i.e., individualism).

Some scholars maintain, however, that the principal of autonomy is congruent with a social structure that favors collectivism over individualism. How is that possible? Individuals exert their autonomous choices when they decide *whether to consult with others or not and how much influence they desire to accept* (Schuman 2012). These thoughts align with the Belmont Report's emphasis on "respect for persons" rather than a primary emphasis on autonomy.

However, a concern with this line of thinking that gives weight to the principle of autonomy amongst societal norms that warrants women to obtain permission from gatekeepers (husband, tribe leaders, etc.) is that it validates inequality and jeopardizes voluntariness. Indeed, Lobato and colleagues showed that women have a greater chance compared to men to have their decision to participate in a clinical trial influenced by their conjugal partner or their families (Lobato et al. 2014). These authors opined that "due to external circumstances, such as lack of power, women should be considered extrinsically vulnerable" (Lobato et al. 2014). Thus, the presence of such differences in context and power relations makes the informed consent process problematic for women on an autonomy based concept.

For researchers to address societal norms that disempower women while ensuring that research participation is nonetheless voluntary, several commentators advocate the use of strategies that involve assessing whether participants understand that they can withdraw at any point without repercussions; commentators also recommend obtaining re-consent several times during the study period to ensure that the women participating in the study are doing so voluntarily (Lobato et al. 2014). Several studies that have assessed the presence of voluntariness of consent among women have shown mixed results (Horwitz et al. 2013; Karim et al. 1998; Onvomaha et al. 2006).

Literacy and Language Whilst Assuring Comprehension

Participants' comprehension of the disclosed information is necessary for consent to be valid. The basic elements of informed consent, as described previously, coupled with extensive legal language as required by pharmaceutical companies and academic sponsors can be quite intimidating and extensive leading to long and complex consent forms. Obtaining informed consent with the use of documents containing complex language remains a challenge when dealing with individuals who are illiterate or who speak a language where research concepts may not be easily translated into the native language (e.g., concepts such as "placebo", "double-blind", "randomization, etc.).

Nakkash and her colleagues in a study that focused on obtaining informed consent from youths in a refugee camp in Lebanon, described their attempt at fulfilling the consent requirements as tedious, time consuming and could even complicate the process when dealing with lower levels of literacy. In addition, certain marginalized populations (e.g., impoverished persons, sex workers, drug addicts, etc.), who might not be familiar with this level of detail- may consider the large amount of information provided in the consent procedure as suspicious. The authors suggest that the social and educational context should be studied to evaluate issues that might affect comprehension and subsequently, consent forms can be written in a manner that addresses the population literacy levels and other needs (Nakkash et al. 2009).

Similarly, Alaei and colleagues from Iran aimed to create a model of how to obtain consent from illiterate populations, particularly in Islamic countries (Alaei et al. 2013). The authors first involved the local religious leaders along with health officials and explained to them the purpose of the research. Afterwards, trained health personnel visited the households of the potential participants and explained the research to them; subsequently participants were allowed one week to ask and discuss with their leaders, families and others the research study until they make their decision on whether they want to participate or not.

Even though such an approach can be time consuming, the authors believed that the process was successful in addressing cultural issues through involving religious leaders and enhancing comprehension of the participants, allowing them enough time to think and discuss their understanding with trained personnel from the same context.

An additional comprehension challenge in informed consent, particularly in international collaborations, involves the need to translate the written document from one language to the other; usually from English to the native language. Inexact translations may affect understanding of the information present in the form and add additional complexity particularly when dealing with persons of low literacy levels. Alaei and colleagues suggested that the presence of a translator who knows the community dialect and understands the terminology of the consent forms is essential to enable comprehension for illiterate populations (Alaei et al. 2013).

When the Culture of Signing Is Problematic

In the CIOMS guidelines, obtaining written signatures is considered the general rule when obtaining an informed consent from competent persons (Council for International Organizations of Medical Sciences (CIOMS) 2002). General exceptions to written signatures exist and are discussed below. However, for many individuals in the Arab region, signing forms is reserved for special transactions. Specifically, signatures in some cultures are used mainly for legal issues or major life events. Thus, asking a participant to sign a document for research purposes may not reflect enough of an important cause for them to do so and hence, might arouse suspicion that they are providing consent for a transaction that may carry some sort of repercussions. Finally, asking for a signature may also be interpreted as lack of trust by the researchers towards the participants (Abdel-Messih et al. 2008a; Nakkash et al. 2009; Killawi et al. 2014).

Killawi and colleagues in their study on informed consent in Qatar noted that participants felt comfortable giving their verbal consent, even though the process was actually being recorded (Killawi et al. 2014). Therefore, in reality, verbal consents are more suitable and acceptable for participants within the Arab region.

From the investigators' point of view, in a study by Hyder and Wali, 40 % of a group of investigators surveyed from low and middle-income countries (LMICs) who collaborated in international studies stated that they did not use written consents in their most recent studies. They even voiced their desire for more flexibility when it comes to documenting informed consent, which would be indicative of appreciating cultural differences (Hyder and Wail 2006).

The Clinical Investigator/Physician and the Therapeutic Misconception

In some Arab countries the doctor is called “El Hakeem”, which is the Arabic word for the wise man; the wording itself reflects how the community sees physicians as somehow more knowledgeable and trustworthy in making decisions. It is a reflection of the amount of respect exhibited by those societies towards the more educated segments (*doctors*), which innately diminishes their own voluntariness and autonomy. Nevertheless, trust actually varies even within those communities depending on factors inherent in the participants themselves; which includes education level, age, gender etc. If the researchers express more knowledge about the culture and context of potential research subjects and shows more respect towards their beliefs, they are more likely to be trusted (Alaei et al. 2013).

A concern with such trust is that patients who are potential participants in health research would enroll in the research study believing that their physician/investigators are advocating specifically for their individual welfare and are recommending therapies that are specifically tailored for them. Such a belief is congruent with the concept of the therapeutic misconception (TM).

At its basic level, TM involves a research participant's failure to recognize the distinction between research and clinical care. There are two ways in which TM can be manifested: (1) when research participants fail to recognize that decisions regarding certain aspects of the research procedures (e.g., randomization, dosages and duration of administered drugs) will not be individualized to their personal needs (TM1); or (2) when research participants hold an unreasonable appraisal of the nature or likelihood of medical benefit from their study participation (TM2) (Appelbaum et al. 2004). Hence, research participants might be mistaken about how the research will be executed (TM1) or may believe that the research is designed in a manner to ensure direct benefits to them (TM2) (Appelbaum et al. 1982).

For more than three decades, commentators have expressed concerns about research participants not distinguishing between research and clinical care (Dresser 2002; Miller and Rosenstein 2003). Indeed, several empirical studies from Western and African countries have shown that individuals participating in clinical research misconstrue a therapeutic intention to the research procedures in a study (Henderson et al. 2006; Molyneux et al. 2004).

Recently, several studies in the Arab region have demonstrated that potential participants in the Middle East are liable to the therapeutic misconception. In a study involving in-depth interviews of 15 lay persons recruited from the outpatient setting of a university hospital Egypt, investigators showed that a majority of participants (11/15) expressed inaccurate beliefs regarding the degree with which individualized care will be maintained in the research setting (TM1) and a smaller number of participants (5/15) manifested an unreasonable belief in the likelihood of benefits to be obtained from a research study (TM2). A total of 12 of the 15 participants were judged to have expressed a TM on either one of these bases (Wazaify et al. 2009). In a cross-sectional study involving 103 participants in ten clinical trials, Mansour and colleagues demonstrated a high rate of the therapeutic misconception. Specifically, they showed that all participants thought the research and the drug would improve their condition; only 46.1% were aware of receiving a non-approved experimental drug and 21.3% were aware of being randomized (Mansour et al. 2015).

The presence of the therapeutic misconception raises several ethical issues. First, failure to appreciate correctly the risks and benefits of research participation raises concerns regarding the validity of informed consent (Appelbaum et al. 1982; Miller and Rosenstein 2003). Second, the presence of TM reflects the very real possibility that research participants will see themselves as patients and conflate the investigator's role with that of the physician. The resulting concern is that patients will be susceptible to exploitation, as investigators might take advantage of the trust patients have for their "doctors" to enroll them in clinical research (de Melo-Martin and Ho 2009). Such investigators might be acting under the influence of a conflict of interest (Abdel-Messih et al. 2008a).

Ethical Issues Involving Refugees and Internally Displaced Persons

Following the Arab Spring, conflict and war emerged in different areas leading to humanitarian emergencies with increasing numbers of internally displaced persons (IDPs) and refugees in need of relief and support (*UNHCR Global Appeal 2015 Update* 2015). Researchers maintain that studies involving refugees and IDPs are important to answer many questions related to their unique condition. These include issues related to distribution of humanitarian aid in the refugee camps, management of mental health due to violence and displacement, and the extent to which their human rights are maintained in such camps. Such studies aim to generate knowledge to enhance their situation.

However, refugees and IDPs have multiple reasons for vulnerability that might compromise the validity of their informed consent and voluntariness to participate in such studies. Suitably described by Leaning, refugees rights are diminished compared to that enjoyed by citizens, as refugees live in an atmosphere with widespread abuse and are commonly threatened by the enemy that made them escape (Leaning 2001). When it comes to performing research involving refugees and IDPs, guidelines have neither provided a specific ethical framework for such research nor provided sufficient information regarding specific measures to provide additional protection.

In general, there are several issues to consider when obtaining informed consent from members of these populations that need investigators to: (1) be cognizant of the backgrounds of the participants and the reasons they fled, (2) consider their level of education, and (3) consider the presence of a language barrier if any and their social framework. Furthermore, during the process of obtaining consent for research purposes, the investigator needs to consider how privacy will be attained in crowded camps, how to establish trust and how to avoid the presence of a power imbalance between researcher and participant (Nakkash et al. 2009). These issues will be further explored in the Chapter in this book involving "Ethical Issues involving research in conflict areas".

Investigators' Awareness and Knowledge in Research Ethics and Its Influence on the Consent Process

Awareness and knowledge among researchers in the Arab region regarding best practices in research ethics, in general, and the importance of informed consent, in particular, have shown to be insufficient (El-Dessouky et al. 2011; Kandeel et al. 2011). Furthermore, senior researchers have often expressed concerns about the limited capacity of their staff in obtaining an informed consent coupled with poor capacities of their overwhelmed research ethic committees to oversee the process (Bhutta 2004; Alahmad et al. 2015; Rab et al. 2008). Thus, training programs need to be developed that focus on enhancing capacities in research ethics in the Arab region (see chapter in this book entitled "Establishing Training Programs for Investigators and Members of Research Ethics Committees"). It might even be advisable to arrange for expert researchers and communication experts to undertake the process of an informed consent (Schuman 2012). For international collaborative research, several commentators believe that different stakeholders representing different backgrounds should be involved in the development of the forms and the procedure of consent obtainment (Rivera et al. 2007).

Methods to Improve Informed Consent

In the light of the challenges described when attempting to obtain an informed consent in the Arab region, the following summarizes several methods that can improve the process:

Community consultation: consulting the community that will be the focus of the research setting before initiating any research establishes trust between the investigators and the potential participants. An important aspect to emphasize is for researchers to engage in discussions with gatekeepers and community leaders with the planning of the informed consent process and with the development of the consent form to ensure that it is written in understandable language that can be readily comprehended for that particular community. Scholars have recommended a tiered consent process consisting of a general informational meeting with the community followed by an individual informed consent process. Such an approach would allow more time for potential participants to think about and discuss with others their willingness to participate in a research study (Alaei et al. 2013; Abdel-Messih et al. 2008a; Nakkash et al. 2009).

Cultural Sensitivity: Aspects of the informed consent process should embrace cultural sensitivity. For example, disclosure of information should take into account the contextual setting of the potential participants and the use of appropriate language and wordings that respect local norms; it might be appropriate to have translators who speak the local language if investigators do not speak the local language themselves. Consent forms should also be written in the local language. In addition, investigators need to embrace a concept of autonomy that is less about individual self-determination and more inclusive of a web of relationships. Nevertheless, obtaining permission from other parties does not by any mean disregard the requirement of a voluntary consent of a potential participant (Abdel-Messih et al. 2008a; Killawi et al. 2014).

Verbal consent: In populations where signatures to enroll in research are viewed with suspicion, it would be more practical to obtain a verbal consent. Alternative ways of documenting the informed consent process may also be applicable. Such measures would include audio-taping and the presence of a witness or the researchers writing on their own notes for documentation. In general, guidelines accept verbal consent only when documentation via a written approach is not feasible (Abdel-Messih et al. 2008b; Killawi et al. 2014).

Addressing literacy levels: Low literacy levels affect the comprehension of potential participants in regards to both the consent dialogue and the informed consent document. Investigators should consider alternative methods that will enhance comprehension; these might include illustrations, video tapes, educational forums or any innovative method that can help clarify the information for those potential participants. Investigators may also involve communication experts in the procedure to facilitate understanding. A method that can enhance and ensure comprehension has been achieved is asking the potential participants questions about the information they received before obtaining consent (Bhutta 2004).

Guidance on obtaining informed consent from refugees and IDPs: Important research needs to be performed that involves the participation of refugees and IDPs. The international community in conjunction with local experts need to develop rigorous guidelines that outline the types of research that can be conducted and that outline the informed consent process from refugees and IDPs. These vulnerable populations are in dire need of protection given their special circumstances. Guidance should aim towards methods of obtaining a valid consent, assurance of voluntariness, and avoidance of exploitation.

Training in research ethics: lack of research ethics training affects the competence of researchers when obtaining informed consent. Such training programs in the Arab region can enhance research ethics capacity, especially among junior researchers. Likewise, the presence of an expert researcher in the field when obtaining an informed consent is advised if the competence of the research staff is in question.

Waivers Involving Informed Consent

There might be occasions when in order to conduct important research, it would be necessary to waive certain aspects of the informed consent process. These situations and the associated criteria includes the following:

Waiver of the Requirement to Obtain a Signed Informed Consent Document.

General exceptions to the obtainment of written signatures to document the informed consent process exists. Research ethics committees (RECs) may waive the requirement to obtain a signed consent form for some or all subjects if it finds that either:

1. The research presents no more than minimal risk of harm to subjects and involves no procedures for which written consent is normally required outside of the research context, or
2. The only record linking the subject and the research would be the informed consent document and the principal risk would be potential harm resulting from a breach of confidentiality.

Alteration or Waiver of Basic Elements of Informed Consent

The REC may approve a consent procedure that alters or does not include some or all of the basic elements of informed consent if it finds and documents that the research activity meets the following criteria:

- The research involves no more than minimal risk to the research participants;
- The waiver or alteration will not adversely affect the rights and welfare of the research participants;
- The research could not practicably be carried out without the waiver or alteration; and
- Whenever appropriate, the research participants will be provided with additional pertinent information after participation.

The concept of being "impracticable" refers to logistical and methodological constraints. An example of the former would be a research study that involves reviewing retrospective records that span over a long period of time from hundreds of participants, many of whom might have died, moved, or changed phone numbers. Examples of methodological constraints would include research in which individuals who might refuse informed consent would lead to consent bias and thus, invalidate the scientific integrity of the research.

Waiver of Consent for Planned Emergency Research

The REC may approve a research study without requiring that informed consent of all research subjects be obtained if it finds and documents that the research activity meets the criteria for an exception to the requirement to obtain informed consent for emergency research as addressed under planned emergency research regulations.

These regulations are summarized at the following website (UCLA Office of the Human Research Protection Program 2011).

Waiver of Parental Consent

In the Arab region where recent conflicts and wars have left many adolescents without parents, important social science research would be hindered if such adolescents are not considered able to provide their own consent. As such, for studies in which parents are not available to give consent, an REC may determine that such adolescents can be considered emancipated minors or mature minors. Such a determination can be made for other types of studies in which parents are not readily available (e.g., studies involving street children).

The REC may also waive the requirement for parental consent if it determines that parental or guardian permission is not a reasonable requirement to protect the participants or obtaining consent would make it impracticable to conduct the study. (e.g., abused or neglected or abused children).

Conclusion

International guidelines present a good framework for researchers around the world when obtaining informed consent. Because such guidelines emanate from western countries, controversies may occur when trying to apply them in social, political, economic, and cultural contexts that differ from the West. Several studies have explored the challenges faced by researchers when applying western regulations in nonwestern regions. For the Arab region, we have highlighted the challenges encountered with the observed differences in culture, religion, economics and politics. Allowing flexibility in the application of guidelines when obtaining an informed consent represents a way forward for a process that is more sensitive to the local setting. Recent issues in the Arab region involving refugees, IDPs, and children without surrogates or guardians need to be considered when current international guidelines are revisited. Informed consent is an integral requirement for ethical conduct of research and should not be jeopardized in any population.

References

Abdel-Messih, I.A., M. El-Setouhy, M.M. Crouch, and K.C. Earhart. 2008a. Developing cultural competence and overcoming ethical challenges in the informed consent process: An experience from Egypt. *The Journal of Research Administration* XXXIX (2): 33–40.

Abdel-Messih, I.A., M. El-Setouhy, M.M. Crouch, and K.D. Earhart. 2008b. Developing cultural competence and overcoming ethical challenges in the informed consent process: An experience from Egypt. *The Journal of Research Administration* XXXIX: 33–40. Available at: http://files.eric.ed.gov/fulltext/EJ888522.pdf.

Rab, Mohammad Abdur, Mohammad Afzal, Alaa Abou-Zeid, and Henry Silverman. 2008. Ethical practices for health research in the eastern Mediterranean region of the World Health Organization: A retrospective data analysis. *PloS One* 3 (5): e2094. https://doi.org/10.1371/journal.pone.0002094.

Alaei, M., A. Pourshams, N. Altaha, G. Goglani, and E. Jafari. 2013. Obtaining informed consent in an illiterate population. *Middle East Journal of Digestive Diseases* 5 (1): 37–40. http://www.ncbi.nlm.nih.gov/pubmed/24829668.

Alahmad, G., M. Al-Jumah, and K. Dierickx. 2015. Confidentiality, informed consent, and children's participation in research involving stored tissue samples: Interviews with medical professionals from the Middle East. *Narrative Inquiry in Bioethics* 5 (1): 53–66.

Appelbaum, P.S., L.H. Roth, and C. Lidz. 1982. The therapeutic misconception: Informed consent in psychiatric research. *International Journal of Law and Psychiatry* 5: 3–4.

Appelbaum, P.S., C.W. Lidz, and T. Grisson. 2004. Therapeutic misconception in clinical research. Frequency and risk factors. *IRB Ethics & Human Research* 26: 1–8.

Bhutta, A.Z. 2004. Beyond informed consent. *Bulletin of the World Health Organization* 82: 771–777.

Council for International Organizations of Medical Sciences (CIOMS). 2002. International ethical guidelines for biomedical research involving human subjects. Geneva. Available at: http://www.cioms.ch/publications/layout_guide2002.pdf.

Council for International Organizations of Medical Sciences (CIOMS). 2016. International Ethical Guidelines for Health-related Research Involving Humans, Fourth Edition. Geneva. Available at: https://cioms.ch/wp-content/uploads/2017/01/WEB-CIOMS-EthicalGuidelines.pdf

de Melo-Martin, I., and A. Ho. 2009. Beyond informed consent: The therapeutic misconception and trust. *Journal of Medical Ethics* 34: 202–205.

Dresser, R. 2002. The ubiquity and utility of the therapeutic misconception. *Social Philosophy & Policy Foundation* 19: 271–294.

El-Dessouky, H.F., A.M. Abdel-Aziz, C. Ibrahim, M. Moni, R. Abul Fadl, and H. Silverman. 2011. Knowledge, awareness, and attitudes about research ethics among dental faculty in the Middle East: A Pilot Study. *International Journal of Dentistry* 2011: 694759. https://doi.org/10.1155/2011/694759.

Henderson, G.E., M.M. Easter, C. Zimmer, M.P. King Nancy, A. Davis, B.B. Rothschild, … D.K. Nelson. 2006. Therapeutic misconception in early phase gene transfer trials. *Social Science & Medicine* 62: 239–253.

Horwitz, R.H., L.W. Roberts, D.W. Seal, P. Joseph, K.J. Maschke, R.I. Verdier,… D.W. Fitzgerald 2013. Assessing whether consent for a clinical trial is voluntary. *Annals of Internal Medicine* 158(3): 222–224. doi:https://doi.org/10.7326/0003-4819-158-3-201302050-00025.

Hyder, A.A., and S.A. Wail. 2006. Informed consent and collaborative research: Perspectives from the developing world. *Developing World Bioethics* 6 (1): 33–40.

Kandeel, N., A. El-Nemer, N.M. Ali, H. Kassem, M. El-Setouhy, M. E. Elgharieb,… H.J. Silverman 2011. A multicenter study of the awareness and attitudes of Egyptian faculty towards research ethics: A pilot study. *Journal of Empirical Research on Human Research Ethics* 6(4): 99–108. doi:https://doi.org/10.1525/jer.2011.6.4.99.

Karim, A.Q., S.S.A. Karim, H.M. Coovadia, and M. Susser. 1998. Informed consent for HIV testing in a South African Hospital: Is it truly informed and truly voluntary? *American Journal of Public Health* 88: 637–640.

Killawi, A., Khidir, A., Elnashar, M., Abdelrahim, H., Hammoud, M., Elliott, H.,… Fetters, M.D. 2014. Procedures of recruiting, obtaining informed consent, and compensating research participants in Qatar: Findings from a qualitative investigation. *BMC Medical Ethics* 15: 9. doi:https://doi.org/10.1186/1472-6939-15-9.

Leaning, J. 2001. Ethics of research in refugee populations. *Lancet* 357 (9266): 1432–1433. https://doi.org/10.1016/S0140-6736(00)04572-4.

Lobato, L., J.M. Bethony, F.B. Pereira, S.L. Grahek, D. Diemert, and M.F. Gazzinelli. 2014. Impact of gender on the decision to participate in a clinical trial: A cross-sectional study. *BMC Public Health* 14: 1156. https://doi.org/10.1186/1471-2458-14-1156.

Mansour, H., N. Zaki, R. Abdelhai, N. Sabry, H. Silverman, and S.S. El-Kamary. 2015. Investigating the informed consent process, therapeutic misconception and motivations of Egyptian research participants: A qualitative pilot study. *Eastern Mediterranean Health Journal* 21 (3): 155–163. http://www.ncbi.nlm.nih.gov/pubmed/26074215.

Miller, F.G., and D.L. Rosenstein. 2003. The therapeutic orientation to clinical trials. *The New England Journal of Medicine* 348: 1383–1386.

Molyneux, C.S., N. Peshu, and K. Marsh. 2004. Understanding of informed consent in a low-income setting: Three case studies from the Kenyan coast. *Social Science & Medicine* 59: 2547–2559.

Nakkash, R., J. Makhoul, and R. Afifi. 2009. Obtaining informed consent: Observations from community research with refugee and impoverished youth. *Journal of Medical Ethics* 35 (10): 638–643. https://doi.org/10.1136/jme.2008.028936.

National Commission for the Protection of Human Subjects of Biomedical and Behavioral Research. 1979. *The Belmont report*. Washington, DC: Department of Health and Human Services. Available at: http://www.hhs.gov/ohrp/humansubjects/guidance/belmont.html.

Nuremberg Code. 1949. *Trials of war criminals before the Nuremberg Military Tribunals under control council law, no. 10*. Washington, DC: U.S. Government Printing Office.

Rivera, R., D. Borasky, R. Rice, F. Carayon, and E. Wong. 2007. Informed consent: An international researchers' perspective. *American Journal of Public Health* 97 (1): 25–30.

Ryan, K.J., J.V. Brady, R.E. Cooke, D.L. Height, A.R. Jonsen, P. King, K. Lebacqz, D.W. Louisell, D.W. Seldin, E. Stellar, R.H. Turtle. 1979. The Belmont report ethical principles and guidelines for the protection of human subjects of research. Retrieved from.

Onvomaha Tindana, P., N. Kass, and P. Akweongo. 2006. The informed consent process in a rural African setting: A case study of the Kassena-Nankana district of Northern Ghana. *IRB* 28 (3): 1–6. Retrieved from http://www.ncbi.nlm.nih.gov/pubmed/17036437.

Schuman, J. 2012. Beyond Nuremberg: A critique of informed consent in Third World Human Subject Research. *Journal of Law and Health* 25: 123–153.

Tindana, P.O., N.E. Kass, and P. Akweongo. 2006. The informed consent process in a Rural African setting: A case study of the Kassena-Nankana District of Northern Ghana. *IRB Ethics & Human Research* 28: 1–6.

U.S. Department of Health and Human Services. 1991. Protection of Human Subjects, 45 Code of Federal Regulations (CFR) 46: Available at: http://www.hhs.gov/ohrp/humansubjects/guidance/45cfr46.html#46.101.

UCLA Office of the Human Research Protection Program. 2011. Guidance: Planned research in emergency settings with waiver of consent. Available at: http://ora.research.ucla.edu/OHRPP/Documents/Policy/8/Emergency_Setting.pdf.

UNHCR Global Appeal 2015 Update. 2015. Retrieved from http://www.unhcr.org/ga15/index.xml.

Wazaify, M., S.S. Khalil, and H.J. Silverman. 2009. Expression of therapeutic misconception amongst Egyptians: A qualitative pilot study. *BMC Medical Ethics* 10: 7. https://doi.org/10.1186/1472-6939-10-7.

World Medical Association. 2013. Declaration of Helsinki. Available at: http://www.wma.net/en/30publications/10policies/b3/.

Children as Research Participants

Henry Silverman

Research involving children has contributed to generalizable knowledge regarding many important illnesses affecting children as well as knowledge regarding their behaviors. However, when considering the potential benefits of involving children in research, one also needs to be aware that children represents a vulnerable group in which additional safeguards to protect their rights and welfare are ncessary.

The history of research involving children demonstrates that their interests were not always considered and they have, in the past, been exploited. For example, the controversial Willowbrook hepatitis experiments involving children that began in 1956 and lasted for 16 years provoked several ethical concerns. In these studies, mentally disabled children were deliberately infected with the hepatitis virus to study the natural course of the illness and to investigate the response to immunoglobulin (Rothman 1982). Furthermore, there were concerns with the informed consent process regarding content as well as the setting that might have served as an undue influence for parents to enroll their children in the research (National Institutes of Health 2016).

A major tenet involving children in research is that children should not be placed at a "disadvantage" by being enrolled in a clinical trial. Children can be "disadvantaged" by the following: (1) being exposed to greater than minimal risk research without the prospect of a compensating benefit, (2) being enrolled as research subjects unnecessarily, (3) participating in research without valid parental permission and without providing their own assent, when applicable.

H. Silverman (✉)
University of Maryland, Baltimore, MD, USA
e-mail: hsilverm@medicine.umaryland.edu

H. Silverman (ed.), *Research Ethics in the Arab Region*, Research Ethics Forum 5,
https://doi.org/10.1007/978-3-319-65266-5_7

Ethical Issues Involving Children in Research in the Arab Region

Research involving children in the Arab region is important for several reasons. First, there are significant childhood illnesses (e.g., malaria and cancer) in which affordable and accessible interventions need to be discovered and management strategies need to be determined (e.g., management of obesity and mental health). Second, children represent a large proportion of the general population in Arab countries. Statistics from 2010 show that approximately 30% of the general population is 15 years old or younger (United Nations Expert Group Meeting On Adolescents 2011). Third, there is an increasing number of "street connected children and youths" (SCCY), many of whom are without parents or guardians due to increasing poverty and recent military conflicts that have occurred in the Arab region. Many live with a variety of behavioral issues and health-related risks that warrant investigations (Woan et al. 2013).

Despite the importance of performing research that investigate childhood diseases, fatwas from the 1990s disallowed research on children (Alahmad and Dierickx 2015). However, the past decade has increasingly witnessed general acceptance that research involving children is important in order to develop new treatment strategies and protect them from non-evidence-based interventions that are nonetheless considered standard of care. In addition, based on a concept of justice, international guidelines discourage the exclusion of vulnerable groups from research. For example, the Declaration of Helsinki states that, "Groups that are underrepresented in medical research should be provided appropriate access to participation in research" (World Medical 2013).

Accordingly, recent fatwas and guidelines from the Islamic Organization of the Medical Sciences allow research involving children. However, of the 14 national guidelines regarding research in the Arab region, only three mention criteria that guide the inclusion of children in research (Saudi Arabia, Qatar, and Morocco) (Alahmad et al. 2012). The previous restrictive fatwas and the paucity of current regulations addressing children research might explain why research involving children in the Arab region has lagged behind the increased research activity seen in other low and middle income countries (Duke and Fuller 2014). Using publication data regarding children research as a benchmark, the Arab region lags behind Africa, Asia, and South Asia during the last decade, as there were less than 20 publications from the Arab region during this time period compared with approximately 800 for Africa (Duke and Fuller 2014).

Recent studies from the Arab region also reveal a continuing reluctance to include children in research. Parental fears of adverse events or of painful procedures encountered in research represents recurring themes serving as barriers for enrollment of children in research (Khalil et al. 2007; Nabulsi et al. 2011). Also, many parents feel that research must be associated with actual benefits, a condition that cannot be guaranteed in research (Khalil et al. 2007).

Vulnerability of Children in the Arab Region

The vulnerability of children stems from the following factors:

- Children commonly lack mature decision making capacity
- They are subject to the authority of others
- They may defer in ways that mask underlying dissent
- Their rights and interests may be socially undervalued
- They may have acute medical conditions requiring immediate decisions without adequate time for education and deliberation

Criteria for the Inclusion of Children in Research

The full range of additional protections for children include the following:

- Scientific Necessity
- Appropriate Balance of Risk and Benefit
- Parental Permission
- Child Assent

Principle of Scientific Necessity

This principle signifies that children should not be enrolled in a clinical investigation unless it is necessary to answer an important scientific question about the health and welfare of children. In addition, the selection of children must be equitable, meaning that participants who are capable of informed consent (adults, if such adult studies can be applicable to children) or assent (e.g., from mature minors) should be enrolled prior to those who cannot provide consent or assent. Additionally, according to the principle of extrapolation, if the course of the disease and the effects of the drug are sufficiently similar in adults and children, then one may conclude that pediatric effectiveness can be appropriately inferred from well-controlled adult studies (Roth-Cline et al. 2011).

Appropriate Balance of Risks and Benefits

Guidelines specify four categories of research based on risk and the appropriate balance between risks and benefits (45 Code of Federal Regulations (CFR) 46, June 18, 1981). All of these categories require that risks be minimized without threatening the scientific integrity of the research. These include eliminating any unnecessary research procedures that do not contribute to any of the scientific objectives, extending the exclusion criteria to prohibit high-risk children from being enrolled in the research, and instituting additional monitoring procedures (e.g., laboratory testing) to identify potential adverse events.

The first category of allowable research, as detailed in the U.S. regulations, entails that research is permitted if the level of risk is no more than minimal risk regardless of whether there is the prospect of direct benefit to the child. Similarly, the ICH Guidelines specify that allowable research requires that the "foreseeable risks to the subjects are low" and that "the negative impact on the subjects' well-being is minimized and low" (International Conference on Harmonization (ICH) 1996). The CIOMS guidelines stipulate that for research interventions or procedures that have no potential individual benefits for participants, the risks must be minimized and be no more than minimal and that the necessary data cannot be obtained without participation of children or adolescents (Council for International Organizations of Medical Sciences (CIOMS) and World Health Organization (WHO) 2016).

The second category of allowable research category regards research that is greater than low or minimal risk, in which case research guidelines worldwide mandate that such research offers a potential for a compensating direct benefit that is comparable to alternatives available outside of the study. In other words, the risk/benefit ratio of the research intervention needs to be as favorable as that offered by treatment alternatives available in clinical care. As such, the research intervention should be in equipoise with alternatives in clinical care. Such a state of equipoise ensures that children are not placed at a disadvantage by being enrolled in the research, as they will be exposed to an intervention that is believed to be comparable to what they would have received if they did not enroll in the research.

Using the concept of "net risks" that is discussed in Chap. 8 on Risks and Benefits, the requirement of equipoise entails that children are not exposed to any "net risks" from the research; that is, the net risks must not be more than zero (net risks for an research intervention is zero when there is equipoise between the research intervention and the alternatives available in clinical care).[1]

In contrast, for adults, the research intervention does not have to be in equipoise to alternatives available outside of the research, and hence, the net risks can be greater than zero. Another way of explaining these situations is to say that when the potential direct benefits from the research intervention, if any, are not enough to justify the risks from the research interventions, then the net risks are greater than zero.[2] These positive net risks to the research participant then need to be justified by the anticipated knowledge to be gained for society. Positive net risks to children should not be justified by knowledge to be gained for society, hence, the requirement of equipoise in children's research. Adults, however, can be "disadvantaged" by the research (i.e., net risks greater than zero), but they do so by giving their own consent for such "net risk" research.

The third type of allowable research category involves greater than minimal risk and no prospect of direct benefits to individual children, but likely to yield

[1]As children can be exposed to risks that are no greater than minimal risk (first risk category), it is more exact to say that children cannot be exposed to net risks that are greater than minimal risks.

[2]In Phase I trials involving healthy adults, there are no potential direct benefits and hence, ALL of the risks of the study represent "net" risks, which then need to be justified by the knowledge to be gained for society.

generalizable knowledge about the participants' disorder or condition. For such research, the following conditions must be present (45 Code of Federal Regulations (CFR) 46, June 18, 1981):

(a) The risk represents a minor increase over minimal risk;
(b) The intervention or procedure presents experiences to subjects that are reasonably commensurate with those inherent in their actual or expected medical, dental, psychological, social, or educational situations;
(c) The intervention or procedure is likely to yield generalizable knowledge about the subjects' disorder or condition that is of vital importance for the understanding or amelioration of the subjects' disorder or condition.

The regulations do not define "minor increase over minimal risk", but such a type of risk, while being more than minimal risk, might be regarded as posing no significant threat to the child's health or well-being. Examples of procedures that generate such risks include:

- Urine collection via catheter
- Lumbar puncture
- Skin punch biopsy with topical pain relief
- Bone marrow aspirate with topical pain relief

The final research risk category involves research not otherwise approvable under any of the above three categories, but has a reasonable opportunity to further the understanding, prevention, or alleviation of a serious problem affecting the health or welfare of children. In the U.S. this type of research can be performed only when reviewed and approved by a panel of experts appointed by a governmental agency (Department of Health and Human Services) and there has been time allowed for public comment.

For all of the above research categories, the following additional safeguards must be present:

- **Permission of a parent or legally authorized representative** in writing, consistent with applicable laws and regulations (Council for International Organizations of Medical Sciences (CIOMS) and World Health Organization (WHO) 2016). Many international guidelines recommend that the permission of one parent is sufficient for research. Studies involving children have documented challenges to parental permission (Nakkash et al. 2014) and several authors have highlighted the importance of cultural considerations when obtaining informed consent (Khalil et al. 2007; Nabulsi et al. 2011; Silverman 2005). Hence, the local laws should govern the exact requirements for parental permission.
- **Theassentof children** should be sought if they have the ability to understand the important aspects of the research (e.g., risks and benefits, purpose of the research,

the procedures to be performed and that participation is voluntary). The research ethics committee (REC) should determine that adequate provisions are present for soliciting the assent of the children, when in the judgment of the REC the children are capable of providing assent. In determining whether children are capable of assenting, the REC shall take into account the age, degree of understanding, maturity, and psychological state of the children involved (World Medical 2013). Assent may be waived if the child's capability is so limited that they cannot be consulted or the prospect of direct benefit important to child's health or well-being is available only in research.

Regarding the age of consent, there may not be an explicit clear legal age of adolescent consent for medical procedures in many countries. In addition, it might not be possible to assume a legal age of consent from what is considered the legal age for other activities, as the legal age can be quite variable between these activities. For example, in Saudi Arabia, adolescents need to be 18 years of age to obtain a permanent driver license, 17 years of age to obtain a job in the ministry, and 21 years old to apply for a passport without parental consent. In Egypt, an individual is considered an adult when above the age of 18 years old according to the Egyptian's child law (2008).

Research Involving Street-Connected Children and Youths (SCCY)

Street children involves those participating in gangs, are homeless due to poverty, or are without parents due to the recent military conflicts occurring in the Arab region. There are many ethical challenges in engaging such children in research, which partly contributes to the significant gaps in knowledge regarding the health of street-connected children and youths (SCCY).

Such ethical challenges include (Embleton et al. 2015):

- the absence of a parent/guardian to provide consent,
- high rates of illiteracy and substance use,
- presence of coercion,
- lack of basic necessities including lack of access to health care, and
- significant human rights violations.

Several safeguards can minimize the above challenges and thus enhance the ethics of research involving SCCYs. First, investigators should engage with local organizations in the community who work with SCCY (where they exist) or inquire about the existence of child protection systems and their potential role in the research process.

Second, investigators should explore potential processes to obtain a valid informed consent. While it is generally not possible to obtain parental consent for SCCY because many either have no identified parent or they frequently live in neglectful and abusive situations, raising issues of safety, several options are available. For example, formal consent can be obtained from the legal guardians of SCCYs, if available, or from stakeholders, such as NGOs, community organizations or SCCY leaders who have increased interaction and involvement in the lives of SCCYs. Alternatively, in certain situations research ethics committees can grant waivers to the requirement for parental permission. Such waivers are usually granted for research involving health reproductive interventions, as adolescents are legally able to consent for these types of treatments/interventions in many countries. Waivers are also granted for certain types of minimal risk research (e.g. survey research) when the requirement for parental consent would make the research impracticable to be performed. Finally, many SCCYs have adequate cognitive capacity to make autonomous decisions about their participation in research without a parent/guardian and depending on the law, may be considered mature minors or emancipated minors to give their own consent. One study that assessed the community's perception of street children's capacity to provide informed consent showed that many believed street children could provide consent for themselves (Vreeman et al. 2012).

Another safeguard for SCCYs can consist of empowering SCCY leaders to serve as peer outreach leaders to support research activities. The use of peer leaders provides additional ethical protection, as they can provide critical feedback about specific research procedures and approaches (Richter et al. 2007).

Finally, any incentive that is offered to enhance participation should be carefully selected to avoid an undue inducement. Since SCCYs lacks necessities and access to care, it might be difficult to determine what, if any type of incentive would be reasonable. Some argue that even the smallest incentive for children and youth living deprived of any possessions is an inducement for participation. Others have opined that compensation for SCCYs' participation in research can be material (a small gift, food, or clothing) or non-material (access to medical care and social services), and should take into consideration the sociocultural context (Richter et al. 2007).

Conclusion

During the past few years, private and public funding for research involving children has increased and there has been growing acceptance by many advocates for children regarding the need for such research. In addition, many now realize that countless drugs administered to children have never been adequately studied in the appropriate children populations. However, others have voiced concerns about allowing research involving children due to apprehensions regarding the present system for protecting human research participants, especially the ethics review system. For example, there is a belief that RECs are not recognizing or requiring additional protections for children. Such a concern is mirrored by the deficiencies with which such protections are mentioned in the present regulations at the national level. These issues warrant enhanced awareness of the ethical requirements for research involving children, additional education of REC members and investigators, assurances of qualified expertise on RECs, and further guidance from the national regulatory bodies. Additionally, all stakeholders involved with such research (e.g., researchers, REC members, institutional officials, and governmental regulators) play an essential role in ensuring excellence in research and assuring the protection of children who participate in such research. Well-designed and properly conducted research involving children is critical to advance the health of children.

References

Alahmad, G., and K. Dierickx. 2015. Pediatric research ethics: Islamic perspectives. *British Journal of Medicine & Medical Research* 5: 1158–1168.

Alahmad, G., M. Al-Jumah, and K. Dierickx. 2012. Review of national research ethics regulations and guidelines in Middle Eastern Arab countries. *BMC Medical Ethics* 13: 34. https://doi.org/10.1186/1472-6939-13-34.

Code of Federal Regulations (CFR) 46. 1981, June 18. Federal Policy for the protection of human subjects: Subpart D: Additional Protections for Children Involved as Subjects in Research.

Council for International Organizations of Medical Sciences (CIOMS), & World Health Organization (WHO). 2016. *International ethical guidelines for health-related research involving humans*. Geneva.

Duke, T., and D. Fuller. 2014. Randomised controlled trials in child health in developing countries: Trends and lessons over 11 years. *Archives of Disease in Childhood* 99 (7): 615–620. https://doi.org/10.1136/archdischild-2013-305702.

Embleton, L., M.A. Ott, J. Wachira, V. Naanyu, A. Kamanda, D. Makori, et al. 2015. Adapting ethical guidelines for adolescent health research to street-connected children and youth in low-and middle-income countries: A case study from western Kenya. *BMC Medical Ethics* 16: 89. https://doi.org/10.1186/s12910-015-0084-y.

International Conference on Harmonization (ICH). 1996. *Good clinical practice*. Available at: http://www.ich.org/products/guidelines/efficacy/article/efficacy-guidelines.html

Khalil, S.S., H.J. Silverman, M. Raafat, S. El-Kamary, and M. El-Setouhy. 2007. Attitudes, understanding, and concerns regarding medical research amongst Egyptians: A qualitative pilot study. *BMC Medical Ethics* 8: 9.

Nabulsi, M., Y. Khalil, and J. Makhoul. 2011. Parental attitudes towards and perceptions of their children's participation in clinical research: A developing-country perspective. *Journal of Medical Ethics* 37 (7): 420–423. https://doi.org/10.1136/jme.2010.035899.

Nakkash, R.T., A. Al Mulla, L. Torossian, R. Karhily, L. Shuayb, Z.R. Mahfoud, et al. 2014. Challenges to obtaining parental permission for child participation in a school-based waterpipe tobacco smoking prevention intervention in Qatar. *BMC Medical Ethics* 15: 70. https://doi.org/10.1186/1472-6939-15-70.

National Institutes of Health. 2016. *Willowbrook hepatitis experiments*. Available at: https://science.education.nih.gov/supplements/nih9/bioethics/guide/pdf/master_5-4.pdf

Richter, M., J.N. Groft, and L. Prinsloo. 2007. Ethical issues surrounding studies with vulnerable populations: A case study of south African street children. *International Journal of Adolescent Medicine and Health* 19: 117–126.

Roth-Cline, M., J. Gerson, P. Bright, C.S. Lee, and R.M. Nelson. 2011. Ethical considerations in conducting pediatric research. *Handbook of Experimental Pharmacology* 205: 219–244. https://doi.org/10.1007/978-3-642-20195-0_11.

Rothman, D.J. 1982. Were Tuskegg & Willowbrook 'Studies in nature? *The Hastings Center* 12: 5–7.

Silverman, H. 2005. Enhancing research ethics capacity: Implications for protection of research subjects, avoiding exploitation and achieving global health. *Middle East Fertil Soc J* 10: 105–109.

United Nations Expert Group Meeting On Adolescents, Y. a. D. 2011. *Youth population and employment in the Middle East and North Africa: Opportunity or challenge?* Available at: http://www.un.org/esa/population/meetings/egm-adolescents/p06_roudi.pdf

Vreeman, R., E. Kamaara, A. Kamanda, D. Ayuku, W. Nyandiko, L. Atwoli, et al. 2012. Community perspectives on research consent involving vulnerable children in Western Kenya. *Journal of Empirical Research on Human Research Ethics* 7 (4): 44–55. https://doi.org/10.1525/jer.2012.7.4.44.

Woan, J., J. Lin, and C. Auerswald. 2013. The health status of street children and youth in low- and middle-income countries: A systematic review of the literature. *The Journal of Adolescent Health* 53 (3): 314–321.e12. e312. https://doi.org/10.1016/j.jadohealth.2013.03.013.

World Medical, A. 2013. World medical association declaration of Helsinki: Ethical principles for medical research involving human subjects. *JAMA* 310 (20): 2191–2194. https://doi.org/10.1001/jama.2013.281053.

Ethical Issues Involved with the Analysis of Risks and Benefits

Mohamed Elhassan Abdalla

Introduction

One of the roles of research ethics committees (RECs) is to ensure that research participants are protected from unnecessary risks. This is accomplished by identifying the risks of the research, minimizing such risks by using procedures that are consistent with sound study design or by using procedures performed clinically, and then determining whether the risks are reasonable to the potential benefits (National Bioethics Advisory Commission (NBAC) 2001b; Wendler and Miller 2007). In evaluating risk and benefits, RECs should consider only those risks and benefits that result from the research procedures.

Judgements as to whether risks are reasonable to benefits represent one of the REC's single most important and difficult determinations regarding whether a research protocol is ethically acceptable. Unfortunately, RECs tend to spend little time discussing the risks and benefits when compared with, for example, reviewing the informed consent form. Furthermore, research ethics guidelines offer little direction on how to weigh risks against potential benefits. As such, this chapter will discuss concepts related to risk and benefits and compare various frameworks offered to provide a systematic approach to assessing when risks are reasonable to benefits.

History of Risks and Benefits in Research Ethics Guidelines

Risks and benefits are mentioned in all of the essential guidelines of research ethics. The Nuremberg Code, which was developed as a result of the trials of war criminals 1946–1949, states that an experiment should yield a productive result for the good of society (beneficence to society), and it should avoid unnecessary physical or

M.E. Abdalla (✉)
College of Medicine, University of Sharjah, Sharjah, UAE
e-mail: melsayed@sharjah.ac.ae

H. Silverman (ed.), *Research Ethics in the Arab Region*, Research Ethics Forum 5,
https://doi.org/10.1007/978-3-319-65266-5_8

mental suffering (non-maleficence) (Nuremberg Code 1949). The Nuremberg Code also states that the degree of risk should never exceed the determined importance of the problem to be solved by the experiment (relationship of risks to benefits). The Helsinki Declaration, first issued by the World Medical Association in 1964 and last updated in 2013, affirms the same concepts, but added two additional requirements: identification of procedures to minimize the research risks and discontinuing the research if the risks are found to outweigh the benefits (World Medical Association 2013). The Belmont report published in 1979 discusses the assessment of risks and benefits and elaborates on the importance of a favorable ratio of risks and benefits (National Commission for the Protection of Human Subjects of Biomedical and Behavioral Research 1979).

Language Meanings

Risk refers to both the probability that a harm might occur and the magnitude of the harm when it occurs. These two constructs, "probability and magnitude", do not always correspond in meaning to each other. For example, a "large" risk might refer to a low probability of a significant magnitude, e.g., death. Similarly, the term "small risk" is ambiguous as it might refer to a small probability of harm or a small magnitude of harm (National Bioethics Advisory Commission (NBAC) 2001b). In contrast, benefits refer only to the magnitude of the outcome without considering the probability, which may lead to an overestimation of benefits, as a significant benefit may also incorporate a small probability of the benefit occurring. When referring to these terms, harms are properly juxtaposed with benefits, and risks (i.e., possible harms) with potential benefits (National Bioethics Advisory Commission (NBAC) 2001b).

Finally, when risks are compared with benefits, the research ethics literature frequently refers to the notion of a favorable "risk-benefit ratio" or that risks and benefits must be "weighed" and balanced. Such concepts imply that there is a quantitative relationship between risks and benefits. Although risks and benefits might be given "weights", but such determinations resist being quantified in an objective manner. Also, as "risks" and "potential benefits" refer to different concepts, it is impossible to "compare" risks and benefits as quantifiable entities, Instead, it would be best to determine whether the risks are 'reasonable' in relation to potential benefits to be gained, if any, to research participants, and to the knowledge to be gain for society". To be sure, the concept of "reasonableness" carries its own subjective ambiguity.

Role of RECs in Assessing Risks and Benefits

In research ethics, the role of RECs in assessing and comparing risks and potential benefits involves the following (i) identification of the risks in the research protocol, (ii) minimization of risks by ensuring that the protocol employs sound research methods or, whenever possible, the research is using procedures that are clinically acceptable, (iii) identification and maximization of benefits, and (iv) justifying the risks relative to the potential benefits.

Identification of Risks: Risks can be categorized as being physical, psychological, social, economic, political, legal, and dignitary (National Bioethics Advisory Commission (NBAC) 2001b). Physical harms include injury, illness, pain, suffering, or discomfort. Psychological harms include adverse emotions generated from answering questions on a survey, responding to an interviewer's questioning, distress and anxiety related to disclosure of a test result, or anxiety and shame related to the disclosure of sensitive or embarrassing information. Social harms include stigma and discrimination that emanate from the disclosure of sensitive information that results in adverse effects in subjects' relationship with others and society; e.g., revelation that one is HIV positive that leads to stigma and employment discrimination. Economic harms occur when research subjects incur financial costs that are not compensated by the research protocol; e.g., travel costs, childcare costs, or time taken off from work. Legal harms occur when legal actions are taken against research participants, such as arrest, conviction, and incarceration when illicit activities are made know to legal authorities. Political harms might occur to members of marginalized groups in society (e.g., refugees and activists) when information about such individuals (medical or social) are revealed and used against them by political forces. Finally, dignitary harms occur when research participants are not treated with respect or as mere means to investigators' interest, e.g., when blood samples are used for purposes other than what were revealed in the informed consent form. Finally, group harms might occur when sensitive information are disclosed about a characteristic of a group, e.g., ancestry data about an ethnic group (Mello and Wolf 2010).

Minimization of Risks: Once risks have been identified, RECs must ensure that such risks are minimized to the extent possible without threatening the scientific integrity of the study design. Minimization of risks can be achieved by the adoption of sound study design that addresses the research objectives, the use of procedures that are already being performed for clinical purposes; avoidance of unnecessary risks, e.g., by eliminating procedures that do not address the objectives, use of qualified personnel, augment confidentiality measures (data security), proper monitoring of participants, expanding exclusion criteria to exclude participants at higher risk, and developing appropriate withdrawal criteria to exclude participants who have already experienced a degree of harm or who are now at higher risk of experiencing harm if they remain in the study.

Identifying and Maximizing Potential Benefits: RECs should identify potential benefits associated with the procedures of a research, which include both potential direct benefits to the research participants and those that will benefit society. Potential direct benefits to research participants include improvement in health status from experimental therapies or from standard interventions that are being assessed, and receipt of clinically significant information from new diagnostic studies that can influence future health. There can also be indirect benefits, such as experiencing increasing social contacts with the research staff or gaining gratification from being part of the acquisition of new knowledge to society (National

Bioethics Advisory Commission (NBAC) 2001b). Such indirect benefits should not be included in the assessment of risks and potential benefits, as they do not relate to any particular research procedure and are likely to be highly variable among research participants. Incentives for participating in research activities should also not be considered in the assessment of benefits. While such "benefits" incentivize individuals to enroll in research, they are not related to any of the study procedures. Additionally, their inclusion in the assessment might bias judgments regarding risks and benefits, as any magnitude of risk from a particular procedure can be counterbalanced merely by increasing the incentives. Similarly, potential direct benefits that emanate from one intervention (e.g., potential benefits from an experimental drug) should not be used to justify the risks association with other procedures.

Finally, RECs need to consider the future benefits to society in the form of the generalizable knowledge to be gained from the research. RECs need to identify the nature of such benefits and to make judgments about the degree of importance of the knowledge to be gained (i.e., social value). As we will discuss, once the risks of all considered interventions are "balanced" against the potential direct benefits to participants, what remains will be the 'net' risks, the magnitude of which needs to be justified by the knowledge to be gained.

Assessing the Relation of Risks Against Benefits

The assessment of whether the risks are justified by the potential benefits when reviewing a research protocol is an integral part of the REC's evaluation of research. However, this is not an easy task for RECs, because of the lack of clear criteria and guidelines for making such judgments in a majority of the current regulations (National Bioethics Advisory Commission (NBAC) 2001b).

RECs frequently perform an assessment of risks in relationship to benefits based on an analysis of the whole protocol (Wendler and Miller 2007). A concern with the "whole protocol" approach is that any procedure or component of the protocol that offers a potential of direct benefit to the participant may be used to justify the risks from a component of the protocol that does not offer a prospect of direct benefit to the participant (e.g., a liver biopsy that is performed merely to obtain research data to address an objective). In other words, the concern is that the risks of non-beneficial procedures may be justified (or offset) by unrelated procedures that hold the prospect of direct benefit to the research participants. In a similar manner, a research intervention that presents considerable risk to participants can be justified by including in the protocol unrelated components to the research, such as free health care (Roth-Cline et al. 2011). This has been referred to as the "fallacy of the package deal" (Institute of Medicine 2004).

Another approach involves a distinct analysis of risks and benefits for each individual component of the protocol without judging the whole protocol as a single unit. This "component" approach categorizes interventions considered to be either therapeutic or non-therapeutic (see Fig. 1) (Weijer and Miller 2004). The

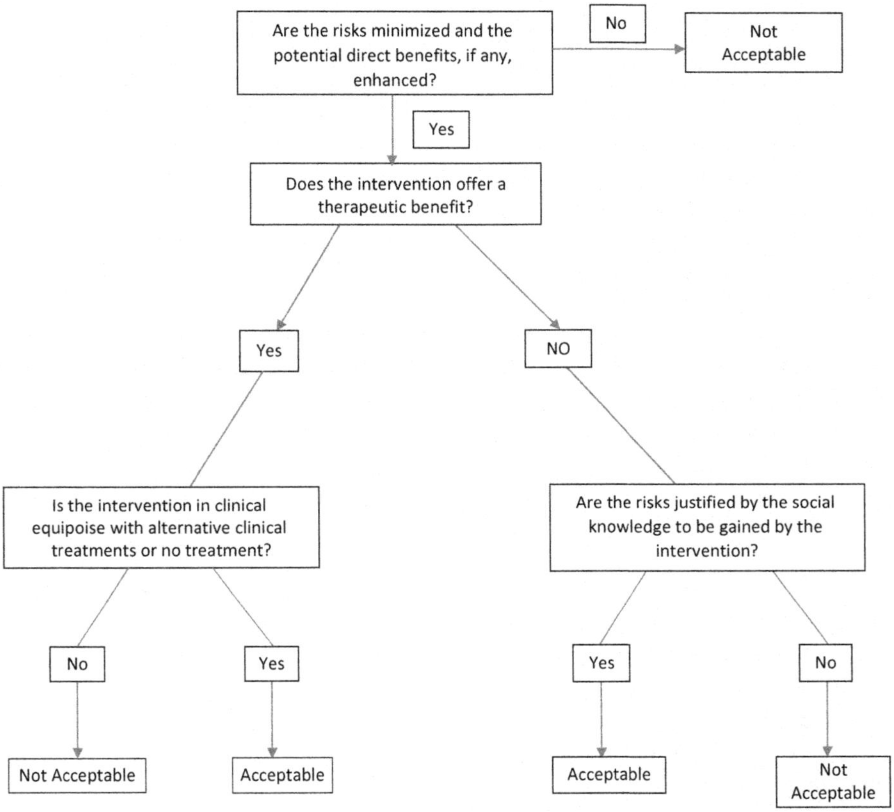

Fig. 1 Dual-track assessment of individual interventions as those that offer potential direct benefits (Adapted from Weijer and Miller 2004)

'component analysis' approach evaluates each component of the research study, some that offer the prospect of direct benefit to research participants (classified as therapeutic procedures) and others with the sole intent of answering the research questions(s) (classified as non-therapeutic). This approach requires RECs to sort the procedures of the research study into these two types of components to determine their ethical acceptability. The analysis of risks and benefits in the children regulations of the U.S. Common Rule (subpart D) incorporates this component analysis approach (45 CFR 46: Protection of Human Subjects, Rev. June 18, 1991).

According to the "component" analysis approach, therapeutic interventions are justified only when they satisfy clinical equipoise, that is, only when there is "uncertainty" in the community of practitioners as to whether the experimental intervention is as favorable as the medical standard of care. As such, the risk-benefit profile of the experimental intervention is at least as promising for the participants as any alternative standard of care that the recipients can receive outside of the study. In contrast, for components that only address a research question (e.g., blood samples that measure circulating mediators) the risks of such non-therapeutic interventions are justified by the social value of the knowledge to be gained.

There are several concerns with the component analysis approach. First, the component analysis uses two different ethical standards to justify therapeutic and non-therapeutic interventions. For example, components designed solely to answer the research question are judged based on an analysis of whether the risks are reasonable in relation to the potential gain in generalizable knowledge, while components that offer the prospect of direct benefit must meet a standard of clinical equipoise. It is unclear as to why different types of procedures (therapeutic and nontherapeutic) should be judged by different standards.

Another concern with component analysis is that the therapeutic/nontherapeutic distinction can be unclear, as seemingly nontherapeutic procedures can at the same time have a prospect of direct benefits. For example, radiological scans performed in healthy volunteers for research purposes can nonetheless offer a benefit to the volunteer if the scans uncover an unsuspecting cancer. Similarly, screening tests used in research to determine whether prospective participants qualify for enrolment can offer some potential for clinical benefit as they can reveal undiagnosed conditions. That many interventions can qualify as both therapeutic and non-therapeutic is problematic for the component analysis approach, as this approach applies conflicting ethical standards for its acceptability.

Another approach used to assess risks relative to benefits is the Net-Risks Test (Wendler and Miller 2007). Similar to component analysis, the REC must consider each intervention in the study by its own, assess the risks and potential direct benefits, and recognize the available clinical alternatives, if any, related to that intervention.

According to Wendler and Miller, there are at least two scenarios in which research interventions pose net risks to participants (Wendler and Miller 2007). The first occurs when the intervention solely addresses a research objective, i.e., it offers participants no potential for clinical benefit and hence, the net research risks is equal to all of the risks that participants face from that intervention. That is, none of the risks is offset by any potential direct benefits to participants, as there are none. For example, for a research study that includes the performance of a positron emission tomography scan for research purposes, such an intervention poses net research risks from the use of low-dose radiation. Interventions that are included to solely address a research objective will always be associated with net risks as there are no associated potential for direct benefits.

The second scenario occurs when an intervention has a prospect of direct benefits, in which case, one determines whether the risk-benefit profile of the research intervention is as favorable for participants as the available alternatives existing in standard of care. In this case, one uses the concept of clinical equipoise as a decision making assessment tool and not as an ethical standard as seen with the component analysis. If clinical equipoise exists between the research intervention and the standard of care alternatives, then there are no net risks associated with the research procedure. If clinical equipoise does not exist and the risk-benefit profile of the research intervention is less favorable to participants than one or more of the available clinical alternatives, then the research intervention pose net research risks. In other words, net risks refer to the extent that the risks and burdens of the intervention exceed its potential for clinical benefit. Examples of research interventions that offer potential direct benefits but can be associated with net risks include experimental interventions in phase II studies /clinical trials in which the intervention is not yet in clinical equipoise with standard of care treatments (i.e., the efficacy and safety of the intervention have not been studied enough for clinicians to consider the intervention to be in equipoise with the standard of care). The lack of clinical equipoise in this instance does not lead to a disapproval of the protocol, as would occur with the component analysis, but rather, one would note the existence of the net risks from this intervention and determine whether it can be justified by the scientific knowledge that will generated from that procedure (Fig. 2).

With the net-risk analysis, RECs calculate the cumulative net risks from all the interventions in the study that pose "net risks" and determine whether the culmulative net risks are "excessive". The cumulative "net risks" are not considered excessive when they are justified by the social value of the study (Fig. 2). For individuals who cannot consent, it is widely agreed that net risks should be minimal or at most a minor increase over minimal. For adults who provide consent for themselve, there is no consensus as to whether there should be a limit to cumulative net risks. With the net-risks test, separate ethical standards are not used for the different types of intervention (those with potential direct benefits and those without) as occurs with the component analysis. The use of clinical equipoise is not used as a standard, but rather as a heuristic device to determine when there is positive net-risks from an intervention that is associated with the prospect of clinical benefit.

It is instructive to ask regarding the component analysis as to why nontherapeutic procedures can be associated with net risks and justified by the social value of the research, yet therapeutic procedures associated with net risks cannot be justified by the social value of the research. Finally, the component analysis does not take into account when there are a series of multiple non-therapeutic interventions that each pose minor risks and hence, fails to determine whether the inclusion of the risks of all of these interventions taken together are excessive.

With the net-risks assessment, RECs need to develop a consistent method of quantifying the net risks of interventions that offer no clinical benefits (e.g., blood draws, chest x-rays, CAT scans, etc.), and the net risks of interventions that offer a potential direct benefit, but whose risk-benefit profile is less favorable than available clinical alternatives. In addition, RECs need to make judgments regarding the comparison of the cumulative net risks to social value. In this regard, RECs need to make sure that they are knowledgeable of the magnitude of the social benefit, in which case they may need to obtain the opinions of clinicians who are experts in subject matter of the protocol, if one is not already present on the REC.

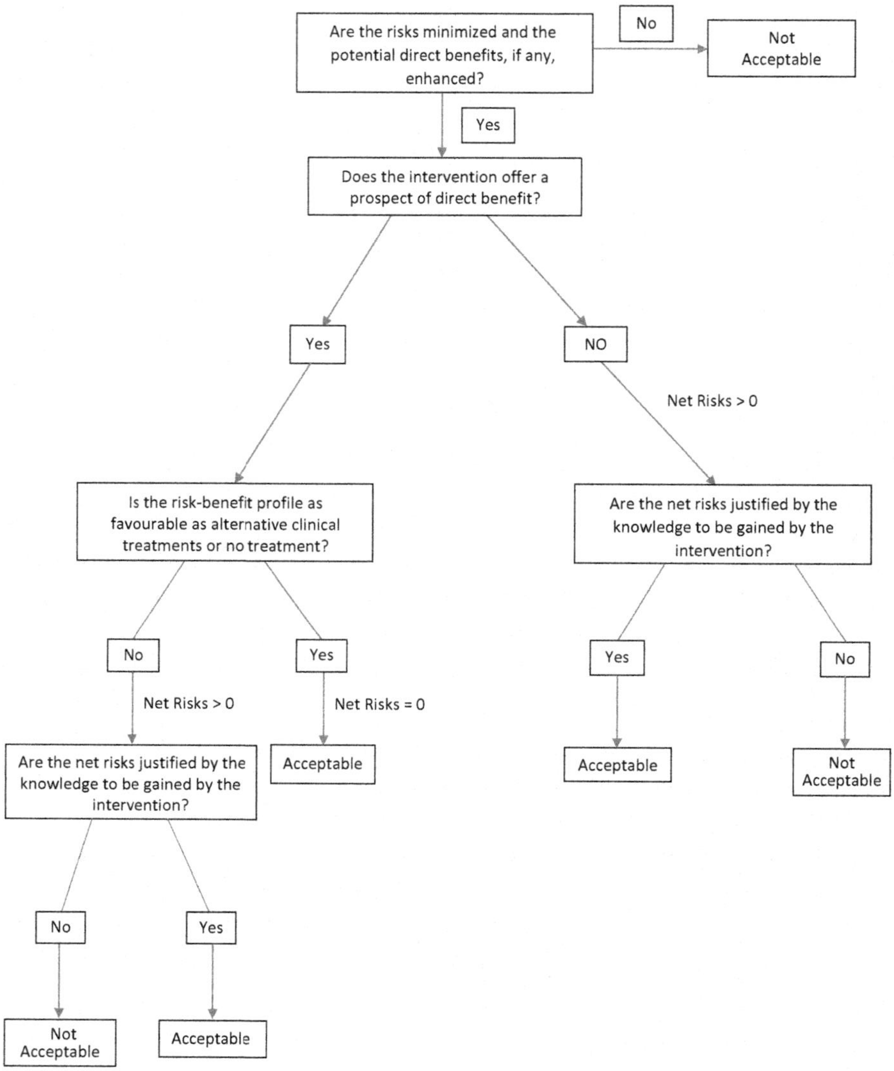

Fig. 2 Net risks test for individual interventions (adapted from Wendler and Miller 2007)

Minimal Risk

The concept of minimal risk also plays an important role in the work of RECs, as it serves as an organizing principle for many determinations. Specifically, the determination of when a waiver of informed consent is allowable depends partly on whether a protocol offers a risk level that is no more than minimal. Similarly, the determination of when a protocol can be considered exempt from the regulations or when a protocol can be reviewed by an expedited process may also depend on whether the risk level is no more than minimal. Finally, some RECs may require that the protocol offers no more than minimal risk in research involving vulnerable subjects.

Federal regulations in the United States define minimal risk as "the probability and magnitude of harm or discomfort anticipated in the research are not greater in and of themselves than those ordinarily encountered in daily life or during the performance of routine physical or psychological examinations or tests" (Department of Health and Human Services 1991).

As written, the definition of minimal risk in federal regulations provides an inconclusive standard by which risks involved in a research study are compared to those encountered in daily life. For example, there may be differences in opinion as to which daily life activities offer no more than minimal risks. The advisory report from the National Bioethics Advisory Commission (NBAC) recommends using a minimal risk standard related to the risks of daily life that are familiar to the general population (National Bioethics Advisory Commission (NBAC) 2001a). Common risks would include, for example:

- Driving to work
- Riding a bike
- Crossing the street
- Getting a blood test
- Answering questions over the telephone

However, how does one compare research procedures with activities in daily life? As such, there is well-documented variability in the interpretation and application of this minimal risk standard (Institute of Medicine 2004; Kopelman 2000).

Another uncertainty lies with whether the definition applies to those risks encountered in the daily lives *of healthy individuals* or in the daily lives of the *potential research participants*. Some RECs have interpreted "daily life" as referring to the daily life of a normal healthy person, a so-called "absolute standard," while others have interpreted "daily lives" as experiences of the "research participant", which refers to a "relative standard of minimal risk", as the standard is indexed to the research participants' own experiences. The relative standard allows research participants with illnesses to be exposed to greater risks, as such research participants are usually exposed to risks that are greater than that for normal healthy participants.

Risks and Benefits in the Arab Region

Countries in the Arab Region either have their own research ethics guidelines or they refer to one or more of the international guidelines (Alahmad et al. 2012). Alahmad and colleagues studied the research ethics guidelines in the Arab regions and concluded that 10 of the 13 countries they studied have their own guidelines. When examining the differences in the ten countries with guidelines, risks and benefits are mentioned in the guidelines of only six countries (Alahmad et al. 2012). All of these guidelines share a common feature: the importance of a favorable risk-benefit ratio, but the guidelines lack clear direction on the method to follow to assess the risks in relationship to the benefits. For example, the guidelines from Saudi Arabia indicate that the expected benefit should "compensate" for the risks identified from research procedures (National Ministry of Health Directorate General of Health Planning and Research 2008). In Kuwait, the guidelines request additional precautions when the risk is more than minimal, but such "precautions" are not specified (Ministry of Health: Kuwait Institute for Medical Specialization 2001). The guidelines for Bahrain and Lebanon only state that it is important to inform participants about the risks and expected benefits to enhance their autonomy to participate (Omran 2009; Lebanon 2012).

In regards to international collaborative research, RECs need to be mindful of the setting in which the research will be conducted as the determination of whether the risk/benefit ratio is as favorable as alternatives outside of the study might be dependent on the local setting. For example, an REC is evaluating a research study assessing the safety and efficacy of an oral rehydration therapy (ORT) in the treatment of acute watery diarrhea caused by cholera. In their analysis, the REC need to consider the side effects of the ORT, which may include vomiting, high blood sodium and high blood potassium. Previous studies have shown that the risk of death from ORT can be as high as 3%. In a country where intravenous fluids can be safely administered via an intravenous line, an REC might refuse to give approval to a study involving the use of ORT. However, in a country where the use of an intravenous solution is not possible and the risk of death from Cholera can be as high as 15%, a research study assessing an ORT solution might be acceptable.

Recommendations

For research to be ethical, risks and benefits must be reviewed according to guidelines existing in the Arab region. However, a clear conceptual framework to guide the process of determining risks and benefits is lacking in the several guidelines that do exist in the region. A precise framework requires clear definitions for the terminologies used and it should be supported by examples. REC members should follow a defined approach in their risk and benefit analysis and they should strive for consistency and transparency.

References

Alahmad, G., M. Al-Jumah, and K. Dierickx. 2012. Review of national research ethics regulations and guidelines in Middle Eastern Arab countries. *BMC Medical Ethics* 13: 34. https://doi.org/10.1186/1472-6939-13-34.

CFR 46: Protection of Human Subjects. Rev. 1991, June 18. Subpart D – additional DHHS protections for children involved as subjects in research.

Department of Health and Human Services. 1991. Federal policy for the protection of human subjects, 45 CFR 46 Subpart A. *Federal Register* 56: 28016.

Institute of Medicine. 2004. Ethical conduct of clinical research involving children. Available at: http://www.nap.edu/catalog/10958/the-ethical-conduct-of-clinical-research-involving-children.

Kopelman, L.M. 2000. Children as research subjects: A dilemma. *The Journal of Medicine and Philosophy* 25 (6): 745–764.

Lebanon. 2012. Code of medical ethics Law No. 240. Available at: https://www.aub.edu.lb/fm/shbpp/ethics/public/Documents/New-Code-of-Medical-Ethics-text-ENGLISH.pdf.

Mello, M.M., and L.E. Wolf. 2010. The Havasupai Indian tribe case – Lessons for research involving stored biologic samples. *The New England Journal of Medicine* 363 (3): 204–207. https://doi.org/10.1056/NEJMp1005203.

Ministry of Health: Kuwait Institute for Medical Specialization. (2001). Ethical guidelines for biomedical research. Available at: http://www.kims.org.kw/Ethical2.doc.

National Bioethics Advisory Commission (NBAC). 2001a. *Ethical and policy issues in research involving human participants*. Retrieved from Rockville, MD.

———. 2001b. *Ethical and policy issues in research involving human participants*. Rockville: U.S. Government Printing Office.

National Commission for the Protection of Human Subjects of Biomedical and Behavioral Research. 1979. *The Belmont report*. Washington, DC: Department of Health and Human Services. Available at: http://www.hhs.gov/ohrp/humansubjects/guidance/belmont.html.

National Ministry of Health Directorate General of Health Planning and Research. 2008. National guidelines for ethical conduct of research involving human subjects. Khartoum.

Nuremberg Code. 1949. *Trials of war criminals before the Nuremberg Military Tribunals Under Control Council Law, No. 10*. Washington, DC: U.S. Government Printing Office.

Omran, A. 2009. Health research structure & procedures. In *Kingdom of Bahrain Ministry of Health* (Ed.). Available at: http://www.moh.gov.bh/PDF/Health. Research Structure and Procedures DRAFT.pdf.

Roth-Cline, M., J. Gerson, P. Bright, C.S. Lee, and R.M. Nelson. 2011. Ethical considerations in conducting pediatric research. *Handbook of Experimental Pharmacology* 205: 219–244. https://doi.org/10.1007/978-3-642-20195-0_11.

Weijer, C., and P.B. Miller. 2004. When are research risks reasonable in relation to anticipated benefits? *Nature Medicine* 10 (6): 570–573. https://doi.org/10.1038/nm0604-570.

Wendler, D., and F.G. Miller. 2007. Assessing research risks systematically: The net risks test. *Journal of Medical Ethics* 33 (8): 481–486. https://doi.org/10.1136/jme.2005.014043.

World Medical Association. 2013. Declaration of Helsinki. Available at: http://www.wma.net/en/30publications/10policies/b3/.

Ethics of Biobanking in the Arab Region

Mamoun Ahram

The Concept of Biobanks

Biobanks represent facilities that collect and store biospecimens and other relevant personal and health information. Biobanks can be classified into private or public facilities. A public biobank is managed with the government. Such biobanks, also known as population-based biobanks, are large repositories of samples collected from healthy and diseased individuals. Private biobanks, on the other hand, are smaller and belong to certain agencies that can be academic, medical, or commercial in nature. These biobanks restrictively share biospecimens with their members or collaborators and have specific interests in terms of diseases or endpoints of research projects. Biobanks can also be classified according to the type of biospecimens they collect. Hence, a biobank can house samples of blood and its derivatives, another can be specific for DNA samples, and a third can be a tissue biobank, and so on.

The Benefits of Biobanks

Biobanks advance biomedical research by enabling researchers to access diverse, high-quality biospecimens, coupled with relevant health information associated of their donors. The growing potential at generating valuable information from such biomedical research is a result of a large number of biospecimens being collected under strict and standardized methodologies allowing for the generation of high-quality and reproducible data. Additionally, the existence of relevant information facilitates linking molecular profiling data to different variables associated with the

M. Ahram (✉)
School of Medicine, The University of Jordan, Amman, Jordan

Office of Research, Jordan University Hospital, The University of Jordan, Amman, Jordan
e-mail: m.ahram@ju.edu.jo; Dr.Ahram@gmail.com

H. Silverman (ed.), *Research Ethics in the Arab Region*, Research Ethics Forum 5,
https://doi.org/10.1007/978-3-319-65266-5_9

donor or biospecimens, which leads to valuable research outcomes. This is particularly true, for example, in regions with differential distribution of diseases due to specified gene pools and environmental exposures, such as occurs in the Arab region. In other words, diseases are not uniformly distributed across and within the different populations. In the Arab region, genetic disorders are common with a high frequency of autosomal recessive disorders (Teebi and Teebi 2005). Egypt is singled out from the other Arab countries in having a high incidence of liver cancer due to exposure to the hepatitis C virus. Therefore, the existence of biobanks in the Arab region facilitates genetic studies that could unravel the etiology of numerous diseases.

Although biobanks require generous funding early on in order to run an effective informatics system, train staff, establish standard operating procedures, and build an infrastructure, it can be argued that a long-term financial benefit can be reached at the national level. Generation of valuable scientific data and identification of novel disease biomarkers can eventually lead to lowering disease burden in a nation and, consequently, reduce costs of diagnosis and treatment (Vora and Thacker 2015). An excellent example is the economic analysis of disease burden in Luxembourg that concluded the need to focus on personalized treatment of lung cancer through the discovery of blood biomarkers, an initiative led by the Integrated Biobank of Luxembourg (Hollricher 2009).

Public Participation in Biobanks

The success of biobanks depends on the participation of individuals. Inclusion of large, diverse groups based on gender, age, ethnicity, etc. is critical in molecular profiling studies, drug-based research, or even molecular evolutionary investigations. Public participation can also provide leverage for official funding and legislative support of research. It is therefore imperative to address the perspectives of potential donors regarding their preferences for participation in biomedical research in order to reach large numbers of potential research participants and to demonstrate respect for their opinions and wishes. For example, the efforts of a national biobank in the UK were initiated via surveying the public in regards to its knowledge and perception of biobanking and the research associated with it. Based on a large body of studies, there is an overall high public interest in biomedical research and willingness to participate in biobanking in different regions of the world. As for the Arab region, reasonably positive attitudes towards biobanking were found in both Jordan and Saudi Arabia (Ahram et al. 2012; Al-Jumah and Abolfotouh 2011).

Ethical Issues Related to Biobanks

Despite the positive attitudes, biobanks are associated with a number of controversial ethical, social, and legal issues that involve the type of consent (e.g., restricted vs. broad, opt-in vs. opt-out), respecting privacy and ensuring confidentiality, returning research results, and the extent of sample and data sharing. These issues must be addressed early in order to run a successful biobanks. In this chapter, major ethical issues related to biobanking will be discussed taking into consideration the cultural and religious background of individuals in the Arab region.

Informed Consent

The informed consent process is an integral part of research that ensures the right of potential participants to make an informed decision regarding their decision to participate. The necessary disclosure of information related to research in general includes its purpose, duration, methodology, benefits and risks, the right to withdraw from the research project without any repercussions, and the right to know the results of the research. As will be explained below, biobanking-based research activities present challenges towards these disclosure requirements.

A specific challenge in the Arab region in regards to informed consent is that it is not a common practice among Arab researchers and is not an expectation among the public. The uncommon practice of informed consent was also reported with those performing genetic testing (Ahram et al. 2015). In addition, in Jordan, for example, the public do not consider the ability to give informed consent an aspect that would influence their decision to donate for a biobank (Ahram et al. 2013). In fact, the latter study revealed that a considerable number of individuals find the existence of a written informed consent as something of a negative value.

Similarly, almost half of a surveyed Saudi public did not believe the use of consent is part of the normal process (Al-Qadire et al. 2010). Even when an informed consent is used, it is deficient of critical information regarding confidentiality protections and information regarding storage of samples, risks, and right of withdrawal (Abdur Rab et al. 2008; Al-Riyami et al. 2011). Part of the problem is the absence of awareness of the important value of informed consent and the overall lack of knowledge of scientific research as a concept among the public as has previously been revealed (Khalil et al. 2007; Wazaify et al. 2009). A possible deterring factor could be the intimidation associated with the need of having the research participant “sign” the consent form. That said, informed consent remains an enduring value in research that needs to be the subject of further awareness campaigns among the public and other stakeholders involved in research.

There has been much debate about the appropriate type of informed consent needed for biobanking. One issue regards the scope of unspecified future research to which donors are giving their consent. Specifically, should the consent form could be broad and, hence, cover multiple uses of biospecimens in future research projects. Several commentators have advocated a broad consent model governed by research ethics guidelines, ethics review, and continued communications with the donors (Hansson et al. 2006; Grady et al. 2015). Broad consent allows for the use of samples in different projects, particularly since re-consenting may not be practicable, can be time-consuming and costly. However, a major concern with broad consent is the lack of knowledge on part of the participant as to the type of future research that might be conducted with the biospecimens. It is difficult to state all potential future projects that might use the collected biospecimens for biobanking, thus preventing the participant from being fully informed. Hence, a traditional format of informed consent is not a practical procedure to implement for biobanking research. Others have argued against a broad consent model due to ethical challenges that can threaten trust in biomedical research (Hofmann 2009; Maschke 2006; Widdows and Cordell 2011).

A number of attempts at formulating informed consents that balance protection of the rights of participants and broad use of samples in biobanks have been presented, taking into consideration national and international regulations (Beskow et al. 2010; da Rocha and Seoane 2008; Porteri and Borry 2008). For example, Stein and Terry (2013) proposed the use of an online dynamic consent process to obtain consent in a quick and inexpensive manner. This method of communication with biobank participants represents an excellent way to actively engage with them, inform them of the current and future states of projects, and, along the way, promote biobanking activities. Although it has a potential to succeed in the Arab region, it is currently not an effective approach due to limited use of the internet in accessing health-related information (Akhu-Zaheya et al. 2014).

Several measures in the informed consent process can be taken to enhance ethical practices and maintain trust, such as the right to withdraw, which is an essential part of any ethical research and has been found to be a favorable option by the Jordanian public (Ahram et al. 2014). Another option involves the inclusion of different levels of consent to choose from that ranges from an open consent, a disease-specific consent, a re-consent requirement, and a one-time consent.

Another debatable informed consent aspect of biobanking regards the conditions for consent required for samples that are either leftover from medical tests or collected previously for research purposes and should consent follow an opt-in or opt-out approach for subsequent secondary use in research. An opt-in approach indicates that a research participant has given explicit consent to include the biospecimen in research, whereas an opt-out approach follows the assumption that all biospecimens can be used in research unless otherwise explicitly stated otherwise. The choice of either approach is dependent on several factors, such as the type of research and its level of risk, the utilized technique, the studied biospecimens, and the individual providing the biospecimen. Giesbertz et al. (2012) offered a recommendation to implement a modified opt-out approach, whereby four conditions must be met to include biospecimens in research (Giesbertz et al. 2012). First, individuals must be aware of the meaning of this approach. Second, the participant must be given the chance to select the preferred approach. Third, competent governance in regards to how decisions are made, the type of research, the control of tissues, etc. must be established. Finally, sufficient information has to be provided to participants about the operation of the biobank.

Privacy and Confidentiality

There are several issues related to privacy and confidentiality that must be addressed in order for a biobank to succeed. An important ethical requirement in research is the need to preserve the confidentiality of participants' data (Saffi and Howard 2015). A biobank might de-identify the biospecimens, yet link the samples to the donors with a code in order to possibly re-contact donors as required for longitudinal studies. However, threats to confidentiality and leakage of information can occur by failure to secure the code.

Another issue regards invasion of third-party privacy, which occurs when donors provide health information about their family members, such as revealing the existence of multifactorial diseases among relatives as a step towards unraveling specific hereditary factors. Hence, a decision to participate in genetic research not only affects the individual, but also the entire family. For example, revealing the existence of an individual with a genetic disease may label the whole family as "diseased." In all events, there are concerns with social discrimination and stigmatization. Hence, an important consideration for any biobank is the choice of informatics systems that limit access coupled with a tight security system involving encryption and passwords.

Returning Research Results

An issue related to re-contacting biobank participants is whether and when to return health-related results to donors. There have been vigorous debates as to the advantages and disadvantages of providing biobank participants with individualized research results. Drawbacks of returning research results include misreporting data, the misinterpretation of genetic results, the association of research data with negative psychological and social burden without clinical benefit, and the need of financial and logistical support such as staffing, training in public communication and genetic counseling (Forsberg et al. 2009; Melas et al. 2010). However, returning research results has many advantages, such as showing respect towards participants, gaining their trust, increasing their interest in research, and providing them with important health-related information, such as the detection of a genetic mutation associated with a certain disease (Forsberg et al. 2009; Melas et al. 2010).

Two types of research results have been defined: individual research results (IRR) and incidental findings (IF); the former refers to results that were expected from the original aims of the intended research, whereas the latter reflects results that are beyond the original aims of the research study, and hence, unexpected (Wolf et al. 2012). For example, a researcher using a genome-wide association study (GWAS) approach in a breast cancer study may find mutations in genes known to be correlated with development of colon cancer. Because the colon cancer genetic association was beyond the aims of the breast cancer study, it is an IF. The aforementioned report offers recommendations in relation to how to deal with such data. First, the biobank must set the criteria that clearly define these findings and, then, confirms their relevance. Before making re-contact, the biobank must have a system to re-identify the donor. The authors suggest that the results must have substantial health benefits, and be validated with beneficial clinical intervention. Nevertheless, even when implementing these recommendations, the situation can be quite murky, since each biobank may develop its own guidelines and criteria in defining data that would have significant impact on the health of individuals. In Jordan, returning research results is highly favored by the public when it comes to participating in a biobank (Ahram et al. 2014). However, it must be cautioned that almost half of the participants did not wish to learn of the possibility of developing cancer by genetic testing (Ahram et al. 2015).

Withdrawal

Autonomy is one of the basic tenets of biomedical research involving human subjects. Giving biobanking donors the right to withdraw is a cornerstone of ethical research and may increase trust in the biobank itself (Helgesson and Johnsson 2005). The option of withdrawal from a biobank ranked third in terms of factors positively influencing participation in biobank among Jordanian respondents (Ahram et al. 2014). Yet, it is with no doubt that, withdrawal may have negative repercussions on the operation of the biobank itself by increasing the cost of sample and data disposal and the effort exerted into it. There is also a concern that withdrawal may affect the scientific outcome of research by creating bias in the data. Furthermore, it is difficult to trace anonymized samples distributed to other researchers or delete data generated from subsequent studies that are based on previous ones (Widdows and Cordell 2011). It gets even more difficult when it comes to defining what withdrawal actually means. Is it discontinuing the further use of biospecimens, the DNA data, or both? Is it only blocking the distribution of the biospecimens and data? Is anonymization of the biospecimens sufficient to satisfy the donor's request for withdrawal? Hug et al. suggested that withdrawal can be permitted, but it can be made a cumbersome process (Hug et al. 2012). Melham et al. later proposed the use of a dynamic consent with multilayer participation and withdrawal options (Melham et al. 2014). The latter two studies also suggested opening a dialogue with the donors about the consequences of withdrawal.

Data Sharing

In 2007, significant progress in the research of multiple sclerosis (MS) was achieved when two genes were identified to be associated with this disease after almost 30 years of reporting the first one. This effort was a result of a consortium of scientists that shared more than a thousand samples and patient information from multiple countries. It was then confirmed that the number of samples presented a limiting factor in genetic research of MS. Four years later, ten times more samples were utilized elucidating the association of 57 genetic markers with MS (International Multiple Sclerosis Genetics et al. 2011). The MS genome projects were part of larger initiatives such as the Welcome Trust Case Control Consortium (WTCCC). The latter initiative relies on the principle of open consent, which allows unrestricted use of biospecimens and disclosure of information and generated data. Such initiatives rely on the existence of biorepositories that house large number of DNA samples for use in multiple projects. They consequently generate large amount genomic data that are often shared among other investigators.

The National Institutes of Health (NIH) recently mandated genetic data sharing in the research it funds in order to promote translational research for improving human health. Therefore, it has established a centralized data repository termed "database for Genotype and Phenotype" (dbGAP). In order to safeguard confidentiality, the NIH established the Genomic Data Sharing (GDS) Policy (Vera-Badillo et al. 2014). The data submitted to dbGAP must be de-identified and consent forms given to research participants must include information about data sharing. A choice is given to the participants whether their data would be available via an unrestricted or controlled access. Whereas unrestricted access indicates that data are publicly available, the controlled-access approach necessitates prior NIH approval. The guidelines set by GDS were the basis of establishing the electronic MEdical Records and GEnomics (eMERGE) Network, a consortium of five institutions that has expanded to nine institutions, each having its own biobank and sharing resources and de-identified medical information to study major chronic conditions (Gottesman et al. 2013).

The issue of data (and biosample) sharing has been extensively analyzed in the Western countries. In general, there is general acceptance to share data for research purposes, but not for commercial purpose. Studies regarding the acceptability of data sharing among participants in the Arab region show different results. In Jordan, when surveyed participants were asked about how the participation of international scientists would affect their decision to participate in biobanking, only approximately 60% of respondents found it to be non-influential. Similarly, a significant minority of Egyptians (20%) surveyed in a study were not in favor of exporting their samples to other Arab scientists, but less eager to do so to Western countries (Abou-Zeid et al. 2010). It is therefore necessary to inform participants of the possibility of having their biospecimens and information shared with other international scientists. Finally, governments of several Arab countries have national security concerns with the exportation of biospecimens to scientists in western countries (e.g., Egypt).

Religion

The influence of religion regarding research involving sample donation can have important implications. For example, a pan-European study found an inverse correlation between belief in God and providing information to a biobank (European Commission 2012). In addition, the UK Human Genetics Commission reported a connection between the degree of religious attachment and negative view of genetic research (Human Genetics Commission 2001). In the Arab region, religion plays an important role in daily affairs of people. A review of the effectiveness of premarital screening and genetic counseling (PMSGC) programs revealed that religious convictions influenced decisions to undergo prenatal genetic testing for β-thalassemia (Saffi and Howard 2015). As for biobanking, Malay-Muslims in Singapore and UK Muslims had a negative perception of donating for a biobank, an opinion influenced by presumed religious teachings (Wong et al. 2004). In Jordan, the role of religion was shown to have the highest positive effect and the strongest correlation towards participating in a biobank (Ahram et al. 2014). In Saudi Arabia, biobanking has been extensively assessed from a religious point of view (Alahmad et al. 2010). It is important to note that the influence of religion may differ in other Arab countries where it plays a lesser role. In addition, the religious factor may not be a determining factor in biobank participation; rather, it is expected to provide psychological comfort into making the decision to enroll in research initiatives.

The Role of Research Ethics Committees

Research Ethics Committees (RECs) play a critical role in the operation of a successful biobanks by ensuring that biobanks embrace ethical practices. RECs review all details related to biobanks, such as the content of consent forms, the collection, processing, storing, and dissemination of biospecimens, as well as plans for data sharing. They may also be involved in reviewing the receipt of biospecimens from other biobanks into their institutional biobanks. However, RECs face a challenging task in making decisions along an ever-changing trend in research involving genetics and biobanking. Today's research does not follow the classical type of one-proposal, one-review type of research. Proposals and consent forms are multi-purpose nowadays where samples and information are involved in several projects with the participation of multiple investigators including international institutions. This trend has changed the way RECs function adding challenges to them. A glaring challenge is the variability that exists among RECs from different institutions in the decision making process of sharing biospecimens among researchers. Variability was based on the institutional source of biospecimens, the involvement of the original investigator who collected the biospecimens, and the required documents (Goldenberg et al. 2015; Rothwell et al. 2015). As a result, several RECs involved in the Clinical and Translational Science Awards (CTSA) consortium of the NIH have decided to implement guidances describing best practices rather than strict policies in order to add flexibility to the decision-making process in this dynamic field (Rothwell et al. 2015).

The Role of an Advisory Committee

It is advisable for a biobank to have an Advisory Committee that consists of members from various backgrounds, such as physicians, scientists, members of non-governmental organizations (NGOs), bioethicists, and laypersons. This committee sets the policies and regulations that govern the operation of the biobank from the point of donor recruitment to sharing of samples and data. The Advisory Committee should also follow any updates regarding ethical considerations of biobanking. The existence of an Access Committee, similar to the REC, is also a crucial part of the operation of a biobank. This committee reviews research applications to determine the suitability of the proposal in terms of scientific value and ethical aspects and decide on the submission of samples and data to researchers. The committee also sets priorities of research proposals to preserve samples for more valuable initiatives. In addition, it can handle critical issues related to sharing research findings that are of health value to the donor. It is advisable that members of this committee are of diverse backgrounds to ensure it evaluates proposal from various angles. The committee can also enroll members of the Advisory Committee to fulfill compliance with the set policies of the biobank. These committees have a critical role in running distinguished biobanks that intricately balance the implementation of ethical guidelines with the promotion of sample and data sharing and the possession of flexibility and speedy decision-making to be appreciated by the public, bioethicists, and researchers.

Recommendations

Establishing a biobank is faced with several ethical challenges, but its development in the Arab region is important due to the increased frequency of genetic disorders in this region. A preliminary step in establishing a biobank in the Arab region is to survey public perceptions. Unexpected outcomes of such surveys are frequently obtained, such as level of public knowledge and support of research initiatives, as well as expectations and concerns. For example, whereas in Western countries, issues related to privacy were of high priority to the public, it was compatibility with religious teachings that are valued in Jordan, based on what influences public decision to donate for biobanks. The public can also be targeted via educational programs that introduce the concept, purpose, and operation of the biobank. Increasing public knowledge reflects respect towards individuals and allows them to make sound decisions. Public engagement, dialogues, and communication are means of establishing public trust among participants. The link with the public is expected to play a critical role in bridging the gap with the scientific community and in illustrating the value of public donations in furthering research for the benefit of the society. Other issues surround the nature of the research itself, the type of collected samples and information and how they are handled, the identity of participating researchers, and storage period of biospecimens and information. Hence, clear biobank governance is instrumental in operating an effective biobank.

References

Abdur Rab, M., M. Afzal, A. Abou-Zeid, and H. Silverman. 2008. Ethical practices for health research in the Eastern Mediterranean region of the World Health Organization: A retrospective data analysis. *PloS One* 3 (5): e2094. https://doi.org/10.1371/journal.pone.0002094.

Abou-Zeid, A., H. Silverman, M. Shehata, M. Shams, M. Elshabrawy, T. Hifnawy,... N. Moharram (2010). Collection, storage and use of blood samples for future research: Views of Egyptian patients expressed in a cross-sectional survey. *Journal of Medical Ethics*, 36(9), 539–547. https://doi.org/10.1136/jme.2009.033100.

Ahram, M., A. Othman, and M. Shahrouri. 2012. Public perception towards biobanking in Jordan. *Biopreservation and Biobanking* 10 (4): 361–365. https://doi.org/10.1089/bio.2012.0010.

———. 2013. Public support and consent preference for biomedical research and biobanking in Jordan. *European Journal of Human Genetics* 21 (5): 567–570. https://doi.org/10.1038/ejhg.2012.213.

Ahram, M., A. Othman, M. Shahrouri, and E. Mustafa. 2014. Factors influencing public participation in biobanking. *European Journal of Human Genetics* 22 (4): 445–451. https://doi.org/10.1038/ejhg.2013.174.

Ahram, M., M. Soubani, L. Abu Salem, H. Saker, and M. Ahmad. 2015. Knowledge, attitudes, and practice regarding genetic testing and genetic counselors in Jordan: A population-based survey. *Journal of Genetic Counseling*. https://doi.org/10.1007/s10897-015-9839-3.

Akhu-Zaheya, L.M., M.T. Jagbir, A. Othman, and M. Ahram. 2014. Media use for seeking health/cancer-related information: Findings from knowledge, attitudes and practices towards cancer prevention and care survey in Jordan. *International Journal of Nursing Practice* 20 (6): 608–615. https://doi.org/10.1111/ijn.12196.

Alahmad, G., M. Al-Juma, A. Alsuwailem. 2010. Research Biobanks and their ethical and Islamic regulations [Al-Bonook Al-Hayawiyya Al-Bahthiyya Dawabitaha Al-Akhlaqiyya wa Al-Shar'iyya]. Retrieved from Saudi Arabia: https://www.researchgate.net/publication/262798001_albnwk_alhywyt_albhthyt_dwabtha_alakhlaqyt_walshryt_ghyath_alahmd_-_mhmd_aljmt_-_bdalzyz_alswylm_alnashr_jamt_alamam_mhmd_bn_swd_alaslamyt_-_alswdyt_-_altbt_bdwn_-_snt_altb_1431h.

Al-Jumah, M.A., and M.A. Abolfotouh. 2011. Public perception and attitude of saudis toward organ and tissue donation. *Biopreservation and Biobanking* 9 (1): 21–27. https://doi.org/10.1089/bio.2010.0025.

Al-Qadire, M.M., M.M. Hammami, H.M. Abdulhameed, and E.A. Al Gaai. 2010. Saudi views on consenting for research on medical records and leftover tissue samples. *BMC Medical Ethics* 11: 18. https://doi.org/10.1186/1472-6939-11-18.

Al-Riyami, A., D. Jaju, S. Jaju, and H.J. Silverman. 2011. The adequacy of informed consent forms in genetic research in Oman: A pilot study. *Developing World Bioethics* 11 (2): 57–62. https://doi.org/10.1111/j.1471-8847.2010.00293.x.

Beskow, L.M., J.Y. Friedman, N.C. Hardy, L. Lin, and K.P. Weinfurt. 2010. Developing a simplified consent form for biobanking. *PloS One* 5 (10): e13302. https://doi.org/10.1371/journal.pone.0013302.

da Rocha, A.C., and J.A. Seoane. 2008. Alternative consent models for biobanks: The new Spanish law on biomedical research. *Bioethics* 22 (8): 440–447. https://doi.org/10.1111/j.1467-8519.2008.00673.x.

European Commission. 2012. *Eurobarometer 73.1 (Jan–Feb 2010)*. Brussels: TNS OPINION & SOCIAL. Retrieved from Cologne: https://dbk.gesis.org/dbksearch/sdesc2.asp?no=5000&db=e&doi=10.4232/1.11428.

Forsberg, J.S., M.G. Hansson, and S. Eriksson. 2009. Changing perspectives in biobank research: From individual rights to concerns about public health regarding the return of results. *European Journal of Human Genetics* 17 (12): 1544–1549. https://doi.org/10.1038/ejhg.2009.87.

Giesbertz, N.A., A.L. Bredenoord, and J.J. van Delden. 2012. Inclusion of residual tissue in biobanks: Opt-in or opt-out? *PLoS Biology* 10 (8): e1001373. https://doi.org/10.1371/journal.pbio.1001373.

Goldenberg, A. J., K. J. Maschke, S. Joffe, J. R. Botkin, E. Rothwell, T. H. Murray,... S. M. Rivera. 2015. IRB practices and policies regarding the secondary research use of biospecimens. *BMC Medical Ethics* 16, 32. doi:https://doi.org/10.1186/s12910-015-0020-1.

Gottesman, O., H. Kuivaniemi, G. Tromp, W.A. Faucett, R. Li, T.A. Manolio, eMERGE Network, et al. 2013. The electronic medical records and genomics (eMERGE) network: Past, present, and future. *Genetics in Medicine* 15 (10): 761–771. https://doi.org/10.1038/gim.2013.72.

Grady, C., L. Eckstein, B. Berkman, D. Brock, R. Cook-Deegan, S.M. Fullerton, et al. 2015. Broad consent for research with biological samples: Workshop conclusions. *The American Journal of Bioethics* 15 (9): 34–42. https://doi.org/10.1080/15265161.2015.1062162.

Hansson, M.G., J. Dillner, C.R. Bartram, J.A. Carlson, and G. Helgesson. 2006. Should donors be allowed to give broad consent to future biobank research? *The Lancet Oncology* 7 (3): 266–269. https://doi.org/10.1016/S1470-2045(06)70618-0.

Helgesson, G., and L. Johnsson. 2005. The right to withdraw consent to research on biobank samples. *Medicine, Health Care, and Philosophy* 8 (3): 315–321. https://doi.org/10.1007/s11019-005-0397-6.

Hofmann, B. 2009. Broadening consent – And diluting ethics? *Journal of Medical Ethics* 35 (2): 125–129. https://doi.org/10.1136/jme.2008.024851.

Hollricher, K. 2009. Life sciences in Luxembourg; A new kid on the block. *Laboratory Times* 6: 16.

Hug, K., G. Hermeren, and M. Johansson. 2012. Withdrawal from biobank research: Considerations and the way forward. *Stem Cell Reviews* 8 (4): 1056–1065. https://doi.org/10.1007/s12015-012-9399-y.

Human Genetics Commission. 2001. Public attitudes to human genetic information. People's panel quantitative study conducted for the human genetic commission. Retrieved from London: http://www.hgc.gov.uk/.

International Multiple Sclerosis Genetics, C, Wellcome Trust Case Control, C, S. Sawcer, G. Hellenthal, M. Pirinen, C.C. Spencer, et al. 2011. Genetic risk and a primary role for cell-mediated immune mechanisms in multiple sclerosis. *Nature* 476 (7359): 214–219. https://doi.org/10.1038/nature10251.

Khalil, S.S., H.J. Silverman, M. Raafat, S. El-Kamary, and M. El-Setouhy. 2007. Attitudes, understanding, and concerns regarding medical research amongst Egyptians: A qualitative pilot study. *BMC Medical Ethics* 8: 9. https://doi.org/10.1186/1472-6939-8-9.

Maschke, K.J. 2006. Alternative consent approaches for biobank research. *The Lancet Oncology* 7 (3): 193–194. https://doi.org/10.1016/S1470-2045(06)70590-3.

Melas, P.A., L.K. Sjoholm, T. Forsner, M. Edhborg, N. Juth, Y. Forsell, and C. Lavebratt. 2010. Examining the public refusal to consent to DNA biobanking: Empirical data from a Swedish population-based study. *Journal of Medical Ethics* 36 (2): 93–98. https://doi.org/10.1136/jme.2009.032367.

Melham, K., L.B. Moraia, C. Mitchell, M. Morrison, H. Teare, and J. Kaye. 2014. The evolution of withdrawal: Negotiating research relationships in biobanking. *Life Science Society Policy* 10: 16. https://doi.org/10.1186/s40504-014-0016-5.

Porteri, C., and P. Borry. 2008. A proposal for a model of informed consent for the collection, storage and use of biological materials for research purposes. *Patient Education and Counseling* 71 (1): 136–142. https://doi.org/10.1016/j.pec.2007.12.003.

Rothwell, E., K.J. Maschke, J.R. Botkin, A. Goldenberg, T.H. Murray, and S.M. Rivera. 2015. Biobanking research and human subjects protections: Perspectives of IRB leaders. *IRB* 37 (2): 8–13.

Saffi, M., and N. Howard. 2015. Exploring the effectiveness of mandatory premarital screening and genetic counselling programmes for beta-thalassaemia in the Middle East: A scoping review. *Public Health Genomics* 18 (4): 193–203. https://doi.org/10.1159/000430837.

Stein, D.T., and S.F. Terry. 2013. Reforming biobank consent policy: A necessary move away from broad consent toward dynamic consent. *Genetic Testing and Molecular Biomarkers* 17 (12): 855–856. https://doi.org/10.1089/gtmb.2013.1550.

Teebi, A.S., and S.A. Teebi. 2005. Genetic diversity among the Arabs. *Community Genetics* 8 (1): 21–26. https://doi.org/10.1159/000083333.

Vera-Badillo, F.E., A.J. Templeton, P. de Gouveia, I. Diaz-Padilla, P.L. Bedard, M. Al-Mubarak, et al. 2014. Androgen receptor expression and outcomes in early breast cancer: A systematic review and meta-analysis. *Journal of the National Cancer Institute* 106 (1): djt319. https://doi.org/10.1093/jnci/djt319.

Vora, T., and N. Thacker. 2015. Impacts of a biobank: Bridging the gap in translational cancer medicine. *Indian Journal Medicine Paediatrica Oncologica* 36 (1): 17–23. https://doi.org/10.4103/0971-5851.151773.

Wazaify, M., S.S. Khalil, and H.J. Silverman. 2009. Expression of therapeutic misconception amongst Egyptians: A qualitative pilot study. *BMC Medical Ethics* 10: 7. https://doi.org/10.1186/1472-6939-10-7.

Widdows, H., and S. Cordell. 2011. The ethics of biobanking: Key issues and controversies. *Health Care Analysis* 19 (3): 207–219. https://doi.org/10.1007/s10728-011-0184-x.

Wolf, S.M., B.N. Crock, B. Van Ness, F. Lawrenz, J.P. Kahn, L.M. Beskow, et al. 2012. Managing incidental findings and research results in genomic research involving biobanks and archived data sets. *Genetics in Medicine* 14 (4): 361–384. https://doi.org/10.1038/gim.2012.23.

Wong, M.L., K.S. Chia, S. Wee, S.E. Chia, J. Lee, W.P. Koh, et al. 2004. Concerns over participation in genetic research among Malay-Muslims, Chinese and Indians in Singapore: A focus group study. *Community Genetics* 7 (1): 44–54. https://doi.org/10.1159/000080303.

Ethics of Stem Cell Research in the Arab Region

Rana Dajani

Only those fear Allah, from among His servants, who have knowledge (Quran 35:28)

Introduction

Stem cell science and associated technologies are rapidly progressing leading to advances in potential therapeutic and clinical applications. While no one denies that the ability to treat or heal suffering is a great good, it must also be recognized that not all methods of achieving a desired good are necessarily morally justifiable (Levine 2010). Indeed, the sources of human stem cells, together with several of its potential applications, result in major ethical issues and challenges for scientists, regulatory bodies, and other stakeholders. When developing regulations and drawing up legislation at either the international or national level, it is important to consider the perspectives of different cultures, philosophies and religions. This chapter will review the science of stem cell technologies, the related ethical issues from Islamic perspectives regarding stem cell applications, and the recent Jordan Law for stem cell research and therapy.

Scientific Background of Stem Cell Biology

Taught man that which he knew not. (Quran 96:5)

Stem cells are defined as cells that have the capacity to divide forever and have the potential to differentiate into all cell types. Until recently, scientists primarily worked with two kinds of stem cells from animals and humans: embryonic stem

R. Dajani (✉)
Biology and Biotechnology Department, Hashemite University, Zarqa, Jordan
e-mail: rdajani@hu.edu.jo

H. Silverman (ed.), *Research Ethics in the Arab Region*, Research Ethics Forum 5,
https://doi.org/10.1007/978-3-319-65266-5_10

cells and non-embryonic "somatic" or "adult" stem cells. This contrasts with muscle cells, blood cells, or nerve cells, which do not normally replicate themselves; whereas, stem cells may replicate many times, or proliferate

Because embryonic cells can proliferate without limit and can contribute to any cell type, human embryonic stem cells offer an unprecedented access to tissues from the human body. They will support basic research on the differentiation and function of human tissues and provide material for testing that may improve the safety and efficacy of human drugs. As such, research on stem cells continues to advance knowledge about how an organism develops from a single cell and how healthy cells replace damaged cells in adult organisms.

Embryonic stem cells are derived from embryos at a developmental stage before the time that implantation would normally occur in the uterus. In the 3- to 5-day-old embryo, called a blastocyst, the inner cells give rise to the entire body of the organism, including all of the many specialized cell types and organs such as the heart, lungs, skin, sperm, eggs and other tissues.

Most embryonic stem cells are derived from leftover embryos that were developed from eggs that were fertilized in vitro in a fertilization clinic and then donated for research purposes with informed consent of the donors. They are not derived from eggs fertilized in a woman's body. Alternatively, embryonic stem cells can be derived from somatic cell nuclear transfer (SCNT). This technique consists of taking an enucleated oocyte (egg cell) and implanting a donor nucleus from virtually any cell of the body (a somatic cell). The resulting nucleated egg (embryo) can then be used for either therapeutic or reproductive cloning. Therapeutic cloning refers to allowing the resulting nucleasted egg to divide repeatedly to form a blastocyst and then, the obtained pluripotent cells (which causes the destruction of the embryo) can potentially treat diseases in any body organ or tissue by replacing damaged and dysfunctional cells. Therapeutic cloning is also important to enhancing our understanding of stem cells and how they and other cells develop. Reproductive cloning occurs by implanted the resulting nucleasted egg (embryo) in a woman's uterus to allow continued development into a fetus and eventually a human being.

Ethical Issues

Ethical Issues involving stem cells consist of the following:

(A) What are ethically permissible sources of human stem cells?

Potential sources include the following (involving both procurement and derivation):

- paying women to donate eggs for stem cell research
- existing stem cell lines regardless of the original source of the embryos
- left-over embryos in fertilization clinics no longer needed for fertilization
- embryos created specifically for research through IVF
- embryos created through cell nuclear transfer into human oocytes or zygotes

- donated gametes
- stem cells from fetal tissues (e.g., from an aborted fetus)
- adult stem cells and cord blood

(B) What are the appropriate uses of human stem cells?

- Human embryonic stem cells and adult stem cells for therapy.
- Therapeutic cloning: Therapeutic cloning occurs when cloned embryos created through somatic cell nuclear transfer (SCNT). The cloned embryos are allowed to grow for a few days and then destroyed for their stem cells to be used for therapy or research.
- Reproductive cloning: Reproductive cloning involves creating a human species that is genetically identical to a donor through somatic cell nuclear transfer (SCNT). In reproductive cloning, the resulting embryo is allowed to grow up to 14 days in a petri dish, and then transplanted into a woman's womb to grow until birth.

Religion and Responsibility

The majority of the population in the Arab region is Muslim and as such, Islam is the predominant religion in the region. There are Muslims in other parts of the world, but Arab-speaking countries in most cases set the standard because the religious texts of Islam are written in Arabic. There is a small percentage of Christians and Jews in the Arab region, however, they usually follow the verdicts of their respective authorities. Much of the controversy and disagreement over activities involving stem cells worldwide arises from the different views of the major religions on the earliest stages of life. Although the use of human embryonic cells is opposed by the Roman Catholic Church and some Protestant denominations, it is generally supported by the Jewish community and accepted in many Muslim countries (Dajani 2014)

How does Islam look at science in general and stem cells in particular? In order to answer this question a few points need to be made in this context, which include the following:

1. In Islam the principles of bioethics are based on the three pillars of Islam legislation: The Holy Quran, Sunnah (the legislative decisions of Prophet Mohammad) and the Ijmaa (consensus of the Muslim scholars) and Ijtihad (every adequately qualified jurist had the right to exercise such original thinking, mainly ra'y (personal judgment) and qiyas (analogical reasoning) (Aksoy 2005).
2. The Quran and Sunnah are not sources of science. They are sources of moral guidelines to assist humans to live in harmony with fellow humans and creatures and the environment and universe. They are not sources of evidence for all scientific discoveries.
3. Islam asks us to observe, think and come up with hypotheses to explain phenomena. In other words, it proposes to Muslims to adopt the scientific method as we call it today in discovering the world around us.

4. Islam requires that we think of the common good because Islam is a religion for the community. The idea that we are all responsible for one another because our livelihoods, resources, and histories are shared is articulated by Prophet Mohammad (peace be upon him): "Everyone is a guardian." (1) In Islam, it is our duty to realize that every one of us is a guardian of God's creation in the world. Everyone from the child just entering adulthood, the student, the mother and the husband to the business owner, the worker, and the politician – all are responsible. Realizing such responsibility is the first step to creating a concrete platform for taking action. Indeed, there are great moments in the history of Islam when the concept was employed in this way. The Muslim scholar Al-Ghazali highlighted the importance of *mahabbah* (love) in his philosophical writings on community. From *mahabbah*, Al-Ghazali derived the idea of *maslaha* (public good). According to *maslaha* one does not think merely of personal benefit when making a decision, but considers, more importantly, the decision's effect on and potential benefit for the public. Global Civics is a new and old concept mirroring Islam. It was developed by Hakan Albany and focuses on the individual responsibility towards all humanity.
5. Science is part of our everyday life. Therefore, Muslims will need guidelines on how to address the ethics of scientific discoveries and their implementations in order to conduct their lives in a manner that is compatible to their religion. This applies to scientists and physicians who are at the forefront of stem cell research and therapy in order to promote and advance science in the Middle East. As the Sacred Sources of Islam do not mention modern technologies, such guidelines will be based only on analogies rather than "explicit doctrines from the Sacred Sources.

The Approach

> And those who have responded to their lord and established prayer and whose affair is [determined by] consultation among themselves, and from what we have provided them, they spend. (Quran 42:38)

The need to address the ethics of all new scientific discoveries using Islam as a guideline becomes essential for research and therapy to move forward in Muslim countries. Usually in such cases, the jurisprudence scholars would read, discuss and render a verdict. In the case of science, this method does not work because of the following reasons:

1. There is not enough information in Arabic for the scholars to read to be able to comprehend the science.
2. It is necessary to discuss the delicate details with scientists specialized in stem cells in addition to all other stakeholders.
3. The science of stem cells is changing every day. Therefore, one verdict in time is not enough. Any verdict should be revisited

Instead, there are several alternative approaches taken to address issues involving new scientific technologies. These include the following:

1. Traditional conferences: There are a number of international and national bodies that have produced guidelines to regulate stem cell research and stem cell therapy (International Society for Stem Cell Research 2016).
2. Regulation by Religious Decrees

   Several countries have used Islamic religious decrees or fatwas to guide this research. A fatwa is an opinion issued by an Islamic scholar or group concerning Islamic law and its interpretation. While these decrees may not be law, they carry great influence they often effectively act as national policy. The Fiqh Council of the Muslim World League in Saudi Arabia issued a fatwa in 2003 detailing the requirements under which stem cell research could be conducted in accordance with Islamic sharia law in the Kingdom. In addition, Iran issued a fatwa in 2002 establishing that human embryonic stem cell research was permissible encouraged scientists to pursue this research with the purpose of advancing technology to save lives (Saniei and De Vries 2008). Stem cell research guidelines created by fatwas may work well within a country, but these decrees are not recognized by many nations as legal or regulatory framework.
3. National Regulations: The proliferation of stem cell research, associated with its ethical and moral implications, has led governments to attempt regulation of both the science and funding of stem cells (Dhar and Hsi-En Ho 2009; Guinn 2006). Governmental stem cell policies, supportive and restrictive, have been directly linked to research performance. Over-performing countries in the field of stem cell research often have long-established, clear, and supportive research policies. In contrast, many underperforming nations are marked by an assortment of varying policies and research environments that are commonly characterized by a combination of prolonged policy debates and hence, uncertainty (Flynn and Matthews 2012). Specifically, in the Muslim world, there are guidelines in regulations in Tunis and Jordan. Tunisia banned the acquisition of embryos for experimental purposes and only allows the preservation of gametes or embryos "for therapeutic purposes to help the couple procreate" (Tebourski and Ben Ammar-Elgaaied 2004). I will describe the law in Jordan below.

The Jordan Law for Stem Cell Research and Therapy

In the process of preparing and approving the Jordan Law, the key to success involved engaging all stakeholders in the discussion, debate, and final formulation of the Jordan Law. Nonetheless, a number of challenges had to be addressed. These challenges were as follows:

1. Terminology: One of the first challenges to address was the confusion between terms used among members of the committees. For example, in many instances the term "stem cells" is used to mean embryonic stem cells. It was important to clarify, through discussion and education, that the two are not exactly the same.

2. Distinguishing Procedures: The therapeutic use of hematopietic stem cell transplantation (HSCT) and bone marrow transplantation (BMT) have been well established in Jordan since 1987. As such, it was important to make a clear distinction between these two standard of care procedures on one hand and stem cell therapy on the other. This allowed for exclusion of HSCT and BMT from the Jordan Law, as both HSCT and BMT are considered standard of care procedures and are governed by the medical practice law.
3. Human embryonic stem cells: the Jordan Iftaa council concurred with the decision (fatwa) of Muslim scholars meeting in 2003 (The Muslim World League's Islamic Jurisprudence Council Conference in December 2003 held in Makkah), which allowed for the use of permissible sources of embryonic stem cells (ESC). The permissible sources included legally produced excess fertilized eggs during IVF. The permission for both therapy and research was limited to public institutions. Several meetings and discussions were held with the Iftaa council to create detailed measures to prevent illegal mixing of genealogy or human cloning, as stated in article seven and nine A and B. The traceability and strict accountability of public institutions facilitated the approval of ESC research in these institutions. The fear of encouraging illegal termination of pregnancies, or commercialization of embryonic cells and tissues was a decisive factor in preventing private institutions to venture into ESC research.
4. Other sources of stem cells: the Iftaa council adopted an open-minded approach to somatic stem cell nuclear transfer (SCNT) and induced pluripotent stem cells (iPSCs). SCNT and iPSCs are specifically mentioned in the Jordan Law, as stated in the definitions and sources of stem cells.

Initial Process

In 2008, a number of initiatives started both at the individual and at the organizational level. Dr. Dajani at the Hashemite University took a proactive novel approach by establishing a group discussion of multiple stakeholders that included scientists, physicians, Arabic language experts and theologians to initiate a discussion around the ethics of stem cell research and therapy. Simultaneously, the Stem Cell Therapy Center (CTC), which was established at the University of Jordan in 2008, established a committee made of multiple stakeholders who included in addition to religious Muslim and Christian scholars, physicians, scientists, legal experts and international experts. The purpose of these committees was to investigate, research, debate, contemplate and explore the various issues related to stem cell research, its therapeutic, as well as its social and ethical issues. Over a period of 4 years, several workshops, meetings and conferences were held. November 2009, the ethics of stem cell research was presented in the fourth scientific research conference in Jordan and the first conference on bioethics was held in November 2009.

The committees adopted the following methodology:

(a) to list all the issues related to stem cell research and therapy
(b) study the verdicts to date for each issue
(c) evaluate the verdicts if realistic
(d) if not reevaluate the evidence and produce new verdicts

Legislation

A national technical committee was formed by Dr. Abdallah Awidi in Jordan to produce a national law for Jordan concerned with stem cell research and therapy. The law decreed the creation of a committee that would meet regularly to evaluate all issues related to stem cell research and therapy. This is the first law in the Arab region and in the Islamic world that is directed specifically to stem cell research and therapy (Dajani 2014). As such, the Stem Cell Research and Therapy by-Law should serve as an example for other countries in the Arab and Muslim world regarding the importance of having national regulations that deal with stem cell research and therapy.

The Ethics of Stem Cell Research from an Islamic Perspective

Determining the permissible sources of the stem cells was essential to developing the law. What follows is a summary of the Islamic position on a number of issues identified by the 2008 committee headed by Dr. Dajani:

(A) Permissible and Impermissible sources of stem cells.

1. Paying women to donate eggs for research

   Currently, this is prohibited in order to prevent taking advantage of humans, based on a concern of exploitation principle of non-permissibility of receiving payments for organs or tissues.
2. Usage of existing stem cell lines is permitted on the condition that the stem cell line was taken from a permissible source originally.
3. Stem cells from embryos.

   One of the fundamental ethical issues regards the procurement of stem cells from embryos thus leading to its destruction. The dilemma involves whether and when the embryo is decreed to be human and thus destroying it means killing a human life. Religious groups have generally been at the forefront of those speaking out publicly for or against stem cell research; particularly embryonic stem cell research. There are very different views held by Christianity, Judaism and Islam. While there is no consensus on when human embryonic life begins, most Muslim scholars consider human life to begin between 40 and 120 days after conception (Daar and al Khitamy 2001; Larijani and Zahedi 2004).

This range of views likely accounts for different levels of acceptance of embryonic stem cell (ESC) research, which is supported by the Jewish community and accepted in many Muslim countries, yet is opposed by the Roman Catholic Church and some Protestant denominations(Guinn 2006).

4. Usage of Remaining embryos no longer needed for fertilization.

   Leftover fertilized embryos from in vitro fertilization that are donated by the couple is permissible. However, leftover embryos cannot be used from the excesses of impermissible pregnancies, e.g., surrogate motherhood (Misha'l 2015).

5. Usage of Embryos created specifically for research through IVF.

   According to Islam, this source is not permissible, as there are concerns regarding the exploitation of women who will serve as the sources (donation) of the eggs (Misha'l 2015).

6. Usage of Embryos created through cell nuclear transfer into human oocytes or zygotes (SCNT).

   A technique in which the nucleus of a somatic cell (any cell of the body except sperm cells and egg cells) is injected, or transferred, into an egg, that has had its nucleus removed. If the new egg is then implanted into the womb of an animal, an individual will be born that is a clone. The clone has the identical genetic material as the somatic cell, which supplied the nucleus that carries the genetic material. This procedure is very inefficient and was first developed for agricultural purposes. However, in human medicine, this technique can be used to isolate embryonic stem cells from eggs that have undergone nuclear transfer. When the somatic cell is supplied from the cells of a person, the stem cells isolated from the developing eggs can be used to make a tissue that will not be rejected by that person, because they have the same genetic material. In this way, 'customized' embryonic stem cells could be made for everyone who needed them.

   Jordan's law takes a more permissive approach to techniques using stem cells that are not derived from human embryos. For example, somatic-cell nuclear transfer (in which a patient's DNA is transplanted into an unfertilized human egg that has no nucleus) and induced pluripotent stem cells, which are made from adult cells, can be worked on by the private sector under the new rules.

7. Embryonic stem cells taken from fetus.

   These cells are taken from embryos or fetuses that have been miscarried of their own accord or aborted for therapeutic reasons allowed by the sharia and with the permission of the parents. Fetuses that are aborted willfully and without a medical reason permitted by Sharia represents an impermissible source.

8. Adult stem cells and cord blood.

   Adults, provided they give permission to do so and if no harm comes to them as a result. Children, if their parents give permission to do so for a permissible reason and if no harm comes to them as a result. The placenta or umbilical cord with the permission of the parents.

(B) Permissible uses of stem cells
1. Therapeutic cloning: Somatic cell nuclear transfer for the isolation of embryonic stem cells. The embryonic stem cells are derived from the blastocyst (before it becomes a fetus) and can be instructed to form particular cell types (e.g. heart muscle) to be implanted into damaged tissue (e.g. heart) to restore its function. If the stem cells are placed back into the individual who gave the DNA for the somatic cell nuclear transfer, the embryonic stem cells and their derivatives are genetically identical and thus immunocompatible (they will not be rejected). Currently, within the Jordanian Law, therapeutic cloning is permissible if the source of the cells is permissible.
2. Reproductive cloning: In reproductive cloning, the DNA of an unfertilized egg is removed and replaced by donor DNA, obtained from cells from another individual. The egg is then coaxed into believing that it has been fertilized and starts dividing, to generate new cells (and form an embryo) in a laboratory culture. Up to this point, the procedure is the same as nuclear transfer to produce stem cells. Once the egg has divided sufficiently, the resulting embryo is then implanted into the uterus of a surrogate mother, where it can develop until birth. In contrast to natural reproduction, reproductive cloning does not create a genetically new and unique individual through the recombination of each chromosome set from each parent. Instead, only the DNA from the DNA donor is present, which makes the newborn a genetic replicate of the DNA donor, a clone (5). Currently, the status of Islam is that reproductive cloning is prohibited.

Conclusion

> Indeed, I will make upon the earth a successive authority. (Quran 2:30)

It is important that there be consistent regulations in the Arab region, i.e., there should be a call for all scientific discoveries that generate ethical issues to be treated in the same way. This would involve a dialogue among stakeholders, most importantly scientists and scholars of religion. An important note to policy makers is to raise public awareness about the potential opportunities, challenges and uncertainties of stem cell research. In addition to raising awareness among the scientific community, Research Councils and policy makers should elicit the views and concerns of the wider public relating to stem cell research, and of the importance of dialogue.

The goal of science is to explore the secrets and laws of nature, which were set by God. Islam has always encouraged man to contemplate, and explore, new horizons. Stem cell research is one of those new horizons, and Islam does not object to this exploration. All of the discussions so far has indicated that stem cell research is permissible in Islam, as long as it is carried out with the purpose of improving human health. This matter still, however, needs to be continually examined and only after this has happened will it be possible to achieve everlasting consensus.

References

Aksoy, S. 2005. Making regulations and drawing up legislation in Islamic countries under conditions of uncertainty, with special reference to embryonic stem cell research. *Journal of Medical Ethics* 31 (7): 399–403. Retrieved from http://www.ncbi.nlm.nih.gov/entrez/query.fcgi?cmd=Retrieve&db=PubMed&dopt=Citation&list_uids=15994358.

Daar, A.S., and A.B. al Khitamy. 2001. Bioethics for clinicians: 21. Islamic bioethics. *CMAJ* 164 (1): 60–63. Retrieved from http://www.ncbi.nlm.nih.gov/pubmed/11202669.

Dajani, R. 2014. Jordan's stem-cell law can guide the Middle East. *Nature* 510 (7504): 189. https://doi.org/10.1038/510189a.

Dhar, D., and J. Hsi-En Ho. 2009. Stem cell research policies around the world. *The Yale Journal of Biology and Medicine* 82 (3): 113–115. Retrieved from http://www.ncbi.nlm.nih.gov/pubmed/19774124.

Flynn, J.M., and K.R.W. Matthews. 2012. Stem cell research in the greater Middle East: The importance of establishing policy and ethics interoperability to foster international collaborations. *Stem Cell Reviews and Reports* 6: 143–150. Available at: http://bakerinstitute.org/media/files/Research/142d211a180/ST-Pub-StemCell-ME-May2010.pdf.

Guinn, D. E. (2006). Handbook of bioethics and religion. Oxford: Oxford University Press.

International Society for Stem Cell Research. (2016). Stem cell policies. Available at: http://www.isscr.org.

Larijani, B., and F. Zahedi. 2004. Islamic perspective on human cloning and stem cell research. *Transplantation Proceedings* 36 (10): 3188–3189. https://doi.org/10.1016/j.transproceed.2004.10.076.

Levine, A.D. 2010. Insights from patients' blogs and the need for systematic data on stem cell tourism. *The American Journal of Bioethics* 10 (5): 28–29. https://doi.org/10.1080/15265161003686571.

Misha'l, A. (2015). Stem cells and human cloning. FIMA year book 2015: Encyclopedia of Islamic medical ethics- part II, pp. 183–192.

Saniei, M., and R. De Vries. 2008. Embryonic stem cell research in Iran: Status and ethics. *Indian Journal of Medical Ethics* 5 (4): 181–184. Retrieved from http://www.ncbi.nlm.nih.gov/pubmed/18988380.

Tebourski, F., and A. Ben Ammar-Elgaaied. 2004. The developing country reactions to biomedical techniques and plant biotechnology: The Tunisian experience. *Journal of Biomedicine Biotechnology* 2004 (3): 124–129.

Ethical Issues in Social and Behavioral Research

Henry Silverman

Social and behavioral research investigates complex issues involving the social, cultural, economic, legal, and political dimensions of human behavior. Methodological approaches range from ethnography to randomized clinical trials, and also includes field experiments, direct observation, interviews, focus groups, surveys, physiological manipulations, descriptive methods, and standardized tests (Levine and Skedsvold 2008).

In general, social and behavioral research pose minimal risks to participants and accordingly, such research can fall under the two review categories of exempt and expedited that exist in many research ethics regulations. However, a large body of social science research can present significant risks due to potential violations of privacy and breaches in confidentiality leading to discrimination and stigmatization (especially for vulnerable and marginalized individuals) as well as psychological distress from a variety of the methodological approaches.

After the 1950s, ethical principles were incorporated into guidelines to govern the conduct of biomedical research. Subsequently, many national regulations expanded the reach of these ethics guidelines to social science research. Social scientists, however, were rarely involved in the drafting of these guidelines, and hence, they claimed that these regulations were are of little relevance to the methodologies and issues that concerned their studies. Additionally, social science researchers questioned the need of external ethical review for their types of studies.

Specifically, social scientists raised several issues regarding the complexities of their research that might make it difficult to conduct ethical review. First, it may be challenging to determine the social value of many types of social science research; for example, many qualitative researchers are exploratory in nature and the focus of the study may change because of the interactions between participants and researchers. Second, the eventual effect of the results on public policy, the aim of many

H. Silverman (✉)
University of Maryland, Baltimore, MD, USA
e-mail: hsilverm@medicine.umaryland.edu

H. Silverman (ed.), *Research Ethics in the Arab Region*, Research Ethics Forum 5,
https://doi.org/10.1007/978-3-319-65266-5_11

social science studies, is largely unknown; hence, it might be difficult to precisely determine the societal benefit that emanates from such research at the outset of the study. Third, unlike biomedical research, it may be difficult to determine the probability and magnitude of harm, e.g., investigators may be unable to prevent spontaneous personal disclosures made by participants and hence, difficult to guarantee confidentiality of personal information that other members participating in focus groups discussion have heard. In addition, much of social and behavioral research is exploratory, and hence, there may be no prior or accurate information about risks. Fourth, social science research is often of little benefit to participants, and hence, determining whether the risks are reasonable to the potential direct benefits may require a standard that differs from biomedical research. Finally, social behavioral research involves methodologies that may not require the fully informed consent of the participants (e.g., deception research) or even their knowledgeable participation (e.g., covert research), which may lead to negative ethical reviews and consequently, disapproval by research ethics committees (Israel 2015).

Researchers raised concerns that external ethical reviews were circumscribing their ability to make their own decisions about ethical issues relating to their specific projects. They argued that how they resolve ethical tensions must depend on the nature of the context, place, situation, technologies, methodologies and research participants. They contend that ethical decisions are often made in the midst of the research study itself, rather than anchored in a more formal ethical review at the beginning of the study. Their contention was that ethics oversight produced a formulaic approach to research ethics that requires one to "tick the right boxes" that might not be relevant once the research is underway.

Beginning in the 1960s, several societies involved with social science research made attempts to develop research ethics codes more appropriate to their work. Nonetheless, ambivalence and tensions occurred amongst the social scientists themselves, as comments ranged from encouraging ethical guidance to completely resisting any regulatory policy for their research. As such, agreement on an ethics code resisted consensus, and hence, the influence of professional associations over ethics largely ceded to the regulations developed for biomedical research (Israel 2015; Levine and Skedsvold 2008).

One valid concern of social scientists is that members of many research ethics committees are not familiar with their study design methods and the implications of such designs on the associated ethical issues and hence, they lack qualifications to review such research. These concerns, however, does not mean that the review of social science research should not be governed by an ethical framework, but rather it makes the case that there be institutional changes in how research ethics committees operate so that they are able to focus on the key ethical issues in social and behavioral studies. In addition, history has shown that the review of research cannot be left to the discretion of researchers, as they have a stake in the research projects they conduct and hence, their bias might cause them to deliberately or inadvertently ignore research risks in order to enroll participants. For all of these reasons, social science research requires ethical review.

Accordingly, the purpose of this chapter is to review the fundamental issues needing attention when reviewing the ethics of social behavioral research. To do this, this chapter will provide an overview of the history of ethical issues in social science research, address the underlying issues that are specific to social science research, and explore the complexity of making ethical determinations, especially in the context of challenging circumstances that occur in the Arab region.

Landmark Cases in the History of Social Science Research

The importance of ethical review for social science research is clear in view of several high profile studies performed in the 1960s that raised ethical issues regarding several types of research methodologies. The following three studies are frequently cited for demonstrating ethical questionable methodologies in social behavioral research.

The Milgram Experiments represented a series of social psychology experiments conducted in the early 1960s by Yale University psychologist Stanley Milgram and addressed the question: "under what conditions will people carry out the commands of an authority figure and when will they refuse to obey?" Research participants were told they were participating in a study on the effect of punishment on memory rather than a study to understand compliance with authority figures under varying conditions. They were asked to assume the role of "teachers" and they would be asking questions of "learners". For each wrong answer, the "teachers" were to give the "learners" electrical shocks, when in reality, there were no shocks. The "learners" were actors, accomplices of the research team, and were physically separated from the teachers. The "learners" had a tape recorder integrated with the electro-shock generator, which played pre-recorded "screams" for each shock level. The research participants or the "teachers" were led to believe that they were causing painful consequences to the learners. If at any time the participants indicated their desire to halt the experiment, they were given verbal encouragement by the research team to continue. Many of the participants obeyed the researcher without questioning and none left the laboratory disgusted or protesting. At the end of each experimental session, the deceit was revealed to participants and they were introduced to the "learners" to demonstrate that they had not received dangerous electric shocks.

Ethical concerns regarding this research involved the deception needed to conduct the study and the potential psychological distress that the participants in the study might have received from the deceit as well as from them realizing that they were being capable of administering increasing shocks to another human being. As such, similar experiments involving deception research was placed under question.

The Stanford Prison Experiment was a landmark study to investigate the psychological effects of perceived power, focusing on the struggle between prisoners and prison guards. Philip Zimbardo of Stanford University conducted this study in 1971. Research participants were randomly assigned to play the role of "prisoner" or "guard". Participants became emotionally involved in their roles as prisoners or guards, as witnessed by psychological aggressive behaviors in the "guards" and submissive behaviors in the "prisoners". Two of the prisoners left mid-experiment, and the whole exercise was abandoned after 6 days following the objections of a graduate student. Although follow-up reports noted no lasting effects on the research participants, the study highlighted the ethical concern of simulating behaviors that ***could*** induce sustained identify stress and potential psychological harm (Levine and Skedsvold 2008).

The Tearoom Trade Study conducted by Laud Humphreys from 1965 to 1968 involved an analysis of homosexual acts taking place in public toilets (the tearoom trade). The study aimed to question some of the stereotypes associated with the men who engaged in male-male sexual encounters that occurred in public places. In order to observe their behavior in the restrooms, Humphreys befriended the men by offering to pose as a lookout for when authorities might enter. Humphreys also wrote down the license plate numbers of the cars belonging to the men whom he observed, enabling him to trace them to their homes, where he had them fill out a questionnaire, pretending that it was for a general "social health survey." From the data he collected with this survey, Humphreys concluded that most of the men he observed were married and had "respectable" lifestyles and that a large proportion of the men were "socially conservative". Hence, the study demonstrated that many of the participants lived otherwise conventional lives as family men and respected members of their communities, and that their activities posed no danger of harassment to heterosexual males. Though The Tearoom Trade study made important contributions to sex research, Humphreys' research methods raised serious concerns. For example, he observed human behavior without the prior knowledge or consent of his subjects (a covert method that violated privacy), the researcher misrepresented his identity and intent (deception), and he gave a survey under false pretenses without later telling the subjects the actual purpose of the research. In addition, he published his findings without the subjects' consent. As such, the *Tearoom Trade* study raised the ethical question as to "whether the value of gaining information about sexual practices justify the violation of people's privacy?" This study is often used as an example of highly controversial social research.

In light of the issues regarding social value, methods, and the need for informed consent that were raised in these three studies, as well as those that have since emerged in other social science research, appeals have been raised for better empirical research regarding existing assumptions regarding participants' notions of privacy and its cultural determinants, what participants consider to be risk or benefits, and what they need to know before they provide informed consent to enroll in certain types of research (Levine and Skedsvold 2008).

What is the Value of Social Science Research?

A major goal of social science research is to generate new knowledge that will inform policy regarding social practices. It aims to determine which "knowledge" is credible, trustworthy, true or legitimate in order to empower people to act to transform society. Research is also concerned with determining the empirical question regarding "who participates" in the production of new knowledge? As such, what paradigm should be followed to ensure that research-generated knowledge emanates from the frame of reference of the research participants and its communities?

This question is crucial because research is never neutral, as stakeholders, which include funders, policy makers, practitioners, researchers and members of the communities influence it. Hence, there can be tension between the ideologies and personal agendas of all parties involved. Dominant Western research paradigms have marginalized developing communities' ways of knowing and have thus led to the design of research that might be irrelevant to the needs of the people. A "positivist" paradigm holds that the scientific method is the only way to establish truth and objective reality.

Alternatively, an "interpretive" paradigm differs with the positivists on assumptions about the nature of reality and what counts as knowledge and its sources. Interpretivists believe that knowledge is subjective because it is socially constructed and mind dependent. Truth lies within the human experience. Statements on what is true and false are therefore culture-bound, and historically and context dependent although some may be universal. Within this context, communities' stories, belief systems and claims of spiritual and earth connections should find space as legitimate knowledge. Often, however, even interpretivist research operates within the mode of a Western historical and culture-bound research framework and treats these belief systems as 'barriers to research or exotic customs with which researchers need to be familiar in order to carry out their work without causing offence' (Chilisa and Preece 2005).

A third paradigm labeled "emancipatory" involves action participatory research with the aim of emancipating and transforming communities through group action (Mertens 1998). On the question of what is truth, researchers within this paradigm maintain that knowledge is true if it can be turned into practice that empowers and transforms the lives of the people. Knowledge is constructed from the participants' frame of reference. The relationship between the 'researcher' and the 'researched' is not based on a power hierarchy as in the interpretive paradigm, but involves the transformation and emancipation of both the 'researcher' and 'researched'. The participatory nature of emancipatory action research involves linking the research processes of systematic data collection and analysis with the purpose of effecting social change. Three distinct links in this kind of research are as follows:

- The process involves collaboration between researchers and the researched community at all stages of the process
- The result is a reciprocal learning experience for researcher and researched
- The intended outcome of the study is new action

Participatory research holds that the knowledge that should be trustworthy comes from the communities themselves and not from an interpretation imposed from above. This does not mean that the researchers have no place in participatory or emancipatory research, but it does mean that the relationship between researcher and researched should be treated more equally. This means seeing the community as co-researchers ensuring dialogue and discussion with community members throughout the process, which involves them in the development of the research question, the design of the study, methods of data collection, analysis and interpretation of the data, dissemination of the data, and implementation of the results in their communities. It is through the emancipatory paradigm that one ensures that the social change is relevant to the needs of the community (Chilisa and Preece 2005).

A Framework for Assessing Risks in Social Behavioral Research

Many of the ethical issues generated in social behavioral research are related to the type and magnitude of the risks, which can range from mere inconvenience to social, economic, psychological, legal, political, and physical risks. The occurrence of wrongs and risks in social behavioral research are mainly due to issues involving informed consent and violations of privacy and breaches of confidentiality. Levine and Skedsvold developed a framework in which risks are related to the following three dimensions of the research:

- the research methods, i.e., the level of methodological intervention.
- The type of vulnerability, which is dependent on the characteristics of the study population coupled with society's attitudes toward the group.
- type of issues being studied, specifically, the degree of substantive sensitivity of the inquiry.

This model, shown in Fig. 1 (adapted from Levine and Skedsvold), is based on the types of vulnerable populations and the types of issues frequently encountered in the Arab region. The categories of methodological interventions that occur in research performed in the Arab region are similar to those in other world regions.

The first dimension of risks involves the methodological interventions, as risks will vary with the type of interaction and intervention, e.g., from no interaction (e.g., use of public data, observation) to indirect or direct contact (e.g., surveys and interviews) to intervention (experimental). Risks also vary in relationship to the degree of actual invasiveness (e.g., video recordings in public places can be more invasive than interviews exploring a relatively mundane issue). Additionally, risks will vary with the magnitude of any manipulation of the environment, e.g., the possible psychological and emotional consequences of any changes in the environment; or the effects of any deception or observation that leads to an invasion of privacy. Finally, there might be physical harms from devices or interventions (e.g., exercise) used in the study or abuse from third parties if they become aware of damaging revelations about them (e.g., gang violence, domestic violence, etc.).

The second dimension represents risks related to the degree of vulnerability of the research participants coupled with their level of social stigmatization, which is dependent on external cultural and social factors. The degree of vulnerability range

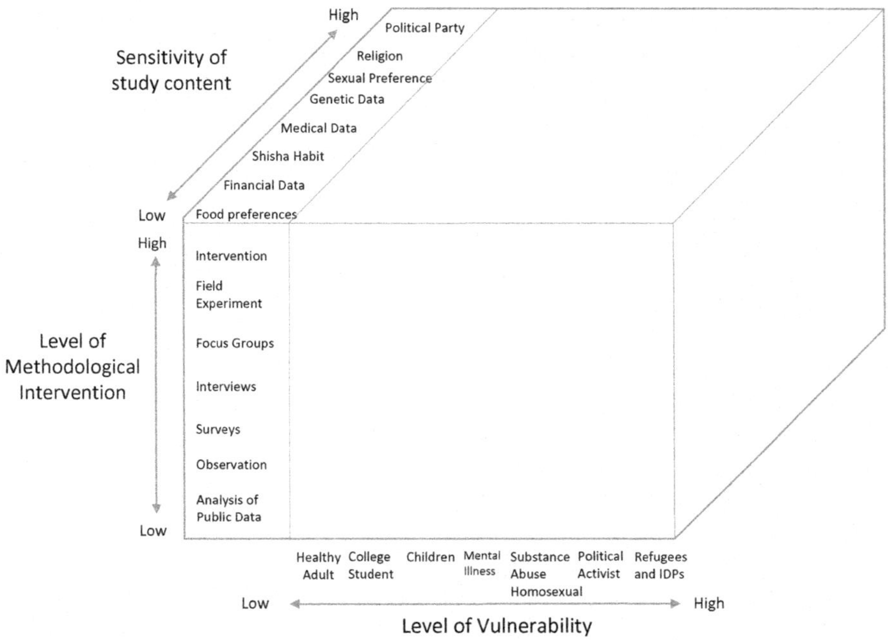

Fig. 1 Dimensions of social science studies that contribute to risks (Adapted from Levine and Skedsvold 2008)

from "healthy adult", to students, children with parental permission, orphans and street children (without guardians), extreme cognitive impairment, poverty, engaging in illegal activities (drug abuse and homosexuality), women, prisoners, refugees and internally displaced persons, and political activists. The potential for risks increases as the degree of vulnerability increases.

The third dimension represents risks from the sensitivity of the study topic, which can range from discomfort or embarrassment to social stigma, legal liability, and political repercussions. The contents of the topics of inquiry may themselves cause psychological stress. For example, a research study on obesity that asks participants about their eating habits may cause minor stress, whereas a study examining domestic violence could cause a great level of stress, as it may evoke tragic memories of verbal and physical abuse.

Cultures differ regarding the degree of the sensitivity of the information. Information considered highly sensitive, particularly in the Arab region, include the following:

- sexual attitudes, preferences or practices
- use of alcohol, drugs or other addictive substances
- illegal behavior

- medical Information (e.g., Hepatitis C status, HIV status, and cancer diagnoses) that, if revealed, could damage people in terms of their financial status, their capacity to pursue employment or their reputation in the community and includes
- mental health of the individual
- genetic information
- religion
- political affiliation

Mechanisms to reduce risk includes methods to protect privacy and prevent breaches in confidentiality. These include the following:

- Restrict unauthorized access to data
- Waive signature documentation of consent
- Require timely scoring review of mental health assessments
- Destroy tapes obtained in qualitative research
- Select location of research participants that enhances privacy

Ethical Challenges from Methodological Approaches

This section focuses on the nature of risks from a range of research methodologies used by social scientists. These methods include field experiments, observation, deception, survey, interview and focus groups, ethnographic, and analysis of public data files. Their effects in producing psychological and moral harms will also be discussed.

Experimental Methods

Experimental methods provide a direct way of testing the cause and effect relationship between variables and can occur in laboratories or in external field settings, e.g., school, community setting, hospital workplace or neighborhood (Levine and Skedsvold 2008). Experiments include randomized control trials and quasi-experimental designs that explore how modification of conditions in the environment affect behaviors or beliefs. An experiment might compare a novel intervention aimed at reducing risky sexual behaviors among teens with a control group that receives a standard educational intervention. Naturalistic experiments can be person-made (e.g., change in legal regulations) or may be naturally occurring (e.g., hurricane or other disaster). Such experiments provide an opportunity to study certain aspects of human behavior with a "before and after design" or through case control comparison.

Unique ethical challenges arise from the introduction of the variable that modifies the environment. First, the mere manipulation of an environmental condition causes research participants to be exposed to an experience they would not otherwise have been exposed. The extent that such manipulations raises ethical issues depend on the intensity and duration of the change variable (Levine and Skedsvold 2008). Other potential ethical issues involve concerns with privacy violations (e.g., can research participants be seen entering an HIV clinic for treatment?); adequate respect for persons (e.g., when participants are not aware of being involved in the research?); and risks from potential emotional trauma (e.g., when participants are interviewed during natural disasters?).

Observation or Covert Research

Observation or covert research is appropriate where it is necessary to achieve a better understanding of certain social phenomena and it is believed that either research participants would change their attitudes or behaviors or might withhold their consent. For example, some researchers have gone undercover to study underground drug cultures and withheld the true nature of their presence to find out about the inner workings of the social life of drug dealers and drug takers, often observing individuals engaging in illegal activities and sometimes finding themselves asked to engage in these same activities (Williams and May 1996). As pointed out by Williams, it is impossible to ask for informed consent from members of such communities, as they do not want to be investigated (Williams and May 1996).

Since observational investigations often functions without the knowledge or consent of the research participants, the level of risk is based on people's expectation of privacy in the particular setting and the level of intrusiveness. As such, research ethics committees will base their determination of risk on whether the setting is public vs. private and whether the nature of the behavior is public or private. Expectations of privacy and hence, whether a setting or behavior can be considered public or private will depend on the culture of the populations. For example, observation of alcohol use or shisha smoking for females or observations of discussions of sexual practices will have different connotations for risk in the Arab region compared with regions in the West.

Observation research conducted without informed consent is only justified if: a) the risk level of the investigation is no more than minimal risk (e.g., minimal possibility of identifying individual subjects at a future time or there is little expectation of privacy in the setting); and b) the information obtained is sufficiently important for science or public health and there is no other methodology that could be used to obtain the information (impracticableness criteria) (Mollet 2001).

Deception Research

In deception research, the true nature of the research is not revealed based on the concern that attitudes and behavior might change if the true purpose was known. The use of deception in social research represents an ethical concern, since the participant cannot give a valid consent.

In general, deceit may be accepted in social investigations when the following three conditions are simultaneously present (Rodriguez et al.):

- Another method cannot be used to achieve the objectives and to reveal the true nature of the study would cause a reasonable person to refuse to participate. (impracticableness criteria)
- The investigation will produce significant knowledge about attitudes or behaviors.
- The deception poses no more than minimal risk.
- Participants will be informed of the deceit once the investigation concludes (if applicable) and the possibility of refusing their data to be included in the study is offered.

Ethical issues with deceit includes an invasion of privacy as well as psychological and moral distress to participants by having been deceived. Essentially, the participant is used as a means to the ends of the investigator, not as a free person capable of making decisions. The damage caused by deceit can be unfixable by revealing to the subject that they have been deceived, since they can feel that their privacy has been invaded and their autonomy not respected.

Deception is difficult to justify on deontological and rule utilitarian grounds. Nevertheless, deception has been justified on the pragmatic grounds that it enables researchers to control stimuli, study low frequency events and gain information that might otherwise be unobtainable. Arguments have been made that the use of deception has not be shown to be a serious issue for research participants (Rodriguez et al.).

Qualitative and Quantitative Methods

These methods are based on the assumption that reality is constructed socially by individuals and by the meaning they give to it, which allows to create a social order. Methods include surveys, interviews, focus groups, and ethnographic studies.

Surveys

The level of risk from surveys is due to following factors:

- Sensitivity of the questionnaire content; for example, health information is more sensitive than consumer preference information. The degree of sensitivity may depend on cultural factors, e.g., information regarding cigarette smoking may be more sensitive among Arab females compared with their counterparts in the West.
- Mode of administration will have implications on the extent of privacy concerns; for example, the following methods have increasing levels of instrusiveness on privacy: mail, internet, telephone, and face-to-face.

- Extent to which individuals can be identified; for example, anonymous surveys obviously does not collect any identifying data and hence, have no risk, whereas if names are collected, breaches in confidentiality can lead to social risks, although strong confidentiality protections (data security and data access plans) can minimize such risks.
- Person or entity collecting the data; for example, in many areas in the Arab region, women are more comfortable when they are approached by women data collectors.

Interviews and Focus Group Methods

The level of risk with interviews are affected by many of same factors as in surveys, such as the sensitivity of the questions and the extent to which identifying information is obtained and stored. Other risk factors specific to the use of interviews include the following:

- Whether the information will be collected in a group setting, in which case, the ability to ensure confidentiality cannot be guaranteed, as participants in a focus group may intentionally or inadvertently disclose another respondent's responses to individuals outside of the focus group.
- The extent of the structure of the interview process: In a structured or semi-structured interview, the questions can be reviewed to determine the level of potential intrusiveness, whereas in an open-ended structure there is less control about what will be discussed. Respondents may reveal unanticipated responses.
- Security in many of the Arab countries has become a crucial issue and hence, there may be a concern for whether participants are able to answer questions freely during the interview.

Ethnographic Methods

These methods involve in-depth observations of as well as interactions with individuals and groups in their own environments. Use of multiple methods include unstructured interviews, semi-structured interviews, unobtrusive observations, participant observation and document or audiovisual analysis.

Risk depends on the issues being studied and the vulnerability of the human participants (see Fig. 1). The method itself may also raise ethical challenges, for example, if the duration of contact with the research participants occurs over long period of time - the researcher and participants may establish strong attachments with each other. The attachment may increase benefits for participants if they feel more at liberty to share information that previously they have found difficult to discuss or disclose; although such disclosures need to be protected by strong measures of confidentiality. On the other hand, if close rapport is not obtained, then the researcher's presence may lead to perceptions of intrusiveness. A methodological issue arises if researchers find it difficult to make objective judgments if they are personally connected with their respondents (Biber 2005).

Analysis of Public Use Data Files

A large amount of information collected about individuals can be used for secondary analysis to examine important research questions. Such data have already been collected and stripped of personal identifiers and hence, such data are usually no longer considered human subject research. Such public use data provide anonymized data for secondary research and hence, risks are essentially non-existent. The most challenging ethical issues associated with such data involves the assurances that the data are appropriately de-identified. Finally, in certain types of research, researchers may want to combine a public data file with a nonpublic data file (not de-identified) and the subsequent data file can increase the risk of identifying individuals.

Informed Consent

While the requirement of obtaining informed consent, based on the principle of respect for persons, is a guiding principle, social researchers argue that in practice, the principle of informed consent is often not straightforward in many of their investigations. They base their claims on several reasons.

First, many social scientists are concerned that the requirement of written informed consent forms can create an artificial, culturally inappropriate and occasionally dangerous bureaucratic process in several types of their researches (Schrag 2010). Researchers have argued against consent forms on several grounds. First, many participants who are illiterate are not able to sign such forms. Second, in many instances, the signed consent form represents the only instance in which a name is linked to the research and hence, the presence of such forms lessens assurances of anonymity from incriminating statements. To be sure, many regulations allow substitution of a witnessed thumbprint for a signature or a verbal consent in situations in which the written signature serves as the only link between a name and a participant's responses.

Social scientists also raise the concern that requiring a signature in many cultures may represent a lack of trust. For example, indigenous communities in Canada wanted nothing to do with the paperwork demanded by the research ethics boards of Canadian universities. Investigators were told:

> If we know you and trust you, we will work with you. Signing a lot of paper that talks about things we might not understand or care about, won't change that. (Israel 2015)

Similarly, in the United States, representatives from an Indian community said the following:

> Indeed, signing a paper may not be perceived as a trustworthy practice, especially in communities with a history of broken treaties and paper based promises. (Israel 2015)

The U.S.'s National Science Foundation (2008) noted that "in most ethnographic projects a request for written, formal consent would seem suspicious, inappropriate, rude and even threatening." As such, the National Research Council has called for the Common Rule to be rewritten to remove any language that might suggest written consent is the 'preferred norm".

Another issue involves "whose consent should be obtained?" and the necessity of obtaining the consent of organizations, community elders or leaders in addition to individual consent. Health researchers working with economically disadvantaged communities in rural sub-Saharan Africa have discussed the importance of seeking approval from formal community leaders. For example, Tindana and colleagues explored the understanding of paramount chiefs, divisional chiefs and community members in one district of Northern Ghana (Tindana et al. 2006). Doumbo reported that the Malaria Research Centre at Bamako in Mali used a stepped approach to gain approval from village elders, heads of extended families, groups of mothers and only then sought consent from individual families who might participate in the study (Doumbo 2005). Similar approaches have been described in Botswanna (Ntseane 2009).

Unfortunately, seeking approval from local leaders may either reinforce local patterns of exclusion, silencing particular voices or conversely, place pressure on members of the community to follow the decision of their leaders to take part. Molyneux and her colleagues explored perception of consent in a rural Kenyan community (Molyneux et al. 2005). While there was widespread agreement that chiefs and elders could give permission for a research project to be conducted within an area, community members reserved the right for households and individuals to make their own decisions. However, there were differences in opinions on the basis of gender, age, status, and educational levels, particularly in relation to who should make decisions about research involving children: 'Simple comments on cultural differences between populations, or description of community views as homogeneous, closed and static makes a far more complex reality" (Molyneux et al. 2005).

Social scientists raise the issue that informed consent is not required in several of their researches. For example, when the research takes place in public spaces or involves public officials, and when the wrong caused by lack of consent might be outweighed by the public benefit obtained, example of such research includes covert and deception methodologies. There is controversy, however, over when the social benefit can justify the degree to which deliberate manipulation of information (deception), misrepresenting one's presence (covert research), or the violation of privacy (observation research) can be justified by the social benefit. In other words, when does potential benefit to society justifies adverse effects on the rights of an individual participant?

Nonetheless, these types of researches have been justified on the pragmatic grounds insofar that it enables researchers to control stimuli, study low frequency events and gain information that might otherwise be unobtainable. In regards to deception research, James Korn maintains that social psychologists do not view their use of deception as a serious matter for research participants, but simply as part of the typical experiences of everyday life (Korn 1997). This equivalence between activities in a research study and "normal activities in everyday life" maintains that such research conforms with the definition of minimal risk. Indeed, deception is commonly used in marketing research, as over 80% of papers published in consumer and marketing research journals used deceptive practices. However, others express the concern that such research harms participants, researchers, research professions and society overall.

Covert research has several alternative rationales. First, it has been justified based on utilitarianism in limited circumstances where it is necessary for the research to remain secret in order to maintain access to the research setting, perhaps in the face of the desire of powerful or secretive interests to block external scrutiny. Second, covert studies have also been defended on the basis of non-maleficence, suggesting that it reduces discomfort of research participants, which would occur if they knew the actual purpose of the research. However, this argument is often dismissed by the charge of unjustified paternalism. Finally, those who collect anonymized data as part of non-participant observation in public spaces have argued that informed consent is not required on the basis that the data involved are publicly accessible or is perceived as public by participants. However, it is not always clear whether or not particular internet sites should be treated as private or public.

Challenges of Performing Social Science Research in the Arab Region

In addition to the above challenges associated with social science research, additional challenges confront international investigators who aim to perform social behavioral research in the Arab Region. First, if the research involves an interview study of political activists or informants, or individuals who engage in illegal activities (e.g., drug abuse or homosexuality),an ethical challenge constitutes determining from whom should the investigator obtain local ethics approval without sacrificing the privacy of the potential participants.

Second, foreign investigators may be required to be accompanied by the police or military escort. This "practice" will question the validity of the obtained data, as participants in the research will not discuss faithfully their thoughts in the presence of police or military personnel.

Third, foreign researchers may require a formal letter of approval from the local authority to conduct research involving the local inhabitants. Such a letter might not be readily obtainable.

Fourth, investigators may encounter situations that require reporting to legal authorities activities/behaviors that are considered illegal in the host country (such as substance abuse and sexual orientation). Such "legal obligations" would threaten confidentiality and the trust between researchers and participants.

Finally, RECs from Western countries are often unfamiliar with the social and political circumstances in low- and middle-income countries and hence, may approve research that proves to be associated with high social risks due to the cultural setting.

References

Biber, H. 2005. *The ethics of social research*. London: Longman.

Chilisa, B., and J. Preece. 2005. *Research methods for adult educators in Africa*. Hamburg: UNESCO and Pearson Education South Africa.

Doumbo, O.K. 2005. It takes a village: Medical research and ethics in Mali. *Science* 307: 680–681. Retrieved from: http://science.sciencemag.org/content/sci/307/5710/5679.full.pdf?ck=nck.

Israel, M. 2015. *Research ethics and integrity for social scientists*. London: Sage.

Korn, J.H. 1997. *Illusions of reality: A history of deception in social psychology*. Albany: State University of New York Press.

Levine, F.J., and P.R. Skedsvold. 2008. Behavioral and social science research. In *The Oxford textbook of research ethics*, ed. E.A. Emmanuel. New York: Oxford.

Mertens, D.B. 1998. *Research methods in educaton and psychology: Integrating diversity with quantitative and qualitative approaches*. Thousand Oaks: Sage Publications.

Mollet, J.A. 2001. Ethical issues in social science research in developing countries: Useful or symbolic. *Australian National University Conference Publications*. Retrieved from: http://hdl.handle.net/1885/8442

Molyneux, C.S., D. Wassenaar, N. Peshu, and K. Marcsh. 2005. "Even if they ask you to stand by a tree all day, you will have to do it!" community voices on the notion and practice of informed consent. *Social Science & Medicine* 61: 443–454.

Ntseane, P.G. 2009. The ethics of the researcher-subject relationship: Experiences from the field. In *Handbook of social research ethics*, ed. D.M. Mertens and P.E. Ginsberg. Thousand Oaks: Sage.

Rodriguez, E., C. Valdebenito, and L. Mondragon. *Ethics of research in social sciences*. Retrieved from: http://www.uchile.cl/documentos/ethics-of-research-in-social-sciences_76704_14_5937.pdf

Schrag Z.M. 2010. *Ethical imperialism: Institutional review boards and the social sciences 1965–2009*. Baltimore: Johns Hopkins University Press.

Tindana, P.O., N.E. Kass, and P. Akweongo. 2006. The informed consent process in a rural African setting: A case study of the Kassena-Nankana District of northern Ghana. *IRb Ethics & Human. Research* 28: 1–6.

Williams, M., and T. May. 1996. *Introduction to the philosophy of social research*. London: University College London Press.

Ethical Issues in Conducting Research in Conflict Settings in the Arab Region

Kaveh Khoshnood, Cindy Sousa, and Kirsty Clark

Introduction

In 2016, the United Nation High Commissioner for Refugees (UNHCR) reported that 65.3 Million people in 2015 were forcibly displaced from their homes, the highest number since World War II (UNHCR 2016). This figure includes about 21.3 Million refugees, 53% of who are from Syria, Afghanistan and Somalia where political violence is a major driver of forced displacement. The Arab region is disproportionately impacted by violent armed conflict. In 2014, the Arab region, home to about 5% of the world's population, contributed to almost 41% (more than 22 million people) of the forcibly displaced population globally (UNHCR 2016). In a 2015 publication, Nygard and colleagues reported that "at least half of the Arab States are affected, directly or indirectly, by armed conflicts of varying intensity" (Nygard et al. 2015). Almost all the forcibly displaced populations from the Arab region come from the conflict-ridden countries of Iraq, Lebanon, Palestine, Somalia, Sudan, Syria and Yemen.

With violent conflicts becoming more focused in major cities, the second decade of the twenty-first century has highlighted that urban environments, including complex facilities like shopping centers, hotels, and factories, are the battlegrounds of the future. The fairly recent transition of conflict and war from relatively isolated regions to particularly urban and populated areas has not only led to an increase in

K. Khoshnood (✉)
Epidemiology of Microbial Diseases, Yale School of Public Health, New Haven, USA

Fogarty International Center/NIH, Bethesda, USA
e-mail: Kaveh.Khoshnood@yale.edu

C. Sousa
Bryn Mawr College, Graduate School of Social Work and Social Research, Bryn Mawr, PA, USA

K. Clark
Chronic Disease Epidemiology, Yale School of Public Health, New Haven, CT, USA

H. Silverman (ed.), *Research Ethics in the Arab Region*, Research Ethics Forum 5,
https://doi.org/10.1007/978-3-319-65266-5_12

the number of civilians who are "caught up in the action" and killed or injured, but also led to an increase in people who face displacement, limited resources, multiple public health threats, and heightened instances of human rights abuses, which are only compounded by a culture of impunity (Pittaway et al. 2010).

On the other hand, the funding available to humanitarian organizations has risen significantly over the last decade. This trend has resulted in a significant increase in the number of research projects conducted in conflict settings, some of which are sponsored by large humanitarian organizations themselves. For example, the number of peer-reviewed articles that Médecins Sans Frontières (MSF) has published involving conflict and crisis settings has increased tenfold since 2002 (Ford et al. 2009). Research in conflict and post-conflict regions, along with areas to which refugees migrate, is necessary and can assess the effectiveness of interventions. As such, humanitarian organizations that provide funding for humanitarian interventions are also requesting research activities that will rigorously evaluate the impact of their programs. However, the conditions of the conflict and the precarious living conditions of people affected by conflict create unique ethical challenges that must be taken into consideration when researchers develop and conduct research. This chapter discusses some of the key ethical and logistical challenges of conducting research in conflict settings and with conflict-affected populations, many of whom are likely to be vulnerable from their traumatized settings. To highlight these issues, we will present and analyze a case study from the West Bank.

The Case for Humanitarian Research

Several reasons justify the conduct of research in conflict settings. First, such research can document the negative health implications of violent conflicts. A 2008 report for investigators working in post-conflict environments highlighted that researchers cannot "wait for the guns to fall silent" before taking action to investigate the health implications of conflict, thus risking the potential health policy outcomes of such research (Thomson 2009). Researchers also argue that it is necessary to produce evidence for health and other social benefits of interventions funded by humanitarian organizations. If independent researchers and humanitarian aid organizations are equipped with an understanding of the complex dynamics of conflict, they are then able to make informed decisions on when, where, and how to conduct health and policy-based research. Furthermore, by failing to draw attention to the plight of vulnerable populations caught up in conflict-based humanitarian crises, we may "contribute to their vulnerability and add to complacency among those who are responsible or contribute to their unfortunate plight" (Ford et al. 2009). This argument highlights that by ignoring conflict-affected populations, the research community is not only turning a blind eye to the victims, but also permitting the actions of the perpetrators of the violence to have a lasting effect.

Some argue, however, that research design issues as well as the lengthy time necessary to approve such research could impede the urgency for immediate emergency health services (Ford et al. 2009). Nonetheless, based on the potential for public health and policy implications, it is not only worthwhile and necessary to conduct research in conflict regions, it is also feasible. With local knowledge, contacts in the specific region, access through organizational partners and gatekeepers, and a flexible approach to adapting research methodologies, it is possible to conduct high-quality research in the midst of conflict-driven humanitarian crises (Goodhand 2000).

We conclude that the current literature suggests that research in conflict-affected regions can shed light on the efficacy of humanitarian interventions, conduct needs assessments for individuals and communities, evaluate health systems, give voice to refugees and internally displaced people (IDPs), and draw attention to post-conflict issues of reconstruction and rehabilitation.

Having made the case for humanitarian research, we now turn to the ethical and logistical challenges that are especially salient when conducting research in regions affected by conflict and crisis. Not only are these environments often politically complex and dangerous, but the research participants are likely to be traumatized and vulnerable. The next several sections will highlight some of the key ethical issues that must be taken into account before and during the research in humanitarian crises.

Ethical Concerns of Research in Conflict Settings

Avoiding the 'Therapeutic Misconception'

Balancing the immediate needs of the populations affected by conflict with the logistical realities of research is often a complex ethical dilemma. The length of time it takes to conduct research and see these results translated into potential programs and policies are longer than what conflict-affected populations often expect, which are immediate actions to alleviate their current situations. Indeed, study populations are often desperate for services and may confuse researchers with humanitarian aid workers and hence, conflate research activities with actual humanitarian aid, thus fostering a "therapeutic misconception." This notion of "therapeutic misconception" is intertwined with the question of what researchers are obligated to "give back" to their research subjects to avoid the charge of exploiting vulnerable subjects. As such, ethical questions emerge around whether or not it is necessary that researchers actually deliver "benefits" to the study populations that are ancillary to the research itself. That is, to have a "positive" impact that goes beyond the objectives of the research itself. However, in the effort to avoid the charge of exploitation, researchers will need to be mindful of the contrary concern of undue inducements that might emerge from these ancillary benefits.

The Moral Hazard of the 'Dual Imperative'

Social scientists doing fieldwork in humanitarian situations often face a dual imperative: research should satisfy high academic standards but also be able help the research populations caught up in humanitarian disasters by being able to influence agencies and governments to develop more effective responses (Jacobsen and Landau 2003). However, in an effort to produce deliverable results for the participants, and take seriously the admonition "that research into others' suffering can only be justified if alleviating that suffering is an explicit objective" (Turton 1996), sound methodology might be compromised. Additionally, when researchers desire their research to be relevant (i.e., "advocacy research") there is a tendency for researchers to "already know what they want to see and say, and come away from the research having 'proved' it" (Jacobsen 2003). In other words, the lens of "advocacy" research might inadvertently bias the outcomes of the research.

The above tension creates a dual imperative: to satisfy the demands of academic peers and to ensure that the knowledge the research generates is able to influence institutions, such as governments and the UN, so that the research populations gain benefits. To be sure, to satisfy the demands of this dual imperative, that the research is both academically rigorous and also leads to policy-generated health benefits, is not necessarily mutually exclusive, as "social scientists trained in logical argument and methodological rigour…can provide a solid empirical basis for policy and advocacy efforts" (Jacobsen). Effective and ethical research requires that methodologies be sound and explicitly recognize and criticize the limits and strengths of approaches to generating both data and the conclusions drawn from them.

Selecting an Appropriate Research Methodology

Research to inform humanitarian action in conflict settings relies on a broad range of evidence, including quantitative data gathered from surveys and routine program monitoring as well as qualitative input gathered through interviews, narrative accounts and oral histories, observation, policy analysis, and expert input. The above considerations regarding the 'dual imperative' make it vital for researchers to choose an appropriate and feasible methodological design that addresses the research question, tends to the local setting, and is responsive to the needs of the population under study. It is imperative that the humanitarian organizations and research group conducting the research design the research in a way that respects the circumstances of the conflict-affected populations while taking in to account the limitations in undertaking the specific research. While there are inherent difficulties in collecting high quality data in conflict settings, there is an obligation to ensure that the research methodology being applied is of the highest standard (Ford et al. 2009).

Additionally, the work of anthropologist Elizabeth Wood with Thai-Burmese refugees catalyzed the "building of a methodology which uses a human rights framework and participatory action research principles to work with refugee groups [and other indigenous groups] in a way which is respectful of their autonomy, agency and capacity." This methodology, borne out of a conflict setting, has been labeled 'reciprocal research', and it allows investigators to conduct ethically-sensitive research "with" conflict-affected populations rather than "on" conflict-affected populations. The multi-step process is based on an ethical framework that positions participants firmly as the leading voices of the research process. Critical to the process of 'reciprocal research' is a confidentiality agreement, in which the researchers ensure that all data and materials collected from participants remain the property of the participants and can only be used with the participants' permission (Pittaway et al. 2010). Conducting research in conflict settings with indigenous and refugee populations is possible; but, it must be conducted within the framework of human rights, and with the participants' best interest always at the forefront of the project.

Challenges for Institutional Review Boards in Reviewing Research in Conflict Settings

A key ethical and logistical challenge in conducting research in humanitarian crisis is the requirement for expedited review and approval from an established ethical review committee or an Institutional review board (IRB). In many countries experiencing violent conflicts IRBs either do not exist or do not function well enough to offer expedited reviews (Mfutso-Bengo et al. 2008). One solution, some have suggested, is that in some situations where humanitarian crises can be anticipated, it may be desirable to request IRB review of a research protocol in advance (Mattox 2001). Others, including Doctors without Borders (MSF) a humanitarian organization that is increasingly engaging in research in partnership with academic institutions and health ministries, have developed its own IRB in 2001 with good success (Schopper et al. 2009).

To further expand upon these points and address others, we now turn to a concrete example in the form of a case study detailing a 2007 health and healthcare delivery project in the West Bank (Sousa 2013). After briefly describing the research project we will use this case to explore the ethical issues and political tensions that arise when research in conflict settings must attend to the twin ethical imperatives of being responsive to the urgency of addressing the immediate needs of the population as well as being relevant enough to influence policy makers and hence, able to make a difference.

Case Study: West Bank

About the Research Project

The West Bank is a region well-known for its history of protracted conflict. The West Bank is the site of persistent military occupation of civilian areas, which began in 1967. Others have written on the effects of conflict zones on health in this area (Becker et al. 2009; Giacaman et al. 2009). In 2007, a collaborative socio-behavioral project began with the Palestinian Medical Relief Society (PMRS), one of the oldest and largest healthcare NGOs in Palestine, to assess how the ongoing conflict in the region affects health and healthcare delivery. The University of Washington's Human Subjects Division approved the data collection processes. Staff from PMRS helped coordinate data collection and provided assistance with translation of all materials (surveys, focus group materials, all consent and recruitment materials). Per data sharing agreements, data belongs jointly to the entire research team.

The lead researcher was a U.S.-based academic. Fieldwork for the project began in 2007, which, in addition to study procedures described below, included traveling around the West Bank and living in a Palestinian village for 12 weeks. The prolonged engagement included two return trips to undertake additional research in 2008 and 2009. This continued commitment to the research endeavor and to the partnership helped both set the stage for the research and helped with the quality of the interpretation (Krefting 1991).

The partnership culminated in two separate investigations. The first was an assessment of how the ongoing conflict and occupation affects healthcare delivery. Procedures to address this assessment included participant observation and interviews. Observations took place within PMRS' mobile clinic visits, as well as group counseling sessions and the accompaniment of health staff in their daily work.

The second investigation explored the relationship between political violence and the health of individuals and communities, as well as individual and collective responses to the stressors of political violence. This was a mixed-method project. Respondents were recruited from general health and women's clinics belonging to PMRS (survey respondents were also drawn from Birzeit University and the Ministry of Health). Staff at these locations approached the potential participants with a prepared script that explained the study and its potential benefits and risks. Participants were recruited if they met the criteria of being a Palestinian woman over the age of 18. Those approached to participate in the study were told it was strictly voluntary and that declining to take part will not affect their services in any way. Those who agreed to participate provided informed consent following a process that included a standard script.

Two hypotheses were examined for this second investigation: (1) rates of exposure to political violence would be related to reports of poorer physical and mental health and (2) processes of coping (including proactive coping; self-reliance; reliance on religious, political and family support; and political/civic engagement) would moderate the effects of political violence, acting as protective factors in the relationship between political violence and health.

For both of these investigations, quantitative data were collected through surveys that were distributed among women in the West Bank (N = 131). Qualitative data were collected via five focus groups (total N = 32) conducted in 2008 with adult Palestinian women in different sectors of the West Bank: Al Khalil (Hebron) (5), Nablus (7), Jerusalem (4), Qalqiliya (10), Tulkarem (6). Focus groups lasted about an hour and were co-facilitated in Arabic by two native Palestinians who were part of the research team. The discussions were taped, and the research team discussed themes immediately following each focus group.

Politics of Partnership and Establishing Community Based Research

In Palestine, historic and modern legacies of colonialism and ongoing control of the geographic and political terrain within the conflict create a dynamic that poses special considerations that researchers must take into account. The health system in Palestine reflects how the strategy of the Israeli occupation moves beyond armed conflicts or military operations to tactics aimed at fundamentally undermining Palestinian infrastructure and thus, sovereignty. This tactic has been described by Sara Roy as de-development: "the deliberate, systematic deconstruction of an indigenous economy by a dominant power." (Roy 1995). In part, de-development of the health sector in Palestine resulted in disjointed efforts among agencies, the gutting of resources and collaborations, and an over-reliance on outside assistance for public health. For example, particularly, though not only, during times of intensive conflict, Palestinian scholars are regularly prevented from reaching their places of work; meetings with colleagues and times for instruction for students are regularly interrupted (Giacaman 2005). Even when there is not active fighting or presence of Israeli military in the West Bank, scholarship is affected by the ongoing occupation due to the ongoing checkpoints and the series of restrictions imposed on Palestinians. These restrictions severely restrict travel both within Palestine and abroad, and thus limit training opportunities and efforts at collaboration. Therefore, in multiple ways, the presence of international partners in the West Bank becomes both particularly important – and particularly dangerous – with regards to the often-troubling dynamics related to the outside researcher.

As Becker and colleagues point out, these legacies make the need for sovereignty and local control of public health all the more important (Becker et al. 2009). The basic tenant of maintaining the control for public health in the hands of the community holds particular ethical importance. Given these dynamics of health within conflict settings, it is clear that international research partnerships, as a form of health solidarity work, should fundamentally work to support sovereignty and self-governance (Summerfield 1999; Weiss et al. 2003). Within conflict settings, however, there is a tendency for researchers, like other development "experts," no matter how well-intentioned, to parachute in with their own agendas to document health as they see it. When so-called "experts" from the outside involve themselves in research and the design of interventions, there is a real risk of emerging with research questions, methods, and implications for practice that are neither culturally appropriate nor sustainable (Summerfield 1999).

The key strategy to counter this disjuncture regarding the priorities of the researcher and that of the community is to approach research in a spirit of partnership and co-learning (Minkler 2005). Establishing mutually beneficial research partnerships within communities who are suffering from conflict is not an easy task, however, and this project brought to light several methodological and ethical dilemmas that reflect how politics of partnership itself contain tensions that reflect the ongoing problems with North-South research partnerships. These dilemmas will be discussed in turn, beginning with attention to issues surrounding the methods and ethics of research that crosses cultural and linguistic borders. We then highlight several complexities of analyzing and interpreting data within conflict zones. This case study ends with a reflection on the obligations researchers must tend to with regards to who benefits from international research partnerships in conflict settings. These topics will be examined below, followed by a discussion about the key lessons learned within this case.

Understanding and Addressing the Power Balance of Research Within Conflict Settings

The "right to define the question".

In addition to dilemmas concerning the data itself, there are also concerns about the questions that are asked in research endeavors, an issue that perhaps above all others illustrates the relations of power between research partners and between the researcher and the researched. As explained by McKnight:

> There is no greater power than the right to define the question. From that right flows a set of necessary answers. If the servicer can effectively assert the right to define the appropriate question, he has the power to determine the need of his neighbor rather than to meet his neighbor's need. While this power allows the professional to use his shiny new remedy, it also defines citizens as people who can't understand whether they have a problem-much less what should be done about it. (p. 48) (McKnight 1995)

In defining the research question itself; it was apparent that the project should not just focus on the pain caused by the conflict. Rather, it was crucial that the project also honored the principles of agency and self-determination, without which, of course health cannot be realized, as scholars in Palestine make clear (Becker et al. 2009). Thus, in line with this principle, the project sought not to only gather information about the health consequences of the occupation, but also to further understand resistance and resilience; how is it that, despite all of the suffering, individuals, families, organizations, and communities in West Bank are able to organize to protect and promote individual and collective wellbeing.

Language: The Ethics and Practice of Cross-Language Research

There are deep epistemological and ontological questions that researchers must grapple with in cross-language research (Temple and Young 2004). When data are collected in one language and subsequently "put" into another language, the process demands attention to researchers' beliefs about the absoluteness of meaning, along with notions of positionality, or where one stands in relation to the project (Herr and Gary 2015). For instance, conversations arose about the choice of words both in the task of translating English into Arabic to conduct the study and the task of translating Arabic into English to analyze the data and write-up the findings. Questions that required pondering included issues about cultural meaning and beliefs related to health (e.g., what words get used for depression and whether people identify and speak of wellness in an individual sense or a collective sense?) along with issues of power (e.g., do people speak more freely in their own language, perhaps to the point where they share things forgetting that it will be translated to audiences in very different contexts?).

These questions, which are laden with ethical implications, require that one contends with the methodological choices regarding translation and interpretation. In our case, the research team consisted of the lead researcher, an American academic woman who does not speak Arabic, but has spent considerable time in Palestine, working alongside Palestinians. In the case of the surveys, Palestinians from both Birzeit University (who were, in this case, professional translators) translated the survey; several PMRS staff members verified this version. The consent forms followed a similar process of translation, and the staff who recruited spoke in Palestinian Arabic when they spoke with potential participants. In the case of the focus group, the lead researcher worked with two Palestinian women: a community psychology graduate student from Birzeit University and a PMRS employee. Although these researchers were familiar with group facilitation and with research, the lead researcher provided some additional training to the Palestinian women.

The conduct of the focus groups represented one instance where new decisions were made once the team critically reflected on the methods; rather than conducting the focus group in English and doing simultaneous translation into Arabic, the team decided to have the Palestinian researchers facilitate the groups in Arabic. The lead researcher listened to each group and helped with the process by working with the other two researchers before, during and after each group. Translations for the focus groups were done in three steps. First, the main moderator of the focus groups provided initial translations and analyses by providing themes for each group. This was done in Palestine so the whole group could discuss the themes in person and decide when data saturation had been reached. Then, more thorough (word for word) translations were conducted by a professional Lebanese translator who was living in the United States. During this process, the lead researcher sat with the professional translator, who interpreted the content verbatim and the lead researcher transcribed and could immediately ask clarifying questions and make notes for follow up with the original team. The lead researcher then took these two translations and compared them, marking any conflicts in interpretations between the two versions. Finally, the team consulted and a final consensus was reached on each transcript.

The multi-phase process described above highlights how decisions about methods (in this case, regarding translation) often coincide with decisions about ethical quandaries. Trying to maintain integrity of meaning across geographies is both laden with tasks that one must attend to in a practical sense; but these tasks also represent ethical imperatives around the complexities of representation.

Ethical Issues with the Use of Local Staff as Recruiters: Ensuring Voluntariness and Confidentiality

PMRS staff approached the potential participants within their organizational settings with a prepared script explaining the purpose of the study, the nature of the partnership (that is, that it is a joint study done by an academic in the United States alongside the local organization), and its potential benefits and risks. Women were informed that participation in the study was strictly voluntary, that they could choose to not answer any questions they wished, and that their services would not be affected by their decision regarding participation. Participants were also informed that the content from the recordings would be transcribed and the recordings would be destroyed. Rather than collect names, participants gave oral consent; nonetheless, participants were informed that if their names came up, there would be no link between their name and the data and if the results of this study were published or presented, their names would not be used. Yet, despite these protections, there remained key considerations regarding confidentiality, particularly around our use of local staff to help recruit participants.

The use of staff to enlist participants had many advantages, including that they had a rapport with participants and might be seen as more open therefore to questions or concerns. Yet, at the same time, despite the involved recruitment and consent process, which was created by the lead researcher (in consultation with PMRS) and her institutional review board, the use of staff to recruit study participants also had some serious ethical issues to be considered. For instance, since much of the data were from clinics in small towns and villages, staff doing the recruiting might not be seen as outsiders, but rather as familiar parts of the community of respondents. While these staff members were not doing the research themselves, there is no doubt that the positive relationships they had with patients made the patients more likely to complete surveys and/or take part in a focus group. Given this, it is important to consider the ethical tensions around using such indigenous research assistants. Critical issues to consider included whether people felt like the research was truly voluntary and whether they felt like the findings really would be confidential (Alexander and Richman 2008). In an attempt to address this, the lead researcher was present when staff conducted the consent processes for both the surveys and the focus groups, and worked to ensure (despite her lack of Arabic) that the full consent process described above was completed. While the lead researcher could not necessarily engage in conversations with the participants (except for those who spoke English), the presence of her alongside the research team was a deliberate attempt to help both the participants and the researcher to have a more intimate connection, to build trust, and for the lead researcher to both build and convey a sense of deep and lasting personal accountability to the women in the study. The lead researcher also spoke regularly with the staff that was doing the recruiting to convey that while gathering an appropriate amount of data was our goal, we also could take the time needed to make sure that participation was not done in a coercive manner.

Using the Process of Analysis, Interpretation, and Presentation of Study Findings to Build Capacity

Building internal capacity is one central feature of engaging in community based research, and an important one when we consider the context of research capacity within most settings of conflict, and particularly in Palestine, where the infrastructure for research has been so deliberately compromised (Giacaman 2005; Roy 1995). Supporting infrastructure for communities (and countries) to retain control over their own individual and collective wellbeing is an important tenant for research in all settings, and the research relationship can be a key mechanism through which outside investigators can apply the process to empower, rather than burden, communities (Minkler 2005). In partnering with an existing agency and in working with and training other researchers (particularly within the focus group project), the lead (US-based) researcher tried to maintain key aspects of the project in the hands of Palestinians, for the individual and collective benefit of Palestinians.

Attention was paid, therefore, to working closely with Palestinians, particularly junior scholars and professionals, to develop and implement the study, and to analyze the findings. Processes around study development were detailed above. Regarding the analysis of the data, the lead researcher led the efforts particularly with the quantitative project. The decision was made to do this because the main people involved in the study in Palestine had moved on to other opportunities (in part, due to the nature of the fact that they were either junior professionals and/or students) and there was some time pressure regarding the analyses. The lead researcher, however, sent drafts of papers to people in the agency for their comments, if they so desired. One key area where tensions remained with regards to this issue was in the decisions around authorship. Despite the huge increase in community based research, journals are still reticent to include a whole agency as a co-author, even though in many cases of community based research (including this one), it is the most accurate way to represent how much collective effort was required to pull off the conceptualization of a study and the collection of appropriate amount of data. In some cases, authorship was shared with the agency, but in other cases, journals required the lead (US-based) researcher to acknowledge the agency rather than including them as an author, concluding that this was more appropriate.

The qualitative data collected through the focus groups provided for a much richer partnership in the analysis of data and the presentations of findings. In the case of the focus group work, authorship was clearer, as the lead facilitator/translator joined the paper as an analyst and a writer. This model was built upon for subsequent work. The lead facilitator/translator and lead researcher have since met at an international conference to talk about the work and to more deliberately create and nurture a small research team that crosses geographic boundaries. This helps to not only assure the trust-worthiness of the interpretation of the qualitative data, and obviously benefits the scholarly development of the lead (US-based) researcher but also allows for a measure of mentorship and professional development for the Palestinian team members. This issue regarding who benefits from research from the standpoint of capacity development of the research team also leads us to our final theme, and that is the question of who benefits from international research in conflict settings.

Ensuring That the Research Holds a Potential of Benefit to Host Communities

A (rightly) central point of tension within this research partnership was the issue of benefit, not only among research team members but also between the research team and the research participants. Particularly when it was clear that an outsider was the lead research partner, participants were often noticeably concerned about whether their time and the information they shared would actually benefit themselves or their communities, rather than just being a scholarly activity (of which they had seen many). As part of an effort to develop a set of research ethics guidelines for Birzeit University in Palestine, there is a recent paper that reviews research ethics and outlines suggestions for research in and on the topic of Palestine (Maira 2013). Among other important issues, this case study presents the issue of research fatigue in Palestine, including how vulnerable communities often become mere laboratories for research, rather than places whose people and issues are considered. In this context, research furthers agendas of control and domination, and the process is little more than another way that outsiders (particularly in the Global North) benefit from the misery of others (particularly in the Global South).

While the lead researcher was aware of this dynamic, it became quite real when the team was asked repeatedly, what are you going to do with this information? And, in particular, participants would often direct comments to the lead researcher with the (justified) demand that the information be brought back to the United States and to the international community. Indeed, the goal of this project was always to assist in advocacy efforts, and findings have been applied to not only scholarly venues like journal articles and conference presentations, but also have been shared and applied to advocacy efforts both in the United States, within the American Public Health Association (APHA), and internationally, with the Lancet Palestinian Health Alliance, launched in 2009 by the Lancet alongside the Institute of Community and Public Health based in Birzeit University, Palestine. This alliance supports research on health conditions by Palestinian public health scientists and leaders. The purpose of this initiative is to support networks between scientists in Palestine and scientists around the world using health as a catalyst to promote peace and justice in the region, and particularly for and with Palestinian people (Horton 2009). Findings have also been shared at non-academic venues, such as community and professional association meetings.

Lessons Learned from the Case and Moving Forward

There has been much written on the dynamics of insiders and outsiders with regards to the research relationship (Clingerman 2007; Minkler 2004; Minkler and Wallerstein 2008; Stoecker 1999). Within international research, we have much to learn from the robust body of work on indigenous research ethics, which, among other lessons, highlight the ways that research often rests on a positivist theory of knowledge wherein everything is easily measurable, neutrality is possible, and the researcher is a divine expert that, through scientific thought, can diagnose and therefore solve problems without the voice of those who are most affected by the problem (Tuhiwai Smith 1999).

However, research in conflict settings should move away from the positivist notion of researcher-researched. In fact, in these settings of massive and human-made hardship, neutrality may not only be unattainable and compromise our ability to truly understand a situation, but it also may be unethical, because these kinds of atrocities must be confronted and resolved (Punamaki 1990).

The alternative to such positivist thinking is research that puts at the center the principle of self-determination – which, it should be noted, is a central demand of health scholars in Palestine, who have noted that without self-determination, a true quest for health is impossible (Becker et al. 2009). To move research within conflict settings away from efforts that further marginalize and disempower populations, researchers from outside of the conflict settings who seek to maintain partnerships must deeply attend to one's place within the historical and modern politics of power that not only surround the research but also the conflict at hand. As scholar Tuhiwai Smith writes, the New Zealand Indigenous Maori alternative framework proposes that to act with respect and humility the researcher must act with caution, deal face to face whenever possible, and look and listen first, and only then speak (Tuhiwai Smith 1999).

References

Alexander, L.B., and K.A. Richman. 2008. Ethical dilemmas in evaluations using indigenous research workers. *American Journal of Evaluation* 29: 73–85.

Becker, A., K. Al Ju'beh, and G. Watt. 2009. Keys to health: Justice, sovereignty, and self-determination. *Lancet* 373 (9668): 985–987.

Clingerman, E. 2007. An insider/outsider team approach in research with migrant farmworker women. *Family & Community Health* 30 (1): S75–S84.

Ford, N., E.J. Mills, R. Zachariah, and R. Upshur. 2009. Ethics of conducting research in conflict settings. *Conflict Health* 3: 7.

Giacaman, R. 2005. Coping with conflict. *Education for Health* 18 (1): 2–4.

Giacaman, R., R. Khatib, L. Shabaneh, A. Ramlawi, B. Sabri, G. Sabatinelli, M. Khawaja, and T. Laurance. 2009. Health status and health services in the occupied Palestinian territory. *The Lancet* 373 (9666): 837–849.

Goodhand, J. 2000. Research in conflict zones: Ethics and accountability. *Forced Migration Review* 8 (4): 12–16.

Herr, K., and A. Gary. 2015. *The action research dissertation: A guide for students and faculty*. Thousand Oaks: Sage.

High Commissioner for Refugees (UNHCR). 2016, June 20. *Global trends: Forced displacement in 2015*. Available at: http://www.refworld.org/docid/57678f3d4.html. Accessed 17 Sept 2017.

Horton, R. 2009. The occupied Palestinian territory: Peace, justice, and health. *Lancet* 373 (9666): 784–788. https://doi.org/10.1016/S0140-6736(09)60100-8.

Jacobsen, Karen, and Loren B. Landau. 2003. The dual imperative in refugee research: Some methodological and ethical considerations in social science research on forced migration. *Disasters* 27 (3).

Krefting, L. 1991. Rigor in qualitative research: The assessment of trustworthiness. *The American Journal of Occupational Therapy* 45 (3): 214–222.

Maira, S. 2013. *Research ethics: A review of relevant research literature*. Retrieved from. Palestine: Birzeit.

Mattox, K. 2001. The world trade center attack, author. Disaster preparedness: Health care is ready, but is the bureaucracy? *Critical Care* 5 (6): 323–325.

McKnight, J. 1995. *The careless society: Community and its counterfeits*. New York: Basic Books.

Mfutso-Bengo, J., F. Masiye, and A. Muula. 2008. Ethical challenges in conducting research in humanitarian crisis situations. *Malawi Medical Journal : The Journal of Medical Association of Malawi*. 20 (2): 46–49.

Minkler, M. 2004. Ethnical challenges for the 'outside' researcher in community-based participatory research. *Health Education & Behavior* 31: 684–697.

———. 2005. Community-based research partnerships: Challenges and opportunities. *Journal of Urban Health* 82 (2): ii3–ii11.

Minkler, M., and N. Wallerstein. 2008. *Community-based participatory research for health: From process to outcomes*. San Francisco: Jossey-Bass.

Nygård, Håvard Mokleiv, and Håvard Hegre. 2015. *Protracted conflict and development in the Arab Region, E/ESCWA/ECRI/2015/2 UNESCWA trends and impacts, 4*. New York: United Nations.

Pittaway, E., L. Bartolomei, and R. Hugman. 2010. 'Stop stealing our stories': The ethics of research with vulnerable groups. *Journal of Human Rights Practice* 2 (2): 229–251.

Punamaki, R.-L. 1990. Relationships between political violence and psychological responses among Palestinian women. *Journal of Peace Research* 271: 75–85.

Roy, S. 1995. *Gaza strip: The political economy of de-development*. Washington, DC: The Institute for Palestine Studies.

Schopper, D., R. Upshur, F. Matthys, et al. 2009. Research ethics review in humanitarian CONTEXTS: The experience of the independent ethics review board of Médecins Sans Frontières. *PLoS Medicine* 6 (7): e1000115. https://doi.org/10.1371/journal.pmed.1000115.

Sousa, C.A. 2013. Political violence, health, and coping among Palestinian women in the West Bank. *The American Journal of Orthopsychiatry* 83 (4): 505–519. https://doi.org/10.1111/ajop.12048.

Stoecker, R. 1999. Are academics irrelevant? Roles for scholars in participatory research. *American Behavioral Scientist* 42 (5): 840–854.

Summerfield, D. 1999. A critique of seven assumptions behind psychological trauma programmes in war-affected areas. *Social Science and Medicine* 48 (10): 1449–1462.

Temple, B., and A. Young. 2004. Qualitative research and translation dilemmas. *Qualitative Research* 4 (2): 161–178.

Thomson, S. 2009. *Developing ethical guidelines for researchers working in post-conflict environments*. Research Report prepared for the Program on States and Security, City University of New York. Available at: http://www.statesandsecurity.org/_pdfs/Thomson.FINAL.9.16.pdf.

Tuhiwai Smith, L. 1999. *Decolonizing methodologies: Research and indigenous peoples*. New York: Zed Books Ltd.

Turton, D. 1996. Migrants and refugees. In *In search of cool ground: War, flight, and homecoming in Northeast Africa*, ed. Tim Allen, 96–110. Trenton: Africa World Press.

———. 2017, June 21. *Global trends: Forced Displacement in 2016*. Available at: http://www.refworld.org/docid/594aa38e0.html. Accessed 17 Sept 2017.

Weiss, M.G., B. Saraceno, S. Saxena, and M. van Ommeren. 2003. Mental health in the aftermath of disasters: Consensus and controversy. *The Journal of Nervous and Mental Disease* 191 (9): 611–615.

An Ethical Framework for Conducting Research Involving Refugees and Internally Displaced Persons in Conflict Settings

Shahd Osman

Introduction

Protracted conflicts worldwide – wars and persecution on the grounds of nationality, race, religion, political opinion or social group – have driven people from their homes (forced migration) without any respite predicted in the near future. Post World War II, the establishment of the United Nations High Commissioner of Refugees (UNHCR) in 1950 was considered a major milestone for addressing refugees' issues. Similarly, to attend to research issues, 'The Association for the Study of the World Refugee Problem' was also established in that same year (Black 2001).

In recent years, there have been a sustained increase in the numbers of victims of such conflicts, refugees and internally displaced persons, (IDPs) being estimated in 2010 to be approximately 11 million and 27.5 million, respectively. Reports from the United Nations High Commissioner of Refugees (UNHCR 2016) show that 86% of the world's refugees are hosted by low- and middle-income (LMICs) countries, with the Americas' hosting approximately 6% and Europe hosting 12% (UNHCR 2016). Regarding internally displaced persons (IDPs), 60% of such individuals exist with five LMICs (Iraq, South Sudan, Syria, Democratic Republic of Congo (DRC) and Nigeria).

Research conducted in conflict settings is undertaken in very complex and dangerous settings coupled with the vulnerability and marginalization of refugees and IDPs, which place these populations at the risk of exploitation and other research harms. Research involving such populations is conducted mostly with an aim to address their health needs, enhance health systems and shape policies (Bilak et al. 2015). Such research can be ethically justified only if the research is designed and conducted in a manner that protects individuals from exploitation and harms and the

S. Osman (✉)
Public Health Institute, Federal Ministry of Health, Khartoum, Sudan
e-mail: Osman.shahd@gmail.com

H. Silverman (ed.), *Research Ethics in the Arab Region*, Research Ethics Forum 5,
https://doi.org/10.1007/978-3-319-65266-5_13

objectives of the research addresses their health needs so that it will contribute to the alleviation of their suffering (Hugman et al. 2011).

Avoiding exploitation is the fundamental ethical challenge of all research with humans, and there are two distinct conceptions of exploitation. The first is the traditional Kantian notion of exploitation that involves "using an individual as means… for an end they do not agree with or to which they have not consented", which violates their autonomy. The presence of poverty, illiteracy, cultural and linguistic differences increase the possibility of such exploitation. This form of exploitation is mitigated by the presence of a valid informed consent and ensuring collaborative partnership with a larger community that not only agrees to the research, but has also influenced and shaped the proposed research.

The second conception of exploitation involves the unfair distribution of the benefits of research between sponsors/researchers and the communities/researchers participating in the research. Addressing this latter type of exploitation requires ensuring social value, i.e., the research addresses important health needs of the community, scientific validity, fair subject selection, and sensitivity to the resources of the host community.

Avoiding the other potential research harms requires the presence of a favorable risk-benefit ratio and respect for enrolled participants, which includes respecting privacy, protecting confidentiality, sensitivity to cultural factors, and safety monitoring. It follows from the above that appropriate attention to sound study methodology coupled with important safeguards are necessary to protect research participants and the associated community from exploitation and harms.

Presently, research in conflict settings lacks a robust ethical framework to guide the avoidance of exploitation and other research harms. Commentators recently performed a qualitative review of existing ethical guidelines for research in disaster settings, of which only four were relevant to conflict settings and the others were pertinent for public health emergencies and natural disasters (Mezinska et al. 2016).

The research ethics framework of Emanuel and colleagues serves as a valuable tool for both researchers and RECs when designing or assessing the ethics of international research studies (Emanuel et al. 2004). The eight requirements described in this framework *(Collaborative partnership, Social value, Scientific validity, Fair selection of study population, Favorable risk-benefit ratio, Independent review, Informed consent, and Respect for recruited participants)* emanate from the ethical principles of respect to persons, beneficence/non-maleficence and justice. While Medecins Sans Frontieres adopted this framework in 2003 to guide its research, it has since moved away from it in "form and content" to address its specific needs (Sheather et al. 2016). Contrarily, we favor the appeal of the framework by Emanuel and colleagues, attributed to its uniqueness in its ability to operationalize ethical principles into research practice. We intend to adopt this framework to refuges and IDPs in conflict settings, but reframe it within a rights-based approach. As such, our aim is to demonstrate the applicability of the Emanuel framework to research in conflict settings and make clear the ethical concerns that might be present when such research is conducted.

Ethical Framework

Collaborative Partnership

Building collaborative partnerships when conducting research in LMICs minimizes exploitation, ensures long term change, and is in itself an act of respect and acknowledgement of cultural and contextual differences. Partnerships commonly occur between the sponsors and researchers on one hand, and with the communities and its policy makers, on the other. Effective collaboration includes engaging representatives of the community with the planning and implementation of the research project, ensuring capacity building opportunities (Jacobsen and Landau 2003) and integrating the results of the research in the health care system of the community (Emanuel et al. 2004).

Challenges in Refugee/IDPs Settings

Developing collaborations is essential when conducting research that involve refugees and IDPs. Research in conflict settings, however, involve multiple levels of stakeholders that create more complex relations. For example, unlike studies that involve citizens, refugees are not residents of the country they reside in, and hence governments might not always know what is best for such populations or guard against their exploitation. Indeed, governments might be the cause of exploitation. Nevertheless, governments act as important gate keepers and hence, access to the refugee population might not occur without establishing some sort of collaboration with the government. Other actors are of equivalent importance, such as local humanitarian organizations, which may represent the ideal partner for researchers to build trust with the community and enhance subsequent recruitment efforts.

Developing partnerships within the refugee community necessitates identifying leaders within the refugee community who can serve as their representatives to the national governments. Occurring in a highly political charged environment, it is not uncommon, however, to forge partnerships with so-called leaders who do not reflect the dominant views of the research participants (who are often subjects of human rights abuses), and instead, might represent a source of threat to the potential participants themselves. Similarly, researchers need to realize that their selection of choices regarding representatives might not represent political choices about "which voices are heard and whose knowledge counts" (Goodhand 2000).

In identifying the "community", several points are worth considering. First, one needs to ask: What makes refugee populations a community? Are we referring to the refugees in the country of refuge (as in even if they are of different nationalities or ethnic groups they are considered one community) or are we referring to the refugee population from a certain country or area of conflict, e.g. Syrian refugees as one community, South Sudanese refugees as a community and Somali refugees as another community? Finally, most researchers will be viewed correctly as the "outsider" with power imbalances between them and the populations they wish to involve in their research. As such, community participatory research will help develop special ethical relationship with participants.

Social Value

Research is designed to answer a valuable question or hypothesis. Studies that lack social value to the community are not worth undertaking and do not justify the risks to the research participants. As it can be very complex to determine whether research will lead to actual social benefits, it is important that communities are involved in determining the type of research that can be socially valuable. Several benchmarks need to be considered to enhance social value. These include: determining what and the extent of the knowledge gap that the research will address; deciding whether alternative research questions are more important; identification of who will be the beneficiaries of the research (the participants themselves, the local community, or communities that extend beyond the immediate borders), the value of the potential benefits for each of the beneficiaries; assurance of the dissemination of research for all beneficiaries (using appropriate languages and platforms for all stakeholders), and consideration of the services already available (Emanuel et al. 2004).

Challenges in Refugee/IDPs Settings

Refugee and IDP studies often conclude with policy recommendations, as researchers in this field usually justify their research by being able to influence future policies (Jacobsen and Landau 2003). However, prospective value is not guaranteed, as research findings may take a long time to turn into practice. As such, it is important for researchers to work with operational agencies to ensure that findings are closely tied to subsequent actions (Goodhand 2000). There is also the risk that researchers might give false hope to communities regarding the extent and likelihood of outcomes and hence, it is crucial that the purpose of the research is clearly explained to community members. Finally, researchers need to ensure that the therapeutic misconception is avoided, as community members may conflate research activities with tangible benefits from humanitarian efforts.

Selection of Research Questions: The research question is supposed to be based on a priority health need of the community (i.e., social value). However, selecting a research question that feeds into advocacy goals or are donor driven raise questions regarding the value of the findings, especially in a field that is dominated by qualitative methods that are subject to biases (see below).

Indeed, many researches are funded by non-profit donors who identify issues simply because they are trendier than others and bring more media attention than others. Such issues may become over-researched and hence, do not lead to the development of new knowledge. Also, donors desire research that can be conducted quickly and cheaply and hence, show results to serve as evidence of their successful funding activities, although such research rarely lead to changes in policies that benefit the host communities. In an effort to please donors and obtain the necessary funds, not-for-profits tend to write proposals with a budget that will most likely be approved and embrace themes that donors are interested in and the trends in the field.

To enhance social value, one must adequately define the community who are to be the recipient of the research results. Organizations commonly describe the community of refugees in their reports using more than one criteria, such as nationality plus the country of refuge, e.g., Syrian refugees in Turkey or Somali refugees in Ethiopia. There may be more levels when tribes affected by the conflict are different, e.g., Dinka refugees from South Sudan in Uganda may have different needs than other South Sudanese tribes.

Not infrequently, social value is determined by local NGOs with or without representatives from refugee communities who are in a better position to identify certain gaps based on the problems they face in the field. But that is problematic as the needs addressed are those of the NGO, which are specific to their mandate rather than the priority needs of the refugee or IDP community.

Another issue regarding social value is that unlike clinical trials, where institutional review boards focus on issues of ensuring that drugs proven to be effective are reasonably available to that community, the situation with social science research is more complex, as social scientists might not have the funds necessary to implement any policy initiatives. This raises the question whether such investigations are ethical if funds to implement these interventions are not available. Hence, while the research might be of social value, its implementation will not be practical or immediately forthcoming. Researchers and humanitarian organization are constantly looking for long range solutions, although they might manage to secure funds to pilot projects. These are questions that need to be answered by ethicists, donors and practitioners in the field.

Dissemination of research results: Another challenge for social accountability involves the dissemination of results to the refugee community. Donors supporting research involving refugees disseminate results to NGOs and humanitarian organizations, but rarely to refugees themselves. Proposals infrequently (if ever) budget monies to deliver results to the refugee population. Accordingly, innovative ways for sharing information should be undertaken and a budget for that purpose needs be allocated even if it requires traveling to those areas. Indeed, refugees will rarely have access to publications in journal articles, attending conferences or reading the reports uploaded to a website.

Scientific Validity

To achieve the potential value of humanitarian research, research must be designed with sufficient methodologic rigor to be able to answer the research question. Poorly designed research does not justify exposing participants to the risks of research.

As such, ethical research requires attention to sound methodological principles. This includes an adequate sample size, as results might not be generalizable to the entire community if the sample selected is not representative of the entire community.

Additionally, there needs to be unbiased interpretation of the data, which is especially important when one performs qualitative research that involves interviews and focus groups that are conducted in the native language and hence, subject to translation errors and inaccuracies.

Challenges in Refugee/IDPs Settings

Dual imperative: Social scientists doing fieldwork in humanitarian situations often face a dual imperative: to satisfy the demands of academic peers and to ensure that the results can influence relevant stakeholders (e.g., governments) that can lead to development of policies that will enhance the plight of refugees. Social scientists trained in logical argument and methodological rigor argue that they can recognize and criticize the limits and strengths of the methodology and hence, the conclusions drawn from the data. However, there is a concern that social scientists are engaging in what has been called 'advocacy research', where researchers already know what they want to see and say, and come away from the research having 'proved' it, which includes widespread acceptance of unsubstantiated facts. Indeed, commentators argue that much of the current research on forced migration is based on unsound methodology, and that the data and subsequent policy conclusions are often flawed or ethically suspect (Jacobsen and Landau 2003). As such, 'Advocacy research' and its associated biased lens can lead to harming refugees more than helping them if the resulting policies do not lead to sustainable changes.

Sampling techniques and sampling frame and selection bias: There might be concerns as to whether the chosen sample is representative of the target population. Imprecise sampling might be due to issues of access to the proper population. Indeed, if the target population represents refugees inside a camp or camp-like setting, there are gatekeepers who will provide researchers the sample frame and sometimes dictate whom researchers will meet. In qualitative exploratory research where researchers are looking for key informants on certain topics, they will most likely partner with NGOs and service providers to identify the sample, who might not select the most representative voices. This is a legitimate problem that is faced by social researchers working on refugee studies with different populations of refugees. Moreover, there are sub-populations among refugees and IDPs that are hidden, e.g., refugees and IDPs who live in urban areas and those who are in areas that are not considered safe for data collectors.

Follow-up data: Another issue involves obtaining follow-up data. Not many longitudinal studies are done among refugees and this is justifiable since longitudinal studies need stable populations. But, with protracted conflicts there are increasingly performance of studies that incorporate follow-up. Researchers are expected to track participants that are lost to follow-up in longitudinal studies to ensure they are not different from those that remain in the study. However, tracking households or individuals lost to follow up in a refugee setting may be deemed unethical due to fears that it might pose a political risk to refugees who chose to hide for safety reasons. Though this is considered a legitimate justification, it still introduces a selection bias and threatens internal validity.

Data collection methods: An added risk comes from local partners in their function as service providers for the researchers. Research participants might fear retaliation from the service provider if the information they provide might be regarded as being inadequate. Also, local partners often act as translators, which requires their presence during data collection generated from interviews and focus groups discussion, which can serve as a risk to confidentiality. In addition, the local partners serving as research assistants might be associated with a group the respondents either fears or despises, which will cause the respondents to be reluctant to provide critical information from fear that the information will be used against them.

The quality of the obtained data from interviews and focus groups discussions may also suffer from the following:

- Interviewing techniques (e.g., conversational tone of the facilitator may prompt particular responses or inadvertently direct the answers, an unconscious process often difficult to avoid)
- Translation inaccuracies due to following sources of bias:
  (a) Use of local researchers
  (b) Avoiding back translations due to costs
  (c) Difficulties with translating dialects
- Biased content and thematic analysis

Fair Selection of Study Population

Fair selection in regards to subject selection typically concerns populations regarded as "vulnerable". Certain types of populations are considered vulnerable because of their inherent characteristics or situation, making them less able to protect their interests. Such practices represent justice issues, as the concern is that vulnerable populations might be susceptible to exploitation. Also, vulnerable populations should not be targeted for research unless their participation is necessary to answer a valuable scientific question. Additionally, fair selection also requires not arbitrarily excluding people from valuable research. Finally, fair subject selection requires that as far as possible, groups and individuals who bear the risks and burdens of research should be in a position to reap its benefits.

Challenges in Refugee/IDPs Settings

Distinctive features of research in conflict settings include the many factors that contribute to the heightened vulnerability of refugees and IDPs in conflict settings. For example, refugees and IDPs tend to include more women and children, persons who are financially disadvantaged, and survivors of a traumatic experience who might be psychologically vulnerable. Presence of other discriminatory factors may complicate things further, e.g., having a disability or being an LGBTI. An additional important characteristic involves having diminished political rights compared to citizens and being subjects of human rights abuses (Leaning 2001). While UNHCR sets some basic standards on how refugees and IDPs should be treated, many countries fall short of enforcing their own laws and refugees are left as standalone communities with minimal protection and loose regulations. The situation involving IDPs has even more vagueness, as they are still within the governance of the system they might be trying to escape (Leaning 2001). One way to address the issue of exploitation is to encourage those involved in the research and their representatives to exercise a greater degree of agency and to influence the terms of engagement and the research process itself. However, such redistributing power might be resisted by some.

Fair selection of participants requires "making political and ethical choices about which voices are heard and whose knowledge counts (Goodhand 2000). The main requirement is that research participants should be chosen based on scientific reasons and not on any other reason, such as accessibility, cost, gender, or malleability (Sumathipala and Jafarey 2010).

Favorable Risk-Benefit Ratio

A favorable risk-benefit ratio requires that risks are minimized to the extent possible and that all unnecessary risks are avoided. Subsequently, risks should be justified by the potential direct benefits to the participants, if any, and by the social value to society. The community should also be able to decide whether the research has a balanced risk benefit ratio (Emanuel 2004).

Challenges in Refugee/IDPs Settings

Various guidelines mention different sources of potential risks to research participants, depending on the research study and the setting itself, which may include the level of security unique in every setting. These issues include the following:

Power Dynamics: In conflict settings involving vulnerable groups, power dynamics play an important role in shaping risks. For example, research participants might fear retaliation if information they share is not well received by the governing bodies. The culture is that if you complain then you are criticizing the governing body.

Security risks: Safety is a fundamental issue for both members of the communities and researchers. Reflection on how researchers conduct research, to whom they talk and what they talk about is essential to avoid putting communities at risk. When choosing issues for discussion, researchers must identify which issues are more sensitive than others and likely to endanger research participants. Researchers need to be constantly aware that while they are present for only a short time, their questions and the discussions they provoke may reverberate for a long time afterwards (Goodhand 2000).

Political risks: The political and legal marginality of refugees and IDPs mean they have few rights and are vulnerable to arbitrary action on the part of state authorities, and sometimes even the international relief community. Many researchers do not adequately consider how their enquiries might put their subjects at risk, particularly in conflict zones or hosting areas where the displaced are highly vulnerable.

Privacy and confidentiality: Basic measures that are needed to protect privacy and enhance confidentiality in humanitarian research can prove to be a challenge. Violations of privacy and breaches of confidential information in conflict settings can produce social risks from resulting discriminatory practices and social stigma, especially in settings of human rights abuses. The challenge is that with the best intentions to respect privacy and secure confidentiality, it might be difficult to achieve. For example, employing local residents to help with focus group interviews may present challenges for maintaining the discussions confidential. Shared housing, shared utilities and aspects of the camp settings in general can make it seem impossible to maintain privacy.

Confidentiality, even though promised by many researchers when obtaining consent, can be easily compromised within camps. For example, in a setting of a relatively small camp, it can be very easy to identify who served as the source of the information even when de-identified. Consequently, research participants may also withhold information in fear that service providers who are used as translators/partners may breach confidentiality (being from the local area). Additionally, researchers need to think carefully about how they bear witness to abuses and pass on information to those trying to address them without endangering the research participants (Goodhand 2000).

Opening old wounds: There might be psychological risks from recounting stories of trauma. For traumatized individuals and groups, silence may be a coping, not just a survival strategy. Researchers might inadvertently re-open wounds by probing into areas of discourse respondents may not wish to discuss (Goodhand 2000).

Independent Review

An independent review by a research ethics committee (REC) in LMICs is necessary when conducting international research to enhance ethical conduct of the research, guard against conflict of interest, and ensure accountability. Transparency about the nature of the research and who are the participating stakeholders is also important to ensure trust. It may sometimes be necessary to gain approval from other regulatory bodies and partners, whether local community committees, NGOs, or ministries of health, depending on the depth of collaboration and the regulatory systems of the country. Ethical reviews need to be both independent and done by competent review boards and hence, performing research in a context where there is questionable competency of the RECs may require training and capacity building in research ethics (Emanuel et al. 2004).

Challenges in Refugee/IDPs Settings

Many of refugee research is performed by humanitarian organizations and unlike academic institutes, it is not standard for them to include ethical review by an REC. Also, since dissemination of research findings is achieved through publishing reports to their websites, the pressure to obtain ethical clearance in order to publish in peer journals is not an issue. Recently, there has been a growing awareness among these organizations about the importance of having an ethical review, but the practice is still sporadic. In general, ethics committees are seen as another layer of bureaucracy that can hold up the start of research and delay the reporting of findings. As such, the time needed to conduct the review comes with opportunity costs. Additionally, many see the overprotection attitudes and paternalistic behavior of RECs as being an obstruction to research that involve the most vulnerable groups. As noted by Northway, safeguards need to be proportionate to potential harm and the unintended results of such safeguards need to be assessed (Northway et al. 2015).

Another issue regards the extent of member training of local or even international RECs. The issue is whether such members have received the required training and experience to make judgments on research involving refugee and IDP. Some of the RECs' requirements might be unhelpful to the refugee population and might even enhance risks. For example, RECs might tend to restrict research away from NGOs in a desire to involve more of the local people. However, at times such local individuals might compromise confidentiality.

Informed Consent

Informed consent is a universal ethical requirement. Disclosure of information should occur in a manner that is comprehensible to the local community. Considering gate keepers and acquiring consent from multiple levels consistent with cultural norms maybe needed through methods considered appropriate by the local community. Participants need to be aware that they are free to participate (or not) in the research and are free to withdraw at any time (Emanuel et al. 2004).

Challenges in Refugee/IDPs Settings

Challenges in informed consent include power relations between researchers and potential participants. The presence of a local partner might affect the decision for participation, whether it is actually voluntary, and whether the participant really understands they can withdraw. Power relations are not only exerted by local partners; humanitarian settings manage to create a social governing system, where leaders also exert some power on other members of the community and there may be a lot of fear from members in the community.

An issue that might threaten the validity of informed consent involves unrealistic expectations and as such, researchers should be "particularly vigilant in ensuring that prospective study participants do not confuse research procedures with clinical care and thus fall prey to the so-called therapeutic misconception" (Collogan et al. 2004). Hence, researchers should "take great care to inform potential research participants [...] that some interventions to which they are subjected might be undertaken primarily for the benefit of the research" (Jennings and Arras 2008).

An issue that might affect voluntariness stems from undue inducement. With scarce resources in refugee settings and the competition between humanitarian organizations, there exists a common culture of financial incentives. In activities such as community awareness or peace building programs, many researchers and sponsors may feel obliged to incentivize participants to participate. Also, in an effort to provide some tangible benefit to the participants, researchers may feel obligated to give incentives to avoid exploitation. Finally, the research participants themselves expect some form of immediate tangible benefits. RECs may consider such ancillary benefits as undue inducement and disallow it.

Furthermore, consideration needs to be given to ensure that consent is obtained in a manner that promotes adequate disclosure of information, ensures comprehension, and allows time for reflection and deliberation of a decision. Such a process should also address the context and needs of the involved community. An innovative example of a stepwise participatory process that combines an informed consent process and action planning to ensure social value has been used by researchers at the Women's Refugee Commission for Children with Disabilities in refugee settings and is presented in Box 1. Such methods are developed to facilitate the consent process and is relevant to Emanuel's proposed benchmarks for informed consent. In conflict settings, time limits might rule out such a staged approach.

Box 1 Staged Approach to Informed Consent and Action Planning

Getting ready for participation

Step 1: Raise awareness in the community

Step 2: Information session for potential participants

Collecting information on GBV and disability

Step 3: Group discussions with parents and caregivers of children with disabilities

Step 4: Participatory activities with children and youth with and without disabilities

Step 5: Home visits

Child and Youth centered action planning

Step 6: Community action planning workshop

What change matters the most to children with disabilities

Evaluation: Collect "stories of change" from children and youth with disabilities

Source: Gender-based Violence and Children and Youth with Disabilities: A Toolkit for Child Protection Actors. Available at http://wrc.ms/GBV-disab-youth-children-toolkit

Another challenging theme that comes up frequently in refugee research involves informed consent for children. In many humanitarian settings many children may be unaccompanied and hence, lack a parent/legal guardian to provide consent. In 2016,

UNICEF published a working paper titled "*What we know about ethical research involving children in humanitarian settings*" that emphasizes the importance of involving children in research in humanitarian settings. However, the paper points out that there are important practical considerations that need to be assessed when conducting such research involving children that include power relations, the consent process, privacy and confidentiality. The working paper presents a good effort towards ensuring ethical research without the need to exclude children from all research activities (Berman et al. 2016).

Respect for Recruited Participants and Communities

Researchers have obligations towards participants and the communities involved in research. Respect to recruited participants entails many of the issues discussed above, e.g., respecting privacy when collecting information and maintaining confidentiality of the data, and attempts at guaranteeing post-study benefits. Other issues include the right to withdraw at any time without repercussions and the dissemination of information to the communities whom participated in the research and inform them about the results. Finally, respect towards participants involve adequate monitoring and assurances of safety.

Conclusion and Recommendations

The analysis presented in this chapter focused on the challenges of conducting ethical research based on a framework informed by the work of Emanuel and colleagues. We have used this framework to present a systematic approach to discussing the problems researchers face in the field when conducting research in conflict settings. Humanitarian researchers are practicing in a unique and difficult environment, resulting from conflict and political settings where the residing population are in dire need for protection and alleviation of suffering. They deserve to be supported by donors' humanitarian organizations, governments and research ethics committees, however by no means should this jeopardize their accountability towards refugees and IDPs and the preservation of ethical values when conducting research among these groups. Conducting research among refugees and IDPs should occur with great planning and efforts in conjunction with stakeholders that include refugees, IDPs and ethicists so that results can be generated and translated into practice and policies.

References

Berman G, J. Hart, D. O'Mathuna, E. Mattellone, A. Potts, C. O'Kane,... T. Tanner. 2016. What we know about ethical research involving children in humanitarian settings: An overview of principles, the literature and case studies. *UNICEF – Working Paper*.

Bilak A., M. Caterina, G. Charron, S. Crozet, L. R. Díaz-Leal, F. Foster et al. 2015. *Global overview 2015 people internally displaced by conflict and violence*. Norwegian Refuge council (NRC). Available at http://www.internal-displacement.org/.

Black, R. 2001. Fifty years of refugee studies: From theory to policy. *International Migration Review* 35 (1): 57–78.

Collogan, L.K., F. Tuma, R. Dolan-Sewell, S. Borja, and A.R. Fleischman. 2004. Ethical issues pertaining to research in the aftermath of disaster. *Journal of Traumatic Stress* 17 (5): 363–372. https://doi.org/10.1023/B:JOTS.0000048949.43570.6a.

Emanuel, E. 2004. What makes clinical research in devleoping countries ethical? The benchmarks of ethical research. *The Journal of Infectious Diseases* 189: 930–937.

Emanuel, E.J., D. Wendler, J. Killen, and C. Grady. 2004. What makes clinical research in developing countries ethical? The benchmarks of ethical research. *The Journal of Infectious Diseases* 189 (5): 930–937. https://doi.org/10.1086/381709.

Goodhand, J. 2000. Research in conflict zones: Ethics and accountability. *Forced Migration Review* 8 (4): 12–16.

Hugman R, E. Pittaway, L. Bartolomei. 2011. When 'Do No Harm' is not enough: The ethics of research with refugees and other vulnerable groups. *British Journal of Social Work*(41).

Jacobsen, K., and L.B. Landau. 2003. The dual imperative in refugee research: Some methodological and ethical considerations in social science research on forced migration. *Disasters* 27 (3): 185–206.

Jennings B, & J. Arras. 2008. Ethical guidance for public health emergency preparedness and response: Highlighting ethics and values in a vital public health service. *Centers for Disease Control and Prevention, Available at:*https://www.cdc.gov/od/science/integrity/phethics/docs/white_paper_final_for_website_2012_4_6_12_final_for_web_508_compliant.pdf.

Leaning, J. 2001. Ethics of research in refugee populations. *Lancet* 357 (9266): 1432–1433. https://doi.org/10.1016/S0140-6736(00)04572-4.

Mezinska, S., P. Kakuk, G. Mijaljica, M. Waligora, and D.P. O'Mathuna. 2016. Research in disaster settings: A systematic qualitative review of ethical guidelines. *BMC Medical Ethics* 17 (1): 62. https://doi.org/10.1186/s12910-016-0148-7.

Northway, R., J. Howarth, and L. Evans. 2015. Participatory research, people with intellectual disabilities and ethical approval: Making reasonable adjustments to enable participation. *Journal of Clinical Nursing* 24 (3–4): 573–581. https://doi.org/10.1111/jocn.12702.

Sheather, J., K. Jobanputra, D. Schopper, J. Pringle, S. Venis, S. Wong, and R. Vincent-Smith. 2016. A Medecins Sans frontieres ethics framework for humanitarian innovation. *PLoS Medicine* 13 (9): e1002111. https://doi.org/10.1371/journal.pmed.1002111.

Sumathipala, A., and A. Jafarey. 2010. Ethics of disaster management, clinical care and research. *Asian Bioethics Review* 2: 124.

United Nations High Commissioner for Refugees (UNHCR). 2016. *Global trends forced displacement in 2015*. Geneva, UNHCR. http://www.unhcr.org/statistics.

Ethical Considerations of Industry-Sponsored Clinical Trials in the Arab Region

Vladimír Mišík, Martin Boleček, and Rachel V. Brady

Introduction

This paper evaluates latest geographic dynamics between 2009 and 2014 in biopharmaceutical clinical trials (BPCTs) and benchmarks accessibility to clinical trials in in the Arab region (Saudi Arabia, UAE, Egypt, Algeria, Kuwait, Oman, Qatar, Bahrain, Lebanon, Jordan, Morocco and Tunisia) against other global regions (# active BPCT sites/capita). In addition, this paper introduces, to our knowledge hitherto never previously published, benchmarks of participation of countries in development of new products (BPCT global market share), relative to the target level of consumption of developed pharmaceutical products (pharmaceutical consumption market share). Our findings imply a potential scientific and ethical challenge: under-representation of patients from Arab region in the development of novel pharmaceutical products relative to the consumption of the developed products. We will discuss the ethical implications for regions with low participation in development of new products (i.e., participation in clinical trials) and yet high consumption of developed products. We encourage that this mismatch between development and consumption of new drugs be addressed by governments, medical institutions and patient organizations in the Arab region as well as biopharmaceutical companies planning to launch new products in these markets.

V. Mišík (✉)
LongTaal, Clinical Trial Analytics, Stare Grunty 61, Bratislava 84104, Slovakia
e-mail: vladimir.misik@longtaal.com

M. Boleček • R.V. Brady
QuintilesIMS, Stella-Klein-Low-Weg 15, Rund 4, Haus B, OG 4, Vienna 1020, Austria

H. Silverman (ed.), *Research Ethics in the Arab Region*, Research Ethics Forum 5,
https://doi.org/10.1007/978-3-319-65266-5_14

Pharmaceutical Sales Growth Compared with Participation in Clinical Trials

During the past three decades, the biopharmaceutical industry (biopharma) enjoyed periods of significant growth in the developed markets, with sales growth outperforming GDP growth, and there was little motivation to look elsewhere. This picture has changed in the past decade and increasingly emerging markets, including those in the Arab region, are outpacing biopharmaceutical sales growth in the developed markets (Pineau and Rink 2013). Due to targeted government investment in healthcare combined with increased healthcare spending of the rising middle class in the emerging markets, biopharma sales growth and healthcare expenditures have been growing ahead of GDP growth in the emerging markets (UBS Investment Research 2010).

Due to such changed dynamics of biopharma growth, in conjunction with significant geographic shifts in consumption of pharmaceuticals to the emerging markets, it would be reasonable to assume that corresponding geographic shifts would occur in the conduct of biopharmaceutical clinical trials (BPCT). Indeed, loss of BPCT market share in the developed markets accompanied by market share gain in emerging markets was reported by several authors (Karlberg 2009, 2014; Misik et al. 2014; Thiers et al. 2008). Comparing market share between the different regions from data obtained from ClinicalTrials.gov, our published data demonstrated that between 2007 and 2012 developed BPCT markets (North America, Western Europe and Australia/New Zealand) lost 3.4% of global market share, while emerging regions gained 2.1% of global market share (Misik et al. 2014). However, among emerging markets only Central and Eastern Europe (CEE) and Emerging Asia (mostly China) experienced growth, while market share of all other emerging markets, including the Arab region, declined from already previously low levels (Misik et al. 2014). Herein, we explore further the data that supports the above generalizations.

Methods, Data Sources, and Model Assumptions

For the purposes of this analysis, we used the following data sources and assumptions:

US clinical trial registry (ClinicalTrials.gov) database has been shown to be reliable data source for analyzing global industry-sponsored clinical trial trends (Karlberg 2010, 2014; Misik et al. 2014).

US clinical trial registry (ClinicalTrials.gov) database was downloaded on 14 April 2015, with the following filters applied: *Phases*: I/II, II, II/III, III, *Recruitment*: Active, Not recruiting; Completed; Enrolling by invitation; Not yet recruiting; Recruiting, *Study types*: Interventional, *Funded By*: Industry. Subsequently the data have been analyzed as described previously (Misik et al. 2014). Customized analyses for this paper were obtained as a courtesy of LongTaal Institute (www.longtaal.com).

Number of Active Clinical Trial Sites

Previous publications that used ClinicalTrials.gov registry to analyze geographic BPCT trends utilized the number of new sites added to the registry over a defined period (Karlberg 2009, 2014; Misik et al. 2014; Thiers et al. 2008). There is a considerable year-on-year variation in terms of new sites added, caused by initiation of studies with large number of sites in some years. For countries with relatively low number of clinical trial sites this can lead to a significant year-on-year under/overestimation of clinical trial market share, and/or market share gains/losses, unless new sites added are aggregated over several years. To enable better year-on-year comparisons of clinical trial market share (as % of active BPCT sites) we developed a novel methodology allowing determination of active sites in each year (rather than only new sites added (Karlberg 2009, 2014; Misik et al. 2014; Thiers et al. 2008).

The following algorithms and assumptions were applied: to determine whether sites in a study were active in a given calendar year, we used the start and completion dates associated with the study record in clinicaltrials.gov. Based on our analysis, less than 3% of studies do not have a completion date entered in their record. For these, the study completion date was replaced with either *study last update* date or start date plus 5 years, whichever is less. Number of active sites in a country represents the sum of all site locations for all active studies in that country.

Global Clinical Trials Market Share

Unless explicitly mentioned differently, any reference to clinical trials trending refers to changes in the number of active industry-sponsored Phase II and III sites in each country/region during any given period, relative to the number of such active sites globally. Country/regional percentage of global BPCT sites (industry-sponsored Phase II and III only) has been assumed equal to BPCT sites market share of those countries/regions. Due to the significant annual variation of the number of Phase II–III industry sponsored clinical trials (partially due to increased adoption of the register use rather than due to the real growth of clinical trial sites), when comparing BPCT market changes between two periods, global market share, rather than absolute number of sites, are being compared to determine the relative market growth in countries/regions.

Accessibility to Clinical Trials[1]

Accessibility to clinical trials has been defined as the number of BPCT sites per one million population. For comparative purposes, BPCT accessibility is expressed

[1] It is conceptually important to understand the difference between the share of the global clinical trial market and the accessibility to clinical trials: whereas share of clinical trials for each country is expressed as a global share of BPCT sites, accessibility is a population-adjusted parameter

relative to the US levels (US BPCT accessibility level being 100%). Source of the population data was the World Bank population databank (The World Bank 2014).

Product Development vs Product Consumption Balance

Participation in biopharma product development versus participation in product consumption balance (Development/Consumption) index is a newly defined parameter introduced by these authors to quantify the balance between participation of countries/regions in development of new pharmaceutical products (i.e., participation in industry-sponsored clinical trials) relative to the consumption of marketed pharmaceutical products.

For the purpose of this paper, this index has been calculated as follows:

$$\frac{\text{Development}}{\text{Consumption}}\text{index} = \frac{\text{Global } \textit{marketshare of BPCTs}}{\text{Global } \textit{marketshare of pharmaceutical consumption}}$$

In this equation, BPCT market share is expressed as a share of active global BPCT Phase II and Phase III sites (see above), and pharmaceutical consumption market share has been calculated based on BMI pharmaceutical sales data (International Federation of Pharmaceutical Manufacturers & Associations 2014).

Results and Discussion

Table 1 shows global trends in BPCTs during the period 2009–2014. The data demonstrate that efforts of many developed countries to protect their share of BPCTs, which they started to lose to the emerging markets following adoption of ICH GCP in year 1996, is beginning to pay off. This is evidenced by stabilization (and even slight increase during the 2013–2014 period) in their BPCT market share at just over 73% total, with a concomitant decline of the market share of emerging markets to below 27%. Developed markets also continued to enjoy high levels of accessibility to clinical trials (with a segment average 70% of the US levels), measured in terms of number of active BPCT sites per capita (see Methods). Among the emerging markets, Central and Eastern Europe managed to retain (and even marginally increase) its emerging market leadership, with 13.4% of global BPCT share, as well as the highest accessibility to clinical trials among emerging markets (30% of US

and refers to the number of BPCT sites per capita in the country relative to the US levels: take example of Bulgaria and the US: US has a 35% share of global clinical trial sites, while Bulgaria has only 0.8% of global market share, but number of industry-sponsored clinical trial sites adjusted per capita (relative to the US) shows US at a 100% and Bulgaria at 96%: i.e. an average Bulgarian has roughly the same chance to participate in an industry-sponsored clinical trial as an average US American. Take Egypt as another example: BPCT market share 0.1% of global BPCT sites, and the accessibility to clinical trials 0.6% of the US levels: i.e., an average Egyptian has ~200× lower accessibility to industry clinical trials relative to an average US American (data not shown).

Table 1 Geographic trending (2009–2014) of clinical trial market share (based on number of biopharmaceutical Phase II and Phase III clinical trial sites), relative market growth (expressed as relative change of clinical trial market share), accessibility to clinical trials (expressed as number of clinical trials sites per capita relative to the US levels) and share of pharmaceutical sales

	Clinical trial market share			Relative market growth	Accessibility to CTs			Share of pharmaceutical sales	Development/ Consumption index
Region	2009–2010	2011–2012	2013–2014 (a)	2009–2010 vs 2013–2014	2009–2010	2011–2012	2013–2014	2014 (b)	2014 (a/b)
Developed Markets	74.4%	72.7%	73.1%	−1.8%	68.0%	68.1%	70.5%	70.0%	1.04
Australia/New Zealand	2.3%	2.3%	2.5%	6.7%	74.3%	75.0%	80.8%	1.3%	1.92
Israel	1.0%	1.0%	1.1%	10.0%	107.8%	108.6%	119.4%	0.2%	6.00
Japan	3.0%	3.6%	3.5%	17.2%	19.9%	24.1%	25.0%	11.2%	0.32
North America	40.5%	39.5%	38.4%	−5.0%	98.9%	98.5%	98.1%	33.9%	1.13
Western Europe	27.6%	26.3%	27.6%	−0.2%	56.0%	54.9%	59.4%	23.4%	1.18
Emerging Markets	25.4%	27.2%	26.8%	5.8%	3.6%	3.9%	3.9%	28.1%	0.96
Asia (excl. Japan)	6.22%	6.83%	6.69%	7.6%	1.4%	1.6%	1.6%	11.6%	0.58
CEE+CIS	12.32%	13.30%	13.44%	9.1%	25.6%	28.4%	29.6%	5.7%	2.35
Latin America	5.17%	5.44%	5.10%	−1.4%	7.3%	7.8%	7.5%	7.2%	0.71
Sub-Saharan Africa	0.97%	0.95%	0.85%	−12.6%	1.0%	0.9%	0.8%	1.0%	0.86
Turkey	0.49%	0.50%	0.60%	22.7%	5.7%	5.9%	7.2%	0.8%	0.72
Arab Region	0.21%	0.19%	0.16%	−21.9%	0.7%	0.6%	0.5%	1.8%	0.09
Algeria	0.001%	0.002%	0.006%		0.0%	0.0%	0.1%	0.30%	0.02
Egypt	0.055%	0.052%	0.057%	2.8%	0.6%	0.6%	0.6%	0.19%	0.29
Jordan	0.006%	0.004%	0.005%	−18.2%	0.9%	0.6%	0.7%	0.08%	0.06

(continued)

Table 1 (continued)

Region	Clinical trial market share			Relative market growth	Accessibility to CTs			Share of pharmaceutical sales	Development/ Consumption index
	2009–2010	2011–2012	2013–2014 (a)	2009–2010 vs 2013–2014	2009–2010	2011–2012	2013–2014	2014 (b)	2014 (a/b)
Kuwait	0.001%	0.002%	0.0005%	−62.8%	0.4%	0.4%	0.1%	0.09%	0.01
Lebanon	0.047%	0.040%	0.036%	−23.6%	9.1%	7.9%	7.2%	0.12%	0.29
Morocco	0.025%	0.010%	0.002%	−90.7%	0.7%	0.3%	0.1%	0.10%	0.02
Oman		0.002%	0.003%		0.2%	0.6%	0.8%	0.04%	0.08
Qatar		0.002%	0.002%		0.0%	0.7%	1.0%	0.04%	0.06
Saudi Arabia	0.019%	0.021%	0.015%	−23.2%	0.6%	0.6%	0.5%	0.53%	0.03
Tunisia	0.050%	0.047%	0.030%	−39.6%	4.0%	3.8%	2.5%	0.08%	0.36
United Arab Emirates	0.006%	0.006%	0.007%	32.2%	0.6%	0.6%	0.7%	0.17%	0.04
Total	100.0%	100.0%	100.0%	0.0%	12%	12%	13%	100%	1.00

The Development/Consumption balance index (i.e. balance between participation in development of new products relative to the participation in the consumption of pharmaceuticals) is calculated only for 2014. See Methods section for details of each definition levels). Collectively, the emerging Asian markets have not shown growth, driven by a significant market share loss in India (Misik et al. 2014), and remained at below 7% of global BPCT share, with accessibility to clinical trials being only 2% of US levels. Latin America fell below their 2009–2010 levels and retained just over 5% of global share and 7% of the US levels of accessibility to clinical trials. Sub-Saharan Africa fell to below 1% global share, with accessibility to clinical trials falling below 1% of the US levels.

The Arab region markets (data from Algeria, Egypt, Jordan, Kuwait, Lebanon, Morocco, Oman, Qatar, Saudi Arabia, Tunisia, and UAE were captured in our analysis) remained the smallest regional market globally, with market share below 0.2%, combined with the lowest accessibility to clinical trials of only 0.5% of the US levels. Egypt, Lebanon, Tunisia, and Saudi Arabia (in that order) remained the largest BPCT markets in the Arab region, but with the exception of Lebanon, accessibility to clinical trials in these countries remained below 1% of the US levels.

Not only has the Arab region remained the smallest BPCT market globally, but its market share declined marginally throughout the period 2009–2014. Presumably, the impact of the Arab Spring (which started in 2011), and subsequent turbulence in some countries in the region, has left a lasting legacy and countries in the Arab region, regardless of whether impacted by these events or not, are not being seriously considered for planning of large BPCTs.

Participation in Clinical Trials Relative to Consumption of Pharmaceuticals

Of note is that while the clinical trial market in the Arab region continues to decline (at least in relative terms) across a majority of the countries in the region, pharmaceutical markets are forecasting growth levels three to four times faster relative to the developed markets (Pineau and Rink 2013).

In order to evaluate and quantify the gaps between participation in development of new products relative to the consumption of marketed pharmaceuticals, we have introduced a Development/Consumption balance index (DCI) expressed as a ratio of BPCT market share and market share of pharmaceutical consumption (see Methods). Thus DCI > 1 implies a research bias (i.e. disproportionally high participation in development of new products relative to their consumption), and DCI < 1 points to a consumption bias (i.e. disproportionally high participation in consumption of pharmaceuticals relative to participation in their development).

As the results in Table 1 show, participation in development of new pharmaceuticals and consumption of pharmaceuticals are remarkably balanced (i.e., DCI is close to 1) across the aggregated sample of the developed markets, as well as emerging markets, with a significant variability between countries/regions. The outliers among the developed markets being Israel (DCI = 6; or 6× research bias), and Japan (DCI = 0.32; or 3.1× consumption bias). Among the emerging regions, the outliers are Central and Eastern Europe (DCI = 2.4; or 2.4× research bias). On the other extreme is the Arab region with DCI <0.1 (i.e. more than 10× consumption bias), the largest consumption bias globally. Among the Arab countries, Kuwait, Algeria, Morocco, Saudi Arabia, UAE, Qatar, Jordan and Oman, with DCI ranging between 0.01 and 0.08 (or 13–100× consumption bias), rank among 25 countries with largest consumption bias globally among 105 countries evaluated: Oman#80, Jordan#83, Qatar#84, UAE #90, Saudi Arabia #95, Morocco #98, Algeria #100, and Kuwait #104 (data not shown).

Implications of such disparity in development versus consumption in the Arab region (largest globally) should be carefully examined, as patients in the region may potentially be treated with medications, the development of which did not include significant sample of patients with similar genetic, dietary, and cultural profile (e.g., understanding impact of Ramadan fasting on the safety and efficacy of the products marketed in the Arab region). An implication of this gap between participation in the development of drugs and the consumption of drugs is that the developed drugs may lack effectiveness or may even be harmful for patients in the Arab region.

In our previous article (Misik et al. 2014), we have advanced the notion that preferential access to clinical trials by certain socioeconomic and ethnic groups, which has been demonstrated within a single hospital or a single country (Noor et al. 2013; Godden et al. 2010), manifests itself also on a much larger geographic scale. The data presented in this paper support this notion and demonstrate a further decline of accessibility to clinical trials to patients in Africa and the AME region, two regions with lowest accessibility to clinical trials globally.

While it was outside the scope of this article to analyze the reasons for the low (and declining) market share of clinical trials in the Arab region, we provide below our views, based on personal observations of the authors as well as anecdotal information shared by regional pharmaceutical managers and healthcare professionals, regarding some of the contributing reasons for the observed trends, many of which stemming from perceptions about the region:

1. Lack of experienced sites and investigators (while certainly pockets of clinical trial experience can be found throughout the region). This should, however, not present a serious limitation, since the bulk of the growth in the emerging regions was fueled via working with inexperienced investigators (properly trained and supported), which clearly has not adversely impacted data quality coming from these regions (Misik et al. 2014).
2. Perception of several sponsors of clinical trials about the absence of or not-well-defined clinical trial processes and infrastructure within the Arab region. This is indeed mostly a perception, as there are a sufficient number of well-trained RECs (several of them registered with the US and with many members trained via the NIH funded Middle East Research Ethics Training Initiative (MERETI)). Several large hospitals have their own clinical trial units staffed with study coordinators, and several global CROs and well as many local CROs operate within the region.
3. Concerns about general safety/security risks in countries experiencing active warfare and/or active military/para-military conflicts (such as Syria, Afghanistan, Libya, and parts of Iraq). Furthermore, the exportation of biospecimens may be regarded as a security concern in some countries. However, the impact of armed

conflict in the other countries is minimal and/or non-existent. Of relevance in this regard is also that the majority of large pharmaceutical companies have substantial and growing numbers of staff located within the region in sales and medical marketing roles.

4. Lack of a regulatory structure for the conduct of clinical trials. As discussed in several chapters in this compendium, many Arab countries lack national regulations for research and well-defined clinical trial regulatory processes and structures for the conduct of clinical trials, which may contribute to long study-site start up times.

Conclusion

Our data demonstrate that across the Arab region there is the largest gap globally between participation in development of new products (expressed as BPCT market share) and consumption of marketed pharmaceuticals (expressed as market share of pharmaceutical sales). Moreover, our data show that this gap is further increasing over time, driven by low BPCT market share with no sign of growth (indeed between 2009 and 2014, the market share of a majority of Arab countries declined marginally from very low levels), against a rapid growth of the pharmaceutical market in the region (2–3× faster growth versus the developed markets). It would therefore be desirable for stakeholders in the Arab Region to enhance research funding, help research institutions to develop their infrastructure for clinical trials, and enhance awareness of clinical trials among patients, all of which are aimed at increasing participation of patients from the Arab countries in the development of new products. Combined efforts of biopharmaceutical companies, national governments, medical institutions, as well as patient organizations in the Arab region, are needed in order to succeed in such endeavors. In the absence of efforts aimed at bridging this gap, patients in the Arab countries may not only be deprived of several benefits of participation in clinical trials, but may potentially be treated with inappropriate medications, as the development of which did not include significant sample of patients with similar genetic, dietary, and cultural profile (e.g., impact of Ramadan fasting on the safety and efficacy of the product).

Acknowledgement Customized clinical trial analytics used in this paper were prepared and provided as a courtesy of LongTaal Institute (www.longtaal.com).

References

Godden, S., G. Ambler, and A.M. Pollack. 2010. Recruitment of minority ethnic groups into clinical cancer research trials to assess adherence to the principles of the Department of Health Research Governance Framework: National sources of data and general issues arising from a study in one hospital in England. *Journal of Medical Ethics* 36: 358–362.

International Federation of Pharmaceutical Manufacturers & Associations. 2014. The pharmaceutical industry and global health, facts and figures 2014. Geneva.

Karlberg, J.P.E. 2009. Uninterrupted globalization of industry sponsored clinical trials. *Clinical Trial Magnifier* 2: 79–94.

———. 2010. WHO international clinical trials registry platform – an in-depth analysis. *Clinical Trial Magnifier* 3: 333–344.

———. 2014. *Globalization of industry-sponsored, clinical trials. Latest insight on shifts in sites among regions. Clinical trial magnifier*, 1–36. Falls Church: FDAnews. ISBN 978–1–60428-140-8.

Misik, V., R.V. Brady, M. Bolecek, and H. Klech. 2014. Current trends in globalization of industry-sponsored clinical trials. *Applied Clinical Research, Clinical Trials & Regulatory Affairs* 1: 56–66.

Noor, A.M., D. Sarker, S. Vizor, B. McLennan, S. Hunter, A. Suder, H. Moller, J.F. Spicer, and S. Papa. 2013. Effect of patient socioeconomic status on access to early-phase cancer trials. *Journal of Clinical Oncology* 31 (2): 224–230.

Pineau, C. and C. Rink. 2013. *Pharmaemerging markets – Picking a pathway to success*. IMS Health White paper. Retrieved from: www.imshealth.com/pharmerging.

The World Bank. 2014. *Data: Population, total* [Data file]. Retrieved from http://data.worldbank.org/indicator/SP.POP.TOTL.

Thiers, F.A., A.J. Sinskey, and E.R. Berndt. 2008. Trends in the globalization of clinical trials. *Nature Reviews: Drug Discovery* 7: 13–14.

UBS Investment Research. 2010. *Global pharma: Doing well by doing good?*, Q-Series: UBS World Pharma Model. Retrieved from: www.ubs.com/investmentresearch

Part II

Research Governance in the Arab Region

Models and Challenges of Research Governance Systems

Henry Silverman

A governance system for research represents the regulatory and ethical oversight mechanisms established for the protection of research participants in a country. Such a system consists of various structures (e.g., governmental bodies as well as regulations, guidelines, policies and decrees) and processes (e.g., ethics review, oversight mechanisms, and accreditation procedures (e.g., for research ethics committees). There are stakeholders at the macro-level who set general parameters (e.g., governmental bodies, such as National Ethics Committees and Drug Regulatory Authorities, and sponsors of research) at the meso-level who set local parameters (e.g., research institutions and clinical trial sites), and at the micro-level who represent the final pathway of compliance (e.g., researchers and their staff) (McDonald et al. 2011). During the last several decades, the regulation and oversight of research in many countries have evolved into complex systems that integrate the stakeholders from these different levels into national regulatory frameworks.

Governance systems for health research represents a response to several factors. These include research scandals that have occurred in many countries during the past several decades and hence, the need to protect the rights and welfare of research participants; the increase in biomedical research activities worldwide; the insistence by international sponsors and organizations that research must comply with standards set out in international regulatory instruments, such as CIOMS, ICH-GCP, Declaration of Helsinki, and the research regulations/guidelines of the sponsoring country; and the need to ensure that international collaborative research addresses the needs of the host country, thus protecting the countries, institutions, and communities from exploitation (Nwabueze 2016).

H. Silverman (✉)
University of Maryland, Baltimore, MD, USA
e-mail: hsilverm@medicine.umaryland.edu

H. Silverman (ed.), *Research Ethics in the Arab Region*, Research Ethics Forum 5,
https://doi.org/10.1007/978-3-319-65266-5_15

Types of Governance Models

As reviewed by Hirtle and colleagues, there are several models of governance systems for research (Hirtle et al. 2000). First, regulation may take the form of professional or industry self-regulation in the absence of any national regulations or guidance. This informal type of regulatory and oversight of research frequently occurs in the initial stages of research activity in a country. Often, in this climate, research ethics review committees may or may not have been established by a high ranking institutional official and hence, an institutional requirement for mandatory ethics review is often lacking.

As the scope and extent of research activity increases in conjunction with the recognition of the potential for abuses that can occur in research, professional self-regulation is often replaced by increasingly complex and formal models of research regulation (Hirtle et al. 2000).

One type of regulatory model at this stage consists of detailed national legislation that makes review of research by research ethics committees (RECs) a legal requirement coupled with oversight and accountability mechanisms at the national and institutional levels to ensure compliance with the rules for governing research and the protection of human research participants. Legal sanctions could accompany noncompliance. This approach reduces variability and possible discrepancies among the RECs in the country at the expense of flexibility and responsibility at the local and institutional levels, as well as sensitivity to the local context.

A second type of regulatory model provides formal legal requirements of accountability and gives research institutions the task of developing its own human subject protection programs that includes a system of ethics review. This model has been described as a legally mandated "self-regulation at the institutional level and a publicly accountable system for protecting the rights and welfare of human subjects" (Hirtle et al. 2000). This model of institutional self-regulation can be supported by centralized mechanisms and is most reflective of the U.S. model, where the Food and Drug Administration (FDA) and the Office of Human Research Protections (OHRP) verify whether regulatory standards are respected, provide standards for RECs, and may investigate potential violations of the regulations.

A third and less stringent regulatory approach consists of governmental bodies (e.g., medical research funding agencies) that adopt guidelines that provide ethical guidance and a framework for the ethics review of government funded research. While this approach proposes an ethical standard for research, it lacks the weight of formal legislation as well as the authority to require compliance or impose sanctions other than funding cuts. Compliance therefore remains largely voluntary.

A fourth approach involves the adoption of framework legislation that integrates, through a cross-reference, other guidelines such as the ICH-GCP guideline. The European Union has favored this model. Reliance on such framework legislation may become problematic if the framework guideline changes (Hirtle et al. 2000).

Challenges of Governance Systems

Goverance systems must address several important issues that enhances it effectiveness. One issue important to its success regards the mechanisms for the enforceability of the regulations and hence, compliance with the regulations. Enforceability usually depends on the source of a particular guideline/regulation. For example, whether the guideline is issued by a professional body or by the government. Guidelines issued by professional bodies do not generally have direct legal force and hence are voluntary. That said, some legal and non legal consequences may accompany a breach of the provisions of such guidelines; for example, discontinuation of funding, termination of employment, or suspension of a research permit issued by the MOH. Finally, guidelines may criminalize a violation of its provisions. In contrast, regulations issued by the government are legally enforceable back up by penal sanctions for the breach of its provisions. For example, the Jordanian Clinical Studies Law specifies fines (up to $30,000) and jail sentences (1–3 years) for failure to comply with the law's requirements, including failure to report adverse events, failure to follow the approved protocol, or failure of a physician to supervise the study. The Moroccan Law specifies that research staff who fails to obtain informed and voluntary consent is liable to sanctions that include 3–5 years of imprisonment and a fine of 500,000 Moroccan dirhams (≈50,000 US dollars). The law in Saudi Arabia specifies that any person violating any provision of the Law shall be subject to one or more of the following penalties:

1. Warning;
2. Suspension of research until the effects of the violation are rectified;
3. Barring the researcher from conducting the research subject of the violation;
4. A fine not exceeding two hundred thousand (200,000) Riyals;
5. Imprisonment for a period not exceeding 6 months.

Another important aspect of a research governance system pertains to the regulation and oversight of local research ethics committees (RECs). As discussed in Part IV: Regulatory Landscape in the Arab Region, the mechanisms instituted by which local RECs are regulated differ between the countries in the Arab region. Such oversight functions exist where formal legal regulations have been issued (e.g., Jordan and Saudi Arabia) and even in countries without formal regulations (e.g., Egypt and Lebanon). A common initial approach involves the requirement for local RECs to register with the Ministry of Health; countries have required different types of information to accompany such registrations. Increasing levels of oversight can include audit and inspections, as well as accreditation mechanisms to ensure that RECs have the necessary structures and processes considered necessary for proper functioning. In lieu of an external accreditation mechanism, RECs can use a self-assessment tool to assess how their structures and processes conform with international guidelines. Such a tool is described in Chap. 29.

A further issue regards the types of research mandated by national legislation to undergo ethics review. Several options exist. First, national legislation can require that all types of human research must comply with the requirement of prior review and approval by an ethics committee. For example, in Saudi Arabia, the "Law of Ethics of Research on Living Creatures" pertain to all research involving humans, including biological samples and retrospective research involving previously collected data.

Alternatively, national regulations may only require ethical review of certain types of research. For example, the Morocco Law only regulates research involving medical interventions that are not ordinarily part of clinical management. The Moroccan Law does not pertain to non-interventional and observational research, as well as retrospective studies involving the analysis of existing health data. The Jordanian Clinical Studies Law regulates only clinical studies involving patients as well as healthy volunteers enrolled in bioequivalence and bioavailability studies.

While the Moroccan and Jordanian regulations are limited in their scope of mandated ethics review, review of non-intervention and observation research are usually dependent on mandates at the institutional level. This is increasingly occurring throughout the Arab region. For example, institutions usually require academic promotions to be dependent on international publications; since international journals require prior ethics review as a criteria for publication, non-intervention and observation research is de facto dependent on the ethics review of research. Finally, in all countries, regardless of the existence of national regulations for research, clinical drug trials cannot be undertaken without the permit or authorization of a central governmental agency (e.g., drug regulatory board), which usually requires prior ethics approval.

A final issue to address regards the strengthening of national medicines regulatory frameworks coupled with a focus towards achieving a balance between advancing the public health interest, the interests of the pharmaceutical industry, and ethical values embraced by society. The goal is to develop robust national medicines regulatory systems that protect the rights and welfare of clinical trial participants, ensure merits of scientific research, maintain consistency of clinical trial assessment, ensure credibility of data for drug regulatory submission, and maintain public trust in the safety of approved drugs. The accomplishment of these goals are largely dependent on the coordinated interactions between the National Ethics Committees (NECs), local Research Ethics Committees, and National Regulatory Authorities (NRAs). The objective is to achieve a balance between the roles and responsibilities of RECs and NRAs that enhances efficiency and effectiveness and avoiding duplication of efforts.

In general, RECs and NRAs have independent and complementary functions. For example, RECs focus mainly on ethical and science issues that include: safeguarding the rights and welfare of research participants, review of clinical trial documents (e.g., the protocol, informed consent, recruitment procedures, etc.), and conduct of continung reivew. NRAs focus on ensuring the quality of the trial product and ensuring that study data are eligible and credible for drug approval. Roles that both parties share include: granting approval/clearance for the protocol to proceed, monitoring/overseeing the study, and receiving and acting on complaints/protocol violations (Slamet 2008). Many of these roles represent broad categories and can have much overlap. As such, within any national medicine regulatory framework, there needs to be specification of the roles and responsibilities of each party reviewing and monitoring a clinical trial. Specifically, roles need to be specified between the local ethics committee versus that of the national ethics committee and between that of the national ethics committee and the national regulatory authority. Figure 1 shows specific areas of focus for RECs and NRAs during review and conduct of clinical trials and post-approval drug monitoring (Sweeney 2010; Ndebele 2017).

Current challenges with establishing coordination between RECs and NRAs include:

(1) understanding each party's function to protect the safety of research participants; (2) sharing responsibilities for the implementation of GCP principles; (3) having similar requirements regarding clinical trial documents and process of review; and (4) enhancing competency on issues of local relevance. Enhanced interactions between RECs and NRAs could lead to: (1) minimization of risks to research participants; (2) increase in the quality of the clinical trial; (3) strengthened

Area of Focus	National Regulatory Authority	Research Ethics Committee
Product safety (investigator brochure	xxx	x
Good manufacturing practices (GMP)	xxx	-
Drug importation	xxx	-
Drug registration	xxx	-
Drug handling and storage	xxx	-
Destruction of leftover drugs	xxx	-
Pharmacy Plan (license of pharmacy and staff)	xxx	-
Drug dispensing	xxx	-
Review of trial's scientific aspects	xx	xxx
Review of ethical aspects of trial (risks and benefits, informed consent, privacy and confidentiality, justice issues, etc.)	-	xxx
Quality, safety, and efficacy	xxxx	--
Human specimen issues (collection, storage, and future use	x	xxx
IRB approval form sponsor country	-	xxx
DSMB establishment and reports	xx	xxx
Qualifications of PI and staff and facilities	xx	xxx
Compensation/indemnity/insurance	x	xxx
Site inspections	XX Drug	XX Ethics
Safety reporting (AEs and SAEs)	Xxx	xx
Continuous monitoring – amendments/deviations/violations	xxx	xxx
Study findings dissemination plans	x	xxx
Post-trial pharmacovigilance	Xxx	-

Fig. 1 Specific areas of focus of National Regulatory Authorities and Research Ethics Committees of Clinical Trials

GCP compliance; (4) enhanced safety of approved drugs; (5) and elimination of overlap between the roles of the RECs and the NRAs.

A common regulatory framework existing in many countries in the Arab region consists of the following:

1. National Ethics Committee provides oversight of local research ethics committees (e.g., registration to ensure proper member constitution and training, availability of resources, monitoring of informed consent processes; and a process of audit/inspection or a system of accreditation).
2. Local REC review of clinical trials.
3. Local and National RECs joint review of complex protocols, (e.g., novel products with potential nation-wide religious, social and security implications).
4. NRA review of clinical trial application package, that includes the following:
   - REC ethics review and approval of protocol
   - Informed consent
   - Trial protocol
   - Investigator Brochure
   - Case Report Form
   - Labeling of study drug
   - Clinical Trial agreement
   - GMP certificate
   - Availability of insurance for reseach injury
   - Financial disclosure of principal investigator
   - Confidentiality agreement
   - Delegation/authorization letter for CRO (if applicable)
   - CVs of PIs and staff
   - GCP certificate of PI

In some countries in the Arab region, both the NREC and the local REC conducts review of all clinical trial protocols. Such double review can result in long approval times and confusion as to when a study can begin. That said, double reviews might be justified for complex protocols and for when the local RECs are in its infancy of development. The goal, however, should be strengthening of the local RECs so that the National REC can focus more on its regulatory and oversight functions of local RECs. Finally, duplication of the ethics review between RECs and the NRA should also be avoided.

Following this chapter, Parts III, IV, and V will examine the various research governance systems existing in the Arab region. Specifically, Part III will survey the national regulations and guidelines currently existing in the Arab countries. Part IV will review the different regulatory systems in several countries, highlighting the interactions between RECs and NRAs in several select countries: Jordan, Saudi Arabia, Egypt, Lebanon, and the United Arab Emirates. Part V will then explore the status of research ethics committees in the region, commenting on challenges of RECs, views of investigators towards RECs, and methods of assessment of RECs. This part will also highlight the structures and processes of the RECs at Cairo

University in Egypt and at the King Hussein Cancer Center in Amman, Jordan. Part IV will conclude with a chapter regarding "Guidance for the Management and Administrative Operations of Research Ethics Committees".

As we review the regulatory landscape in the Arab region, one will quickly notice the large variability in the regulatory and oversight structures and processes that exist in the countries of the Arab region. Such variability emanates from the different pathways of regulatory and ethics development that has occurred in each country and will include governance systems that range from well-developed decentralized ethics review systems (i.e., dependent on local or regional ethical review) to more centralized systems whereby health research is reviewed by a national committee.

References

Hirtle, M., T. Lemmens, and D. Sprumont. 2000. A comparative analysis of research ethics review mechanisms and the ICH good clinical practice guideline. *European Journal of Health Law* 7: 265–292.

McDonald, M., D. Pullman, N.P. Anderson, and H. Sampson. 2011. Research ethics in 2020: Strengths, weaknesses, opportunities, and threats. *Health Law Review* 19 (3): 36–55.

Ndebele, P. 2017. *A review of national ethical review systems in selected African countries: What lessons can we learn for strengthening national health research oversight?* Presented at: Enhancing ethics of clinical trials. Khartoum University, Sudan.

Nwabueze, R.N. 2016. *Legal and ethical regulation of biomedical research in developing countries*. New York: Routledge/Taylor & Francis Group.

Slamet, L. S. 2008. *Communications between regulators (NRA) and ethics committees on clinical trials*. In: The 13th international conference for drug regulatory authority, Bern, Switzerland.

Sweeney, F. 2010. *Introduction to ICH-GCP: Role of regulatory agencies and ethics committees. Inspection approach*. European Medicines Agency. Presented at the: International Workshop on ethical and GCP aspects of the acceptance of clinical trials submitted in Marketing Authorisation Applications to EMA; London.

Part III

National Regulations and Guidelines in the Arab Region

Introduction: National Regulations and Guidelines

Henry Silverman and Farida Lada

The importance of having frameworks for ethics in research became clear after a variety of ethical abuses and controversies involving research participants occurred during the last several decades in several countries (Kim 2012; Okonta 2014). As such, several international organizations developed documents describing broad standards that govern research involving human participants. Standards for the protection of human research participants is an ethical responsibility and have been mandated by national governance bodies and operationalized at both the national and institutional levels. The international standards for the ethical conduct of human subject research include:

(i) the World Medical Association's Declaration of Helsinki, which sets forth "ethical principles for medical research involving human subjects" (World Medical Association 2013);
(ii) the Council for International Organizations of Medical Sciences' (CIOMS) International Ethical Guidelines for Health-Related Research Involving Humans, which "provide internationally vetted ethical principles and detailed commentary on how these principles should be applied, with particular attention to conducting research in low-and middle-income countries". ((Council for International Organizations of Medical Sciences (CIOMS) 2002);
(iii) the International Conference on Harmonisation's (ICH) Good Clinical Practices (GCP) guidelines, which describe the responsibilities and expectations of all stakeholders in the conduct of clinical trials (International Conference on Harmonization (ICH) 1996); and

H. Silverman (✉)
University of Maryland, Baltimore, MD, USA
e-mail: hsilverm@medicine.umaryland.edu

F. Lada
The City University of New York, New York, NY, USA
e-mail: farida.lada@cuny.edu

H. Silverman (ed.), *Research Ethics in the Arab Region*, Research Ethics Forum 5,
https://doi.org/10.1007/978-3-319-65266-5_16

(iv) the World Health Organization's Standards and Operational Guidance for Ethics Review of Health-Related Research with Human Participants, which provides "guidance to the research ethics committees (RECs) on which organizations rely to review and oversee the ethical aspects of research"(World Health Organization 2011).

These documents are routinely cited in international policies for the protection of human participants – but they have no binding or regulatory power. As such, many countries have developed their own national regulations that have the force of law, which then can impose legal sanctions for non-compliance.

At the national level, at least 107 countries have issued some combination of laws, regulations, guidelines, and codes governing human subject research (Office for Human Research Protections (OHRP) 2016). Rules defined at the national level differ in their scope based on the type of research (biomedical, health-related, behavioral, clinical trials, etc.) and on the source of funding. For example, the United States Office for Human Research Protections regulations apply to "all research involving human subjects conducted, supported or otherwise subject to regulation by any federal department or agency…"(U.S. Department of Health and Human Services, June 18, 1991); the Sudanese "National Guidelines for Ethical Conduct of Research Involving Human Subjects" applies to "medical and behavioural studies pertaining to human health" (National Ministry of Health Directorate General of Health Planning and Research 2008); Morocco's Law only applies to interventional research; and Jordan's Clinical Studies Law only applies to clinical trials.

All of the international standards and most of those at the national levels include a mandate for the establishment of Research Ethics Committees (REC) to provide a review of the ethics of research. The RECs are responsible for reviewing research and thereby ensuring that the rights and welfare of human participants are protected in such research, which may require the monitoring of approved research. In countries that have not enacted legislation to govern research, RECs usually rely on guidelines adopted by a competent authority, such as the state's health or medical research council or a professional association. Alternatively, RECs can rely on international research guidelines (Alahmad et al. 2012). These include the Declaration of Helsinki; CIOMS guidelines; the ICH Harmonized Tripartite Guidelines: Guideline for Good Clinical Practice, which regulates the conduct of clinical trial; and the US Federal Regulations (Common Rule) (Sleem et al. 2010).

Reliance on international guidelines is not necessarily problematic and can be useful in several ways. These instruments can serve as a rich source of information for research participants on the level of professional conduct expected of the investigators, they can provide a useful resource for members of RECs, and they can provide an excellent model for the eventual development of national legal standards.

Nevertheless, for several reasons, countries in the Arab region need to promulgate national regulations. First, the multiplicity of existing international research guidelines and their often-conflicting provisions create a situation in which the formulation of national guidance assumes particular importance. Second, by developing its own national regulations, countries can take account of its particular needs and cultural context; otherwise, Arab countries would continue to go through the difficult process of interpreting and applying international research guidelines against the background and cultural contexts of Arabia, a process that is not free from controversy. In other words, there can be a disconnect between ideal ethical standards that are embodied in international guidelines and how they are applied in a world of social, political, and economic inequities. Accordingly, different ethics committees may agree on the principle of informed consent, but disagree on its correct application to research in their particular local setting. The issue, therefore, is the correct interpretation, specification, and application of international guidelines, in light of cultural and local circumstances. The most appropriate way forward, however, is for countries in the Arab region to develop their own regulations that take into account the local setting that might be influenced by cultural and religious values.

A third reason to develop research regulations is that such directives will have the force of law and are legally enforceable with legal and sometimes penal sanctions for non-compliance.

There has been scarce analytical focus on the existence, substance, and operation of research regulations in individual countries in the Arab region. As such, Part III aims to address this gap by first presenting an overview of the landscape of regulations and guidelines that currently exist in the region and then providing an in depth examination of the regulations in Saudi Arabia and Morocco, both of which can serve as models for the Arab region.

References

Alahmad, G., M. Al-Jumah, and K. Dierickx. 2012. Review of national research ethics regulations and guidelines in Middle Eastern Arab countries. *BMC medical ethics 13*: 34. https://doi.org/10.1186/1472-6939-13-34.

Council for International Organizations of Medical Sciences (CIOMS). 2002. *International ethical guidelines for biomedical research involving human subjects*. Geneva: CIOMS.

International Conference on Harmonization (ICH). 1996. *Good clinical practice*: Available at http://www.ich.org/products/guidelines/efficacy/article/efficacy-guidelines.html.

Kim, W.O. 2012. Institutional review board (IRB) and ethical issues in clinical research. *Korean J Anesthesiol 62* (1): 3–12. https://doi.org/10.4097/kjae.2012.62.1.3.

National Ministry of Health Directorate General of Health Planning and Research. 2008. *National guidelines for ethical conduct of research involving human subjects*. Khartoum.

Office for Human Research Protections (OHRP). 2016. *International compilation of human research standards*. Washington, DC: U.S. Department of Health and Human Services.

Okonta, P.I. 2014. Ethics of clinical trials in Nigeria. *Niger Med J 55* (3): 188–194. https://doi.org/10.4103/0300-1652.132035.

Sleem, H., S. El-Kamary, and H.J. Silverman. 2010. Identifying structures, processes, resources and needs of research ethics committees in Egypt. *BMC Med Ethics 11*: 12.
U.S. Department of Health and Human Services. 1991, June 18. Protection of human subjects, 45 Code of Federal Regulations (CFR) 46: Available at http://www.hhs.gov/ohrp/humansubjects/guidance/45cfr46.html – 46.101.
World Health Organization. 2011. *Standards and operational guidance for ethics review of health-related research with human participants*. Available at http://www.who.int/ethics/research/en/
World Medical Association. 2013. Declaration of Helsinki: Available at http://www.wma.net/en/30publications/10policies/b3/.

National Guidelines Regarding Research Ethics in the Arab Countries: An Overview

Ghiath Alahmad

Introduction: Evolution of Research Ethics Guidelines

Ethical violations have occurred in medical experiments throughout history. As such, philosophers, bioethicists, legal scholars and other stakeholders have developed ethics guidelines, especially in the last 60 years, to regulate the ethical conduct of medical research. This is especially true in the Western world, but is missing in many of the low and middle income countries (LMICs).

Major ethical guidelines from the West have included the Nuremberg Code that was issued in 1947, which highlighted the need to obtain the consent of participants in research, as well as requiring that research be conducted by qualified researchers and be based on a solid scientific basis (Nuremberg Code 1949). In 1964, one of the most important international ethical guidelines, the Declaration of Helsinki (adopted, 1964; latest revision, 2013), was issued by the World Medical Association (WMA) (World Medical Association 1964). This document continues to serve as an international standard for conducting medical research. Many countries apply the Declaration of Helsinki as their official regulations in the absence of their own national regulations and has served as the basis of national guidelines for other countries. For the conduct of international collaborative research in LMICs, The Council for International Organizations of Medical Sciences (CIOMS) issued in 2002 the International Ethical Guidelines for Biomedical Research Involving Human Subjects (Council for International Organizations of Medical Sciences (CIOMS) 2002). This guideline was recently updated in 2016 (Council for International Organizations of Medical Sciences (CIOMS) & World Health Organization (WHO) 2016).

G. Alahmad (✉)
King Abdullah International Medical Research Center (KAIMRC), King Saud bin Abdulaziz University For Health Sciences (KSAU-HS), King Abdulaziz Medical City, Ministry of National Guard – Health Affairs, P.O. Box 22490, Riyadh 11426, Saudi Arabia
e-mail: ghiathalahmad@hotmail.com

H. Silverman (ed.), *Research Ethics in the Arab Region*, Research Ethics Forum 5,
https://doi.org/10.1007/978-3-319-65266-5_17

In 1996, the International Conference of Harmonization (ICH) issued Good Clinical Practice guidelines (participation of the United States, the European Union, and Japan) with the aim to harmonize standards for the conduct of clinical trials (International Conference on Harmonization (ICH) 1996). These guidelines define the role and responsibilities of sponsors, investigators, monitors and research ethics committees (RECs). The ICH's mission is to achieve "greater harmonization worldwide to ensure that safe, effective, and high quality medicines are developed and registered in the most resource-efficient manner." The World Health Organization (WHO) developed standards to guide the operations of research ethics committees in 2000 that was expanded in 2013 (World Health Organization 2011).

In response to a series of ethical violations that occurred in U.S. research, as documented by Henry Beecher (1966), and as occurred in the Tuskegee Study (Tuskegee Syphilis Study Ad Hoc Advisory Panel 1973), the U.S. passed the National Research Act in 1979 that established the National Commission to develop regulations to govern research. Subsequently, the Belmont Report was written, which described three main research principles to protect research participants: respect for persons, beneficence, and justice (The National Commission for the Protection of Human Subjects of Biomedical and Behavioral Research 1979). In 1991, the US federal law for protection of research participants was issued (45 Code of Federal Regulations (CFR) 46. 116 1991). Many countries have since used these regulations as a basis for their own national regulations governing research.

Research Guidelines in the Arab Region

Due to the increasing number of research and clinical trials being performed in the Arab region, regional ethicists have well-defined the many ethical issues involving human participants in research. These issues have been brought to the attention of officials of national governments, universities, research centers, and other stakeholders. The use of international codes of ethics to guide local research reflects the initial response. But the local application of international guidelines fails to account for cultural, economic, social, religious, and political aspects that often influence research practice. Indeed, in a study conducted among members of RECs in Egypt, 92% ranked that the lack of appropriate national guidelines represents a major challenge for RECs and investigators (Sleem et al. 2010).

To better map the situation regarding the existence of national regulations in the Arab region, we accessed the websites of various governmental agencies in the Arab countries and conducted a review of the online sources for clinical research laws and research ethics guidelines, as well as codes of ethics that addressed research ethics (Alahmad et al. 2012). We also reviewed the extent to which these documents incorporated the ethical requirements for research (Emanuel et al. 2000). These requirements include social value, scientific validity, fair subject selection, favorable risk benefit assessment, informed consent, independent review of research, and respect for enrolled subjects.

Table 1 lists the countries that have regulations or guidelines and the associated characteristics of these documents. Many countries do not have any national regulations or guidelines related specifically to research involving human participants. These countries include: Egypt, Lebanon, Syria, Iraq, Palestine, Oman, Yemen, Algeria and Libya. This chapter will survey and analyze all research ethics guidelines, as well as general ethics and professional codes that refer to research in the countries of the Arab region.

Bahrain

In 2009 the "Health Research Structure & Procedures" was issued by the Bahrain Ministry of Health's research committee (draft) (Omran 2009). This document addressed the presence of scientific merit, no known risks to human subjects, and the need for informed consent and ethics committee approval. Many other points were not mentioned, especially safeguards for the inclusion of vulnerable groups, confidentiality assurances, and the need for safety monitoring.

Egypt

No national guidelines exist in Egypt, although a draft law was recently developed. Consideration of approval will occur after a Parliament is chosen. Currently, what does exist include the "Profession Ethics Regulations" issued by the resolution of the Minister of Health & Population No. 238/2003 (Egypt 2003). The fourth part of this law pertains to regulating the conduct of medical research and experiments on human beings and has three parts. The first requires that doctors shall comply with implementation of moral criteria and guidelines, as well as the social and religious values. The second part discusses procedures prior to conducting any research, and the third relates to the procedures during and after the research. The Egyptian constitution also contains a provision requiring the informed consent from research participants (Egyptian Government 1971).

Jordan

The Clinical Studies Law (CSL) issued in 2001 (Jordan Food & Drug Administration 2001) as a draft and passed as a law in 2011, serves as the only document about clinical research in Jordan. This law points to the "Declaration of Helsinki" as a reference of ethical standard of clinical research; clinical studies must comply with the principles of "ICH-GCP" and "Good Laboratory Practice (GLP)".

The CSL covers clinical studies involving patients as well as healthy volunteers enrolled in bioequivalence and bioavailability studies. According to the CSL,

Table 1 Research ethics regulations and guidelines in the ARAB Region- 2015

Country	Sudan	Saudi Arabia	UAE	Qatar	Kuwait	Bahrain	Jordan	Morocco
Name of document	National guidelines for Ethical Conduct of Research Involving Human Subjects	The Law of ethics of research on living creatures & SFDA clinical trial requirements	Federal law No. (10) concerning medical liability (2008) The cabinet decision No. (33) of 2009	Guidelines, regulations and policies for research	Ethical guidelines for biomedical research	Ethical guidelines for health research (draft)	Clinical Studies Law	Protection of persons participating in biomedical research
Date of issue	2008	2010, 2011 (revised 2015)	2008, 2009	2009	2001	2009	2001	2015
The issuing organization	National Ministry of Health	Council of Ministries	Ministry of Health	Ministry of Health	Kuwait Institute for Medical Specialization	Ministry of Health	Prime Minister's Council	Parliament
Ethical requirements for research								
Independent review of research	✓	✓	✓	✓	✓	√	√	√
Social value	✓	✓	x	x	x	√	x	√
Scientific validity	✓	✓	x	✓	✓	x	√	√

(continued)

Fair subject selection, safeguards for vulnerable groups	✓	✓	x	✓	✓	x	x	√
Assessment of risks and benefits	✓	✓	x	✓	✓	√	x	√
Informed consent	✓	✓	✓	✓	✓	√	√	√
Respect for research subjects	✓	✓	✓	✓	✓	x	x	√

clinical studies must be authorized by the Minister of Health upon a recommendation from the Clinical Studies Committee of the Jordanian Food & Drug Administration. Informed consent, scientific justifications, and insurance coverage for research injury are essential items that need to be addressed before conducting any clinical study. The CSL also requires ethical review by an "Institutional Review Board Committee"; the structure, and the role of these review committees are also detailed in the CSL.

In 2014, a Stem Cell By-law was issued, which regulate all aspects related to use of stem cells (2014). Rana Dajani recently reviewed highlights of this law (2014).

Kuwait

The only official document about research ethics guidance in Kuwait is the "Ethical Guidelines for Biomedical Research" released by the "Kuwait Institute for Medical Specialization" established in 2001 (Ministry of Health: Kuwait Institute for Medical Specialization 2001). These guidelines give details about the ethics committee, its structure and function, and requirement for informed consent. The guidelines also include a worksheet titled "Ethical Evaluation of the Research Protocol, Consent Form and Letter of Information". The Nuremberg Code, Belmont Report and Declaration of Helsinki were used as international references for these guidelines.

Lebanon

There are no national guidelines regarding medical research in Lebanon. Clinical research is briefly mentioned in the "Law of Medical Ethics, No. (288)", which was issued in 1994 (renewed in 2012) (Lebanon 2012). It is a general law regulating the duties and ethics of medical practitioners in Lebanon. It discusses confidentiality and informed consent as essential requirements for medical practice. According to the article 30 of this law, it is not allowed to conduct any clinical trial unless it provides a direct benefit to research subjects and does not cause any harm or put them at risk. Informed consent is essential and when the research participant is a child or an individual who lacks decision making capacity, guardian consent is required.

Qatar

Qatar's Policies, Regulations and Guidelines Involving Human, approved by the Qatar's Supreme Council for Health in 2009, is responsible for regulating clinical trials (Qatar Supreme Council of Health 2009). These regulations outline ethical guidelines in conducting research involving human subjects. It also covers research performed in collaboration with non-Qatari institutions.

These regulations relied predominantly on several international documents, e.g., "The Belmont Report", "Declaration of Helsinki", and "CIOMS" Guidelines. The contents of this Qatari document include the basic policy for protection of human research subjects, along with additional protections for different groups involved in research, such as pregnant women, human fetuses and neonates, prisoners, and children. Also included are the structure and functions of RECs and the basic and additional elements of the informed consent, including the process of informed consent involving adults and minors.

Saudi Arabia

Saudi Arabia's "The Law of Ethics of Research on Living Creatures" was passed in 2010 (National Committee of Bioethics – King Abdulaziz City of Science and Technology 2010). In 2011, the "Implementing Regulations of the Law of Ethics of Research on Living Creatures" was issued (revised in 2015) and explains many of the points in this Law, as well as instructions for its implementation (National Committee of Bioethics – King Abdulaziz City of Science and Technology 2011). It also explains the role of the National Committee in regulating research, which includes periodic inspection by the National Committee in accordance with the Implementing Regulations. Both documents are considered the official research guidelines in Saudi Arabia. The Law and the Implementing Regulations together form one unit. No research entity is allowed to conduct research involving humans until required procedures are completed according to both the Law and the Implementing Regulations.

The Saudi law and its Implementing Regulations discuss important points in research ethics, including mandating informed consent and voluntariness of participants and ensuring confidentiality. Cloning and conducting research on fertilized eggs and fetuses are not allowed. Special protections must be implemented when performing research involving prisoners, minors, mentally ill, people with handicaps, and pregnant women. Items regarding research involving animals and plants are mentioned as well.

The Saudi Food and Drug Authority (SFDA), which was established in March 2003, provides oversight for clinical trials in Saudi Arabia. The SFDA issued The Clinical Trial Requirement Guidelines in 2015, using the same structure of ICH-GCP (Saudi Food and Drug Administration 2015).

Sudan

The "National Guidelines for Ethical Conduct of Research Involving Human Subjects" was issued in 2008 by the Federal Ministry of Health Directorate General of Health Planning and Research (Federal Ministry of Health 2008). It highlights many important issues, such as the principles of ethics for research involving human subjects, the roles of research ethics committee, and the requirement for informed consent. These guidelines do not have the force of law, although there are current efforts underway to draft a law and ensure harmonization between the National Ethics Committee and the National Poisons Board, which regulates drug clinical trials.

Tunisia

In 2014 the Decree n° 2014–3657 dated 3 October 2014, amending and completing decree n° 1990–1401 dated 3 September 1990, fixed the methods of medical or scientific experimentation intended for human medicines (Official Gazette 2014). According to this decree, experimentation can be conducted involving minors and those who are mentally disadvantaged only when it targets their diseases and only after obtaining the consent from a legally authorized individual. Financial incentives are not allowed to be provided to research participants except for reimbursement for expenses and compensation for any research injury that might have occurred. Informed consent in necessary and risks should be justified by the potential benefits. When research involves vulnerable individuals, risks should not exceed a minimal risk threshold. This decree is followed by two orders of the Minister of Health in 2015; the first regards fixing the fees and amounts of compensation, while the second order involves developing protection committees of research participants (Official Gazette 2015).

United Arab Emirates (UAE)

The "Federal Law No. (10) of 2008 Concerning Medical Liability" contains in its Article 10 two sections: the first one prohibits human cloning and the second prohibits "researches or medical experiments on human beings… without obtaining the proper approval of the concerned authority". Further specification came when the Cabinet Decision No. (33) of 2009 issued the Implementing Regulation of Federal Law No. (10), which contained Articles 8, 9, and 10 regarding medical research (Health Authority – Abu Dhabi 2008).

Article 8 prohibits medical research or experiments involving humans unless one obtains the necessary license from a governing body, such as Ministry of Health of the UAE, Health Authority of Abu Dhabi or Dubai, the Dubai Healthcare City, or a public university.

Article 9 includes conditional requirements for the conduct of research, such as: (1) research shall take place in a licensed health facility equipped with all required capabilities; (2) research shall be performed by competent and licensed persons; (3) all research shall be conducted according to international standards with respect to all related legal and Sharia aspects; (4) the research shall respect the rights and dignity of research participants, preserve their health and ensure confidentiality of private information; (5) informed consent shall be obtained from participants or from a legal guardian if they are incapacitated; and (6) informed consent shall not be given in return for a tangible or intangible benefit or under material or moral duress and may not be based on fraud or deceit. Additionally, research protocols must contain the background scientific information, objectives, the potential benefits, research setting, approval of official authority, expected research period, resumes of the members of the research team, and particulars of the financial resources for the research.

Finally, Article 10 gives the Ministry of Health the authority to regulate research and develop consent forms for research.

Other Countries

National guidelines for conducting clinical research in Syria do not exist. Instead, the Syrian Ministry of Health refers to both the Declaration of Helsinki and CIOMS Guidelines, to which every researcher must follow. In Iraq, mention regarding clinical research is found in the "Iraqi Medical Association" modified law No. 6 of 1985. This document states that research is not allowed if there is any possible harm to research subjects and any trials involving drugs must be performed on animals first. Research not considered to be scientifically justified will be considered criminal act.

The Omani Ministry of Health only refers to the need to comply with the ethical regulations for medical research without reference to any specific rules. Recently, interest in research ethics has surfaced in Libya, however no guidelines have been established (Bugaighis et al. 2016). There is no mention of any guidelines for research conducted in Palestine or Yemen. Finally, Morocco recently passed a law regulating research and its ethical review, which is reviewed in the next chapter by Latifa Adarmouch.

Conclusion

Our review of the existing regulations and guidelines for research in the Arab countries show a wide range of established regulations for research. For example, several countries have issued regulations codified in the form of a law while others have guidelines; several countries do not have special guidelines regarding research, but the ethics of research is mentioned in other documents, such as the code of ethics in Egypt, and in Lebanon; other countries such as Syria and Iraq use the international guidelines (e.g., Helsinki Declaration or CIOMS); and finally, other countries make no references to clinical research (Palestine and Yemen).

Our analysis of the existing national regulations and guidelines shown in Table 1 reveal that all documents include independent review of research and the securing the informed consent. However, there are important missing requirements in several of these documents, such as: social value in the Emirati, Qatari and Kuwaiti guidelines; and fair selection of research subjects in the Emirati and Bahraini guidelines.

References

Code of Federal Regulations(CFR) 46. 116. 1991. Protection of human subjects; Rev. June 18.

Alahmad, G., M. Al-Jumah, and K. Dierickx. 2012. Review of national research ethics regulations and guidelines in Middle Eastern Arab countries. *BMC Medical Ethics* 13: 34. https://doi.org/10.1186/1472-6939-13-34.

Bugaighis, I., A. El-Howati, A.S.A. Elmusrati, and A. Arheiam. 2016. The establishment of ethical guidelines for biomedical research in Libya. *The Libyan journal of medicine* 11 (1): 33424.

Beecher, J.K. 1966. Ethics and clinical research. *The New England Journal of Medicine* 274: 1354–1360.

Council for International Organizations of Medical Sciences (CIOMS). 2002. International ethical guidelines for biomedical research involving human subjects.

Council for International Organizations of Medical Sciences (CIOMS), & World Health Organization (WHO). 2016. *International ethical guidelines for health-related research involving humans*. Geneva: CIOMS.

Dajani, R. 2014. Jordan's stem-cell law can guide the Middle East. *Nature* 510 (7504): 189. https://doi.org/10.1038/510189a.

Egyptian Government. 1971. Constitution of the Arab Republic of Egypt *Article 43* (pp.): Available at: http://aceproject.org/ero-en/regions/mideast/EG/Egyptian%20Constitution%20-%20english.pdf.

Emanuel, E.J., D. Wendler, and C. Grady. 2000. What makes clinical research ethical? *JAMA* 283: 2701–2711.

Federal Ministry of Health. 2008. National guidelines for ethical conduct of research involving human subjects (Vol. Available at: http://sites.google.com/site/healthresearchlibrary/national-guidelines).

Health Authority – Abu Dhabi. 2008. Federal law No. (10) of 2008 Concerning medical liability and cabinet decision No. (33) of 2009.

Issuing the Implementing Regulation of Federal Law No. (10) of 2008 n.d. Concerning medical liability: Available at: http://www.haad.ae/HAAD/LinkClick.aspx?fileticket=_-p5s8m9xvU=&tabid=1159.

International Conference on Harmonization (ICH). 1996. Good Clinical Practice: Available at: http://www.ich.org/products/guidelines/efficacy/article/efficacy-guidelines.html.

Jordan Food & Drug Administration. 2001. Law of clinical studies provisional law No. 97 for the Year 2001. *Retrieved at:*http://www.menareti.net/uploadfiles/Mereti/Clinical_trial_law_jordan_provisional_law_97_2001.pdf.

Lebanon. 2012. Code of medical ethics. *Law No. 240*: Available at: https://www.aub.edu.lb/fm/shbpp/ethics/public/Documents/New-Code-of-Medical-Ethics-text-ENGLISH.pdf.

Ministry of Health: Kuwait Institute for Medical Specialization. 2001. Ethical guidelines for biomedical research: Available at: http://www.kims.org.kw/Ethical%202.doc.

National Committee of Bioethics – King Abdulaziz City of Science and Technology. 2010. Law of ethics of research on living creatures (Arabic): Available at: http://bioethics.kacst.edu.sa/getattachment/4bd0d4e2-1b93-4c32-b483-57902227fae2/Bioethic-Rgl-fin-bks.aspx

———. 2011. Implementing regulations of the law of ethics of research on living creatures: Available at: http://bioethics.kacst.edu.sa/getattachment/9bc41471-034a-482c-8afe-a7a3348f6c16/Implementing-Regulations-research-ethics-on-living.aspx.

Nuremberg Code. 1949. *Trials of war criminals before the nuremberg military tribunals under control council law, No. 10*. Washington, DC: U.S. Government Printing Office.

Omran, A. 2009. Health research structure & procedures. In: Kingdom of Bahrain Ministry of Health (Ed.). Available at: http://www.moh.gov.bh/PDF/Health%20Research%20Structure%20and%20Procedures%20%20DRAFT.pdf.

Qatar Supreme Council of Health. 2009. *Policies, regulations and guidelines involving human*. Available at: http://www.moph.qa/app/media/24.

Republic of Tunisia. 2014. *Official Gazette*, N° 84 (17 October 2014) Page 855.

———. 2015. *Official Gazette*, N° 9 (30 January 2015) Page 115.

Saudi Food and Drug Administration. 2015. *The clinical trial requirement guidelines*. Available at: http://www.fdanews.com/ext/resources/files/08-15/8-15-SaudiTrials.pdf?1441030524.

Sleem, H., S. El-Kamary, and H.J. Silverman. 2010. Identifying structures, processes, resources and needs of research ethics committees in Egypt. *BMC Medical Ethics* 11: 12.

The National Commission for the Protection of Human Subjects of Biomedical and Behavioral Research. 1979. *Ethical principles and guidelines for the protection of human subjects of research.* Available at: http://www.hhs.gov/ohrp/humansubjects/guidance/belmont.html.

Tuskegee Syphilis Study Ad Hoc Advisory Panel. 1973. *Final Report of the Tuskegee Syphilis Study Ad Hoc Panel*. U.S. Department of Health, Education and Welfare, Public Health Service.

World Health Organization. 2011. Standards and operational guidance for ethics review of health-related research with human participants (Vol. Available at: http://www.who.int/ethics/research/en/).

World Medical Association. 1964. *Declaration of Helsinki: Ethical principles for medical research involving human subjects*. Ferney-Voltaire: World Health Organization.

National Guidelines Regarding Research Ethics in Saudi Arabia

Ghiath Alahmad

Introduction

Saudi Arabia is one of the largest Arab countries with a population of more than 32 million and with high standard of living ($25,961 GDP per capita). The age of the population is skewed towards a young demographic, as the percentage of people younger than 15 years old is 34.8%, whereas the percentage of people above 65 years old is 3.2%. It has a tribal social structure with strong extended family relationships (General Authority Statistics 2016). Saudi Arabia is ruled by a royal family and the King is the head of the Council of Ministers, which issues the laws in Saudi Arabia. These laws must not contradict Islam, which is considered the official religion of the country (Council of Ministers 1412H 1991).

The huge discoveries of oil contributed to raising the standard of living in Saudi Arabia as well as the construction of universities, tertiary hospitals and research centers. This accounts for the increase in research output that has occurred in Saudi Arabia; both in government and in the private area. The governmental entities where research is conducted include research centers of the Ministry of Health, the National Guard, the Defense Ministry, and in many governmental tertiary hospitals. Also, research is conducted in many large private hospitals.

To establish research ethics guidelines with this expansion in medical research, the government established the National Committee on Bioethics (NCBE) in 2001. The NCBE took the responsibility to develop research ethics guidelines, (National Committee of Bioethics 2015) and subsequently, local ethics committees were established; presently, there are 45 registered local

G. Alahmad (✉)
King Abdullah International Medical Research Center (KAIMRC), King Saud bin Abdulaziz University For Health Sciences (KSAU-HS), King Abdulaziz Medical City, Ministry of National Guard – Health Affairs, P.O. Box 22490, Riyadh 11426, Saudi Arabia
e-mail: ghiathalahmad@hotmail.com

H. Silverman (ed.), *Research Ethics in the Arab Region*, Research Ethics Forum 5,
https://doi.org/10.1007/978-3-319-65266-5_18

ethics committees nationwide (http://bioethics.kacst.edu.sa/LocalCommittees/registered-IRB.aspx). Associated with these regulatory activities were educational initiatives in research ethics, including the establishment of the "Research Ethics Course" at King Saud bin Abdulaziz University of Health Sciences in 2012 http://www.ksau-hs.edu.sa/English/Media/Events/Pages/ResearchEthics2.aspx.

In this chapter, I aim to give a brief description of the National Committee of Bioethics, which is the official authorized entity assigned to prepare the standards for the Ethics of Research on Living Creatures and associated Implementing Regulations. Following this, I will discuss the substance of the Law in conjunction with an analysis of the law.

The National Committee of Bioethics (NCBE)

The National Committee of Bioethics was established according to Royal Decree Number 7/B/9012 in 18/5/1422H (08 August 2001). Its task was to develop ethical standards for conducting research on living creatures and to monitor compliance with these regulations (National Committee of Bioethics 2015).

The objectives of the National Committee cover all the entities interested in medical research in the entire Kingdom. A later decree issued by the Ministers' Council approved this law, in decision number 321 dated 13/9/1431H (National Committee of Bioethics 2010). The NCBE has four (4) different sub-committees. The first one is the Legal Sub-Committee, which reviews all guidelines and recommendations by other sub-committees concentrating on the legal, religious and judicial aspects. The second sub-committee is the Human Research Sub-Committee, which specialized in ethics related to research involving humans, which includes the Genetic and Biobanking Sub-Committee and the Clinical Research Sub-Committee. The third sub-committee is the Animal Research Sub-Committee, which is focused on the ethics of research on animals and pertinent methods of research; the fourth sub-committee is the Education and Media Sub-Committee, which is focused on developing supporting plans and educational programs.

The NCBE is considered the national reference of research ethics and has many duties, including developing the Research Ethics standards, implementing them, and also registering local institutional review boards and researchers. The NCBE also supervises and monitors local institutional review boards, and to build a database and a national bank of genetic materials. Moreover, it developed the ethical requirements of research labs and monitors these labs' compliance with the ethical standards. It also collaborates with international institutions concerned with research ethics. The NCBE conducts educational activities such as workshops, courses and seminars regarding ethical aspects on many issues, such as stem cells, genetic distinctiveness, gene ownership, biobanks, and animal cloning, as well as training courses for members of local committees.

Table 1 Ethical requirements of research laboratories

Supervision by a licensed governmental institution or a private agency
Presence of qualified specialists
Laboratories not affiliated with a governmental institution should satisfy conditions set forth in the "Law of Private Laboratories"
Ability to meet legal liability arising from damage caused by practices
Meet safety conditions and preventive measures
Respect confidentiality and privacy

Structure of Law of Ethics of Research

The Law of Ethics of Research on Living Creatures is considered an outcome of efforts over the course of several years from the beginning of the establishment of the NCBE in 2001 until the issuance of the law in 2010, followed by issuing the Implementing Regulations in 2011. To address several deficiencies in the Law, a second edition was issued in 20/4/1436H (9/2/2015). This second revised version includes topics such as ethics related to stem cells and exporting samples outside the Kingdom.

The first chapter provides definitions and general provisions, such as informed consent, minimum risk, research, guardianship and others. This chapter contends that the law covers all research activities in the Kingdom and it is not allowed to conduct any research outside authorized and permitted institutions. The second chapter (Article 2) explains the objectives of research ethics law and the general standards and rules for conducting research. The standards include protecting human rights, maintaining research participant safety, respecting human dignity, and not causing unnecessary harm to research participants. Article 3 states that all ethical rules and precautions should be completed before allowing the researcher to conduct research.

The third chapter (Articles 3, 4, 5 and 6) explains the structure of the NCBE and how the committee members are chosen, their qualifications, and the period of their membership, as well as the characteristics of the committee chair and the duties of the general council of the NCBE, how meetings are held and how decisions are made. In Article 6, rules for exporting samples outside the country for research purposes are detailed. This includes granting the local committees the right to issue approval for exporting samples and notifying the national committee, but without a need to get its approval, as it was one of the requirements before the law was modified. The conditions for exporting samples outside the country include that they be sent to a well-known scientific institution and according to a contract that guarantees the confidentiality and the safety of samples and that no previous similar research has been done before. This chapter explains that KASCT will build a database of national information on genetic materials in Saudi society. Moreover, it explains the conditions of research labs, see Table 1.

Chapter 4 (Article 7) explains the financial issues of the work of the NCBE, while Chapter 5 (Articles 8 and 9) explains the structure of the research ethics

Table 2 Full board review and expedited review according to Saudi law

	Expedited	Full Board
Structure of board	Chairman or an expert	Members from different specialties, and chairperson or co-chairman should be interested in bioethics
Who takes decision	Chairman	5 members minimum
Voting	No voting	Majority
If research includes more than minimum risk	Research should not include more than minimum risk	Research includes more than minimum risks.
Research on vulnerable people	Research should not include vulnerable people	Research involves vulnerable people
Type of decision	Approve only	Approve or disapprove
Research includes evaluating new drug	May not evaluate new drug	Research involves a new drug
Research includes evaluating new equipment	My not evaluate new equipment	Research involves new equipment
Research includes evaluating changed dosage.	May not evaluate changed dosage	Evaluate changed dosage
Informed consent	informed consent should include all elements	Informed consent should include all elements; research may waive consent under appropriate criteria

monitoring office, its duties and mechanisms of work. The Monitoring Office is responsible for registering the local committees and monitor their compliance with the law and its regulations.

Chapter 6 (Article 10) discusses the requirements for creating local research ethics committees, their functions and their procedures. It also explains how the research ethics committee should evaluate research proposals and the mechanisms of granting approvals, including but not limited to expedited review approvals (Table 2).

Chapter 7 (Articles 11, 12, 13 and 14) discusses the requirement of informed consent, including the necessary elements that should be included in the informed consent (Table 3). Moreover, this chapter explains the correct mechanism for obtaining informed consent and how it should be documented. It also explains the conditions for allowing research without having informed consent.

Chapter 8 (Articles 15, 16, 17, 18, 19, 20, 21, 22 and 23) explains the requirements for conducting research involving humans. Article 15 states that scientific objectives of the research should be clear and that approval should be granted before allowing the researcher to start the research. The benefits should outweigh the risks (Article 16); the research should not involve exploitation or coercion (17); and the research should respect Shari'a boundaries (Article 18).

Article 19 prohibits the use of gametes, zygotes and organs. However, it allows conducting research on organs after getting informed consent (20) and allows doing

Table 3 The informed consent elements

Invitation to participate in research	Research title
Name of institution	Research objectives
Presence of Benefits	Presence of risk or harm
Alternative treatments	Confidentiality
Procedures related to the research	Duration of the research project
Requirements to be fulfilled by the human participantt	Type, quantity and method of use of samples taken from the human participant
Participation is voluntary, refusal to participate shall not entail penalty or loss of benefits	Right to withdraw
Risks or harms that might ensue due to withdrawal from research	The investigator's pledge
Contact numbers and addresses	Signature of the human participant or guardian, the researcher, and any other person whose signature on the form is required
Date and place of the "Informed Consent"	Compensation for research injury

Table 4 Ethical criteria for genetic research

A written approval shall be obtained from the National Committee
Gene therapy research shall be subject to controls set forth in the Law and Regulations of NCBE
Be consistent with the provisions of Shari'a
Comply with the criteria set forth in international agreements without prejudice to Shari'a
Be limited to incurable diseases affecting human life, which have not yet been successfully treated by conventional medical methods
All available treatment options have been exhausted prior to approval of research
The local committee evaluating this type of research shall comprise at least two persons with scientific competence to evaluate gene therapy research
Be conducted in qualified hospitals and research centers
The research plan shall include all necessary research proposal elements
The research shall be based on scientific principles and preceded by sufficient laboratory experiments and animal testing
Expected benefit from the research shall outweigh any potential risks
The research shall be conducted by a qualified investigators specialized in genetic medicine
Gene therapy may not be carried out for research purposes on gametes or stem cells obtained from fertilized zygotes or related to reproductive cloning
All research stages should be in accordance with the controls set forth in the Law and Regulations.

research on fetuses and gametes according to specific regulations (Article 21). Table 4 explains the ethical criteria for conducting genetic research.

Article 22 of the law forbids human cloning, but allows doing research on stem cells if certain requirements are met. The law also allows establishing a stem cell biobank after obtaining approval from the NCBE and local research committees and informed consent from the participants. This biobank should belong to a governmental entity and storage should guarantee confidentiality (23).

Chapter 9 (Article 24) explains the requirements for doing research involving prisoners and prohibits any exploitation of the prisoners or forcing them to participate in research without full informed consent. All research on prisoners should target prison diseases and prisoners' health and how to improve it.

Chapter 10 (Article 25) regulates research involving certain special groups, specifically minors, pregnant women, fetuses and incompetent persons. It mandates obtaining a guardian to provide informed consent to allow research, that the research will not contradict the interests of the child, and that the risk should be minimal and the expected potential benefits should be similar to the benefits of the available methods available elsewhere.

Article 26 explains the restrictions regarding research involving pregnant women and requires that risks should be minimized and the research should not involve procedures that interfere with or threaten to end the pregnancy or change the way a pregnancy is ended, especially if it leads to increased risk; approval is required from the wife and the husband.

Research involving fetuses is prohibited if it does not target the health needs of fetuses or if it has the possibility of causing harm. It is not allowed to use gametes, zygotes, tissues or any part of the developing organism unless it is according to requirements that will be developed later.

It is forbidden to use cloning to produce genetic stem cells for research purposes (28). Moreover, it is not allowed to establish banks for male or female reproductive cells (29). However, it is allowed to use the tissues and the organs of voluntarily aborted fetuses.

Chapter 11 provides requirements for dealing with genetic materials and biobanks. According to Article 21, the King Abdulaziz City of Science and Technology will build a central information bank where all information about genetic material will be stored. This bank will provide necessary information to researchers for their research. Information will include personal and familial and social data, respecting privacy and confidentiality, without providing any genetic material. The law mandates respecting Shari'a rules and respecting ethical guidelines in dealing with any genetic material. The results of research are considered the property of the state and are not allowed to be sold, although financial and scientific rights are given to researchers. All local biobanks should write annual reports on the central biobanks about the status of genetic materials and all research conducted on these materials. All genetic research should aim to study genetic diseases and not to change human characteristics. It is allowed only to conduct research involving somatic and stem cells, but not reproductive cells (Article 32).

The law allows doing research involving genetic samples in multiple research projects of different purposes without obtaining an "Informed Consent" for each purpose under two conditions. The first is that the sample was previously obtained for diagnostic purposes and was retained for a time sufficient to preclude identification of the source by the investigator; secondly, the local research office committee (Article 33) approves it. The local committee may restrict the researcher's use of results on genetic material if the results may harm public interest (article 35) and may cause racial discrimination (Article 36).

Chapter 12 (Article 38) explains the ethical requirements for conducting research on animals and plants. The researcher needs to employ experimental procedures that do not cause "unusual pain" to animals, conduct the research according to scientific principles of research, and proceed only with the approval of the local ethics committee. Animal research should be limited to the smallest number of animals needed to carry out the research objectives, and should limit pain to its minimum level.

The local research ethics committee should observe several conditions before issuing its approval, such as reviewing the researcher's qualifications, scientific validity, plans dealing with risks. The law forbids artificial hybridization among animals unless they are of the same species. It allows cloning if at least two specialists guarantee the safety of animals.

The law forbids use of plants for research that causes harm to environmental balance; moreover, it is not allowed to use rare plants for research (Article 39).

Chapter 13 regards the formation of a Violation Review Committee in charge of detecting violations of the provisions of the Law. It mentions the membership composition, how members are selected, its processes, and when the violation can be raised to court.

Chapter 14 explains penalties for violating ethics regulations, which includes warnings, suspension of research privileges, forbidding the researcher to continue the research, fines, and imprisonment for a period not exceeding 6 months.

Analysis

The Saudi law regarding ethics of research on living creatures presents an inclusive framework that includes all ethical requirements to conduct medical research according to international guidelines (the Nuremberg code (Nuremberg Code 1949), the Declaration of Helsinki (World Medical Association 1964), or the International Ethical Guidelines for Biomedical Research Involving Human Subjects in 2002, (Council for International Organizations of Medical Sciences (CIOMS) 2002), and the ethical conditions that have been outlined by scholars (such as the framework provided by Emmanuel and colleagues (Emanuel 2000).

Saudi Law requires an independent review of research through local research committees through their structures or procedures or methods of decision making (Articles 4 & 10). Moreover, it establishes the necessary conditions for ensuring social values from medical research through requiring it to be conducted in a way that maximizes benefits and through preventing research that negatively affects society and individuals (Articles 16, 18, 19, 21, 22, 23, 31, 36, 37 and 38).

Scientific validity is also considered one of the important issues that Saudi Law takes in account in order to approve research proposals (Article 15). Fair subject selection is also mentioned in the law in items 24, 25 and 26 as a necessary requirement for doing medical research, including how to select research participants in general and also among vulnerable groups such as pregnant women (Article 27). Favorable assessment of risks and benefits is one of the major points in the law (Article 16). The law assures that risk is kept to the minimum possible level when conducting research involving children, pregnant women and other vulnerable groups (Articles 24, 25 and 26).

Saudi law also considers informed consent as an obligation to conduct research. All informed consent elements have been detailed in the law, and the correct procedures are explained (Articles 11, 12, 13 and 14). The law insists that respect of research participants is important in many places (Articles 8, 9, 10, 11, 12 and 34). Specifically, it guarantees that participation is completely voluntary, and that safety is respected. Although the Saudi Law incorporates many of the important ethical requirements, at the same time, some other points need more expansion, such as doing research involving children, handicapped individuals and research involving plants and animals, which are expected to be expanded in future editions (Alahmad et al. 2012).

References

Alahmad, G., M. Al-Jumah, and K. Dierickx. 2012. Review of national research ethics regulations and guidelines in Middle Eastern Arab countries. *BMC Medical Ethics* 13: 34. https://doi.org/10.1186/1472-6939-13-34.

Council for International Organizations of Medical Sciences (CIOMS). 2002. *International ethical guidelines for biomedical research involving human subjects*. Geneva: Switzerland. Available at: http://www.cioms.ch/publications/layout_guide2002.pdf.

Council of Ministers. (1412H) [1991]. Ruling system. Available at: https://www.saudi.gov.sa/wps/portal/saudi/aboutKingdom

Emanuel, E.J., D. Wendler, and C. Grady. 2000. What makes clinical research ethical? *JAMA* 283: 2701–2711.

General Authority Statistics. 2016. Demographic research bulletin (Demography Survey). Available at: https://www.stats.gov.sa/en/4522.

National Committee of Bioethics – King Abdulaziz City of Science and Technology. 2010. Law of ethics of research on living creatures (Arabic): Available at: http://bioethics.kacst.edu.sa/getattachment/4bd0d4e2-1b93-4c32-b483-57902227fae2/Bioethic-Rgl-fin-bks.aspx.

———. 2015. Implementing regulations of the law of ethics of research on living creatures: Available at: http://bioethics.kacst.edu.sa/getattachment/9bc41471-034a-482c-8afe-a7a3348f6c16/Implementing-Regulations-research-ethics-on-living.aspx.

Nuremberg Code. 1949. *Trials of war criminals before the nuremberg military tribunals under Control Council Law, No. 10*. Washington, DC: U.S. Government Printing Office.

World Medical Association. 1964. *Declaration of Helsinki: Ethical principles for medical research involving human subjects*. Ferney-Voltaire: World Health Organization.

Biomedical Research Law in Morocco

Latifa Adarmouch

Introduction

The need for a biomedical research law in Morocco became more urgent due to two developments; first, the number of research studies was increasing, including collaborative international research that requires compliance with international ethical standards; and second, there was a growing commitment to promote research to enhance the health of the country.

Previously, in order to conduct clinical trials in Morocco, authorization and approval was required from the Ministry of Health (MoH). Also, a ministerial decree stipulated that approval from a local research ethics committee (REC) was required before submitting documents for approval by the MoH. Following this decree, a law was drafted and eventually gained the approval of the Moroccan Parliament in August 2015. This law is referred to as Law Number 28–13 and is entitled *Protection of Persons Participating in Biomedical Research* (Bulletin Officiel 2015).

The law consists of 79 articles, organized in the following chapters:

- Preliminary title: scope and definitions
- Title I: provisions concerning persons participating in biomedical research
- Title II: provisions concerning the conduct of biomedical research
- Title III: finding of infringement and sanctions
- Title IV: transitional and final provisions

The aim of this chapter is to perform an ethical analysis of the Moroccan law using a framework based on the seven ethical requirements for clinical research that

L. Adarmouch (✉)
Community Medicine and Public Health Department, School of Medicine, Cadi Ayyad University, Marrakech, Morocco

Clinical Research Center, Mohammed VI University Hospital, Marrakech, Morocco
e-mail: l.adarmouch@hotmail.com

H. Silverman (ed.), *Research Ethics in the Arab Region*, Research Ethics Forum 5,
https://doi.org/10.1007/978-3-319-65266-5_19

were developed by Emanuel and colleagues (Emanuel et al. 2000). These commentators synthesized from available international codes, declarations and guidelines a set of seven ethical requirements for ethical clinical research that constitutes a normative framework to analyze biomedical research.

The first requirement is social value, which corresponds to the importance and relevance of the generalizable knowledge generated by the research to the population's health and welfare. Social value justifies the allocation of scarce financial and scientific resources devoted to the research, as well as justifies the risks assumed by individuals enrolled in the research. In a similar fashion, the second requirement, scientific validity, requires that the methodological aspects of the study ensure that the research will be able to generate results. The third requirement of fair participants' selection obligates that the target population for enrollment is guided by scientific objectives rather than convenience and easy availability of vulnerable persons. Also, there should be a fair distribution of risks and benefits among those in society.

The fourth requirement of a favorable risk-benefit ratio entails three conditions: identification of risks and benefits, minimization of the risks and maximization of the benefits, followed by an assessment as to whether the risks are reasonable to the potential direct benefits, if any, to the participants, and to the knowledge to be gained to society.

The fifth requirement refers to review of research by an independent body, which ensures that research is performed with minimal conflicts of interests either from investigators or from the institution itself. This requirement ensures "social accountability" and public trust in the research enterprise.

The sixth requirement entails that informed consent is grounded in the principle of respect for persons. Individuals' decisions to enroll in research should be guided by their preferences, interests and values that lead to an autonomous authorization to participate. To protect those with diminished autonomy, a legally authorized representative needs to give informed consent.

Finally, the seventh requirement for "respect for potential and enrolled partiicpants" embodies the principle of respect for persons beyond informed consent. Specifically, there should be respect for participants' right to withdrawal, their right for privacy, assurances of confidentiality, monitoring of safety throughout the study, and disclosure of new information that might affect continued participation in the study.

Analysis of the Biomedical Research Law in Morocco

Scope of the Law

The present law distinguishes between interventional and non-interventional research. Interventional research includes:

- Research involving a "medical intervention" that is not ordinarily part of medical management.

- Intervention research not involving drugs and representing only negligible risks.
- Clinical investigations involving experimental drugs or medical devices

The Moroccan Law does not regulate non-interventional and observational research, and retrospective studies involving the analysis of existing health data. The determination of whether the research study is classified as being "interventional" is to be performed by the director of the institution at which the research will take place, e.g., director of the hospital. If the research is deemed non-interventional, it does not require approval from a regional ethics committee, as described in this law, although approval by a local ethics committee may be required as per the policy of the institution. Nonetheless, in the case of a disagreement between the sponsor and the institution regarding the nature of research, an evaluation by a regional ethics committee is required to make this determination (article 26).

Social Value

There are two references in the law that address the requirement of social value of research. In the chapter dedicated to research ethics committees, it is stated that these committees will base their decisions on their analysis of the relevance of research (article 22). The second reference to social value appears in article 27, which states that the research should aim to "expand scientific knowledge of the human being and the means of improving his condition".

Scientific Validity

Parallel to social value, reference to scientific validity appears in articles 22 and 27. Areas that should be examined by research ethics committees include the adequacy of the alignment between the research aims and methodology. Moreover, the law requires that research should be based on available scientific knowledge.

Fair Participant's Selection

Addressing concerns related to the involvement of vulnerable populations are present in the third chapter of title I entitled: "specific provisions for certain persons".

Minors and adults under legal protection should be considered for participation in research only if the research holds the prospect of potential direct benefit for the individuals. In the absence of a potential direct benefit, such research can be authorized under three conditions:

- There is no serious foreseeable risk
- There is a prospect of future potential benefit for persons with the same age or disease patterns
- The research cannot be performed otherwise.

Once the research is approvable, consent should be sought from the subject's legal representative. Nonetheless, if prospective participants are "able to express [their] will", then they should provide consent. The law includes a category of "minors over the age of discernment and persons of unsound mind during a moment of clarity". The first category refers to emancipated minors and the second category refers to individuals with psychiatric disorders who, nonetheless, have capacity to provide their own consent.

The Moroccan Law also specifies that the category of "certain persons" includes pregnant women, post-partum mothers, and breastfeeding women. Research cannot be performed among these groups unless it is necessary and the prospects of direct benefits for the woman, the fetus or newborn outweigh the foreseeable risks. Prisoners as well as unauthorized immigrants cannot be involved in biomedical research. Although not considered a vulnerable group, the Moroccan Law does not permit the participation of healthy individuals in research.

Favorable Risk Benefit Ratio

The concept of risk minimization is frequently encountered in the law. For example, there is an emphasis on the adequacy of research setting, the experience of investigators and research staff, quality control and sponsor responsibilities. Article 7 stipulates that study sponsors, investigators and intervening persons need to ensure all "necessary measures to reduce research negative repercussions on physical integrity and psychological equilibrium of research participants". In article 3, a basic principle for research is to comply with Good Clinical Practices guidelines. Prior to the study participation, potential participants should undergo screening in order to ensure that they do not present any contraindication to the study. Finally, an individual cannot be enrolled in several biomedical studies at the same time. An "exclusion period", during which the subject cannot be enrolled in another research, should be specified in the study protocol.

In regards to benefits, the Moroccan Law states that if any study drug is shown to have a benefit, but participants are not able to access the medicine, e.g., if unavailable due to the length of time it takes for the medicine to gain approval, then sponsors are responsible to ensure that research participants have access to the drugs.

Reference to the concept of risk-benefit assessment is found in two places:

- Research ethics committee approval will depend on a "satisfactory evaluation of expected benefits and foreseeable risks; and on the grounded conclusions of this evaluation".
- Governmental authority that approves research will ensure that foreseeable risks for participants are not disproportionate with regard to expected potential direct benefits for participants or the community.

Independent Review

The Moroccan law mandates the establishment of regional ethics committees for the Protection of Persons Participating in biomedical research (CPP), according to the administrative regions in Morocco. A research cannot be authorized without the approval from a CPP (article 27). Since 2015, there are 12 administrative regions in Morocco. Typically, the approval is sought from the regional committee in the region to which the principal investigator's institution belongs. In case of an unfavorable decision, the sponsor or investigator can request from the governmental authority to designate a CPP from another region to re-review the protocol.

There are no details regarding the composition of these committees, although article 18 emphasizes the multidisciplinary make-up of the committee members and specifies the various disciplines: medicine, biology, ethics, social, psychology, religion and legal. There is also reference in the law to the professional integrity of members and there is specification that members cannot delegate their responsibilities to others. Finally, article 19 underlines the concept of independency in the functioning of ethics committees.

Secrecy regarding all information related to the research is also emphasized. A "conflicts of interests" disclosure is to be addressed to the chair of the committee each time a member is involved in a protocol submitted for approval. As a general rule, an investigator whose protocol is under review and is also a member of a review committee cannot take part in the deliberations. Furthermore, sponsors or their representatives cannot be members of the ethics committee.

Informed Consent

The requirement for informed consent is mentioned within the chapter entitled: "dispositions related to persons participating in biomedical research". The consent should be "voluntary, informed and on purpose". The investigator or another physician should provide information, verbally and by a written document, in the language of the potential subject.

Article 4 specifies the following information that should be disclosed:

- Participants' rights under the present law
- Research aim, methodology and duration
- Foreseeable constraints and risks
- Expected benefits
- Available medical alternatives

In order for participants to better understand the disclosed information, they may "appeal to any person of their choice". The law also guarantees the right to refuse participation and to withdraw from the study (article 5). The consent needs to be documented by a written and signed document.

In "the case of a clinical situation preventing from obtaining consent from the concerned person", surrogate consent may be obtained from a family member. The law specifies family members from whom the consent needs to be sought. Participants should be informed regarding their participation in research as soon as their health condition allows it. Their consent is needed to continue the research. Nevertheless, what constitutes such clinical situations is not specified.

Respect for Potential and Enrolled Participants

The second chapter of the title I is related to the rights of the research participants. This part emphasizes participants' rights for the protection of their "life, health, physical integrity, psychological equilibrium and dignity". Article 5 emphasizes the right of participants to receive continued medical monitoring after withdrawal if they are still sick. The privacy of the person involved in biomedical research must be respected and the confidentiality of data must be ensured by the sponsor, investigator and stakeholders in accordance with the laws and regulations of Morocco.

Payment for study participants is not permitted; reimbursements are allowed for extra costs incurred by research participation or healthcare. More importantly, the law stipulates that sponsors are responsible to cover any injury that is determined to have been caused by research participation, regardless of the delay of its onset. Thus, the sponsor should maintain insurance for the entire period of the study.

Finding of Violations and Sanctions

Title III contains articles that mention violations and corresponding sanctions. The first article states that leaders of healthcare facilities, the sponsor, investigator and stakeholders involved in the implementation of biomedical research, are subject to periodic inspections designed to verify compliance with the provisions of this Act. Inspectors upon uncovering a violation shall notify the appropriate government authority to suspend authorization of the research in question and transmit the minutes of the said infringement to the public prosecutor.

The Law mentions specific types of violations. For example, anyone who includes an individual in a biomedical (interventional) research without obtaining informed and voluntary consent or anyone who fails to obtain a new consent after a protocol amendment is liable to sanctions that include 3–5 years of imprisonment and a fine of 500,000 Moroccan dirhams (≈50,000 US dollars). The same sanctions apply when research is performed among vulnerable groups without respecting the appropriate provisions the law. Moreover, individuals guilty of the last infringement are prohibited from professional activity for a period of 5–10 years.

Excluding the reimbursement of expenses incurred by or the compensation of constraints due to research participation, any person involved in the paymentfrom individuals in return of their participation in research is punishable by 3–5 years of imprisonment and a fine of 500,000 dirhams. Sanctions extend to the participants themselves; anyone perceived or attempted to receive a financial contribution for participating in a research is punishable by imprisonment of 1–3 years and or a fine of 2,000–20,000 dirhams. Another example of sanctions concerns post-trial access; a sponsor who refuses to facilitate access to the drug or medical device to the participants is punishable by a fine of 500,000 dirhams.

Discussion

The Moroccan Law recognizes that while research performed previously in Morocco was guided by international guidelines, such guidance did not have the legal force needed to secure and guarantee the ethical practice of research in Morocco. What follows is a discussion of the major constructive aspects of the Law, as well as controversial aspects.

The Scope

The Moroccan law only applies to interventional research. This might represent an unintended consequence of the law if the failure to include non-interventional research in the Law is interpreted to mean that such research does not require ethics review. Such researches would include socio-behavioral research, which can carry significant social risks to participants. For instance, a qualitative study consisting of observing intravenous drug users would carry risks that include stigmatization and criminal liability if there is noncompliance with ethical guidelines that would mandate privacy and confidentiality assurances. Another example would include a study that uses a questionnaire with the aim of identifying factors associated with treatment compliance among HIV patients, a highly stigmatizing disease in many contexts. Even if there is no intervention, there is still a need for ethical oversight for such studies in order to protect privacy and ensure confidentiality protections of participants' data.

As the Moroccan Law only applies to interventional studies, there will be greater reliance on local research ethics committee to review research protocols that are interpreted as being observational or non-interventional studies.

A Central Research Ethics Committee Model

The Law provides an interesting model for ethical oversight for biomedical research based on CPPs or central research ethics committees established for each region. These central ethics committees present several advantages. First, they will ensure the consideration of regional specificities in a country with much cultural diversity between regions. Second, these committees can provide a single approval for research being performed at multiple institutions within a specified region, thus enhancing efficiency and consistency.

However, the present law omits details as to how these committees will interact with any future National Ethics Committee. Such a committee is anticipated, as

Article 21 introduces the role of a "governmental authority" in designating a CPP for a second evaluation, when a sponsor requests it after disapproval from the first CPP.

Vulnerable Participants

The Moroccan Law includes criteria for when it might be appropriate to enroll "certain persons" who might be vulnerable and identifies who might be considered vulnerable. It also identifies associated protection mechanisms. The law emphasizes the principle of scientific necessity when considering the inclusion of these "certain persons" in research. The mentioning of concepts regarding vulnerable participants represents an important inclusion, as details regarding vulnerable populations have been omitted from other regulations in the Arab region (Alahmad et al. 2012).

International Research

The Moroccan Law makes reference to international research and requires that foreign sponsors need to have local representatives in Morocco, in which case they need to delegate to their representatives all activities related to the research conduct. These articles describe the categories of sponsors' legal representatives and their duties, especially with regard to the importation and handling of experimental drugs and devices. Two major strengths are to be emphasized regarding the consideration of international research in this law. First, standardized provisions and protections should allow for a better control of such research activity within the country. Second, research needs to be responsive to the population health needs, as every research has to prove its social value in order to be authorized.

Payment for Research Participants

It appears that the Moroccan law is overprotective regarding payment for research participants, as it adopts a reimbursement model for payment. It prohibits payments that can act as an incentive to enroll, which would occur under a wage payment model or a market model (Dickert and Grady 1999). While a reimbursement model is probably adequate for studies that present a prospect of direct benefit to participant, such a model might be controversial for research studies that hold no benefits, but present potential risks, such as phase I clinical trials. In such instance, a reimbursement model of payment may be considered exploitative for the subject. However, as the Law prohibit the inclusion of healthy participants, a reimbursement model might be sufficient.

Some would argue that this overprotective approach might be justified at this initial stage of enforcing regulations and that once oversight mechanisms are in place and there are functioning RECs operating in the country, then the research enterprise will be able to accept a broadening of professional sanctions in place of restrictions. This is similar to other regulations in the region, such as the Jordan's Clinical Studies Law (Jordan Food and Drug Administration 2001).

The sanctions include fines as well as imprisonment and they apply to sponsors, investigators, and other involved persons in research. They even extend to research participants if they accept payments intended to obtain their participation in the research, i.e., payment exceeding reimbursements.

We can assume that such a system of sanctions will enhance compliance with the law. But whether it will negatively or positively impact the conduct of research in our country will be determined in the future, especially in regards to our ability to attract international research. Ensuring a balanced system that protects the rights and welfare of human participants while promoting research represents a difficult challenge.

Waiver of Informed Consent

The law does not provide criteria for when it might be acceptable to waive consent or waive the need to have written documentation of consent. This can be justified as the scope of the law only includes interventional research (e.g., clinical trials) where a waiver of consent would not be applicable. This contrasts with types of retrospective or observational research (not covered in the Law), in which a waiver might be applicable.

Biobanks

Details for biobanks are addressed as part of the conduct of interventional research. Donation of samples to a biobank requires a separate consent specifying the aim of the sample use. Any future change in this aim requires obtaining a new consent along with a new reporting to the authority.

Conclusion

The Moroccan law constitutes an important step towards ensuring the protection of the rights and welfare of research participants. It also provides an ethical framework that will ensure the ethical conduct of research. Main components of this framework include regional review committees, requirements that need to be satisfied for participants' involvement, general guidelines for research conduct and stakeholders' duties and responsibilities. Finally, it will ensure that local and international research will be responsive to the health care needs of the population.

That said, there are important omissions. For example, there needs to be more details regarding the operations of local institutional review boards, a better definition of oversight at the national level, and requirements for the conduct of other types of research not included in the present law. In parallel, the law needs to specify training requirements of persons involved in research and for members of ethics committees, which represent key steps to promote ethical conduct and compliance. Finally, there is a need for the establishment of an accreditation system for the CPPs.

It is also necessary to inform the entire population and especially potential research participants about the law. Hospitals and more specifically, teaching hospitals, may be the first step for such awareness campaigns. Raising awareness among stakeholders and the community concerning the development of ethical and responsible biomedical research is a cornerstone for protecting the rights and the welfare of our population and also maintaining public trust in the research enterprise.

References

Alahmad, G., M. Al-Jumah, and K. Dierickx. 2012. Review of national research ethics regulations and guidelines in Middle Eastern Arab countries. *BMC Medical Ethics* 13: 34. https://doi.org/10.1186/1472-6939-13-34.

Bulletin Officiel. 2015. Loi n° 28-13 relative à la protection des personnes participants aux recherches biomédicales. Numéro 6396 (p3458–67).

Dickert, N., and C. Grady. 1999. What's the price of a research subject? Approaches to payment for research participation. *The New England Journal of Medicine* 341 (3): 198–203. https://doi.org/10.1056/NEJM199907153410312.

Emanuel, E.J., D. Wendler, and C. Grady. 2000. What makes clinical research ethical? *JAMA* 283: 2701–2711.

Jordan Food & Drug Administration. 2001. Clinical research law. Available at: http://www.jfda.jo/EN/Laws/LawInfo.aspx?id=507.

Part IV

Regulatory Landscape in the Arab Region

Regulatory Landscape in the Arab Region: Introduction

Henry Silverman

Current Regulatory Situation in the Arab Region

Research governance systems vary between the different countries in the Arab Region and embrace some variant of the models discussed in Chapter 15. In those countries who operate a "loose" regulatory climate, concerns will exist regarding the adequacy of the protection of the rights and welfare of research participants. Such concerns will suggest the need for the development of robust national regulatory systems that include adequate oversight mechanisms and robust ethics review of research. The aim of Part IV is to describe the regulatory systems that exist in several countries in the Arab region.

The case studies in this section serve several purposes. First, to show the range of the regulatory frameworks governing research in several of the Arabic countries. This review will show that several countries lack robust systems, but several have reached a level of sophistication that conform with international standards and are comparable to the systems in many western countries. Second, those countries who have achieved a robust regulatory system can thus provide a "model" to which other Arabic countries with developing research governance systems can emulate.

H. Silverman (✉)
University of Maryland, Baltimore, MD, USA
e-mail: hsilverm@medicine.umaryland.edu

H. Silverman (ed.), *Research Ethics in the Arab Region*, Research Ethics Forum 5,
https://doi.org/10.1007/978-3-319-65266-5_20

Research Ethics Governance in the Arab Region: Jordan

Amal Al-Omari and Maysa Al-Hussaini

Jordan was the first Arab country to enact clinical research regulations and its subsequent regulatory environment makes it among the most important potential markets for clinical trials in the Arab region. Several aspects of Jordan's clinical research environment are considered in this section.

Health Care System

Jordan has of population of 9.532 million (year 2015) that is relatively young, as the median age is 23 years. According to the World Bank classification, Jordan is an upper middle-income country. In 2014, the gross domestic product (GDP) was estimated at $35.83 billion and gross national income (GNI) per capita at $5160 (The World Bank 2015).

The country has a well- developed and reputable healthcare system, which is attributed mainly to a relatively high physician to population ratio, well-equipped hospitals, and high level of technology (World Health Organization Regional Office for the Eastern Mediterranean 2006). Furthermore, Jordan has a fairly advanced domestic pharmaceutical industry, dedicated mainly to the manufacturing of generics. As such, bioavailability and bioequivalence (BA/BE) studies constitute much of the research performed in Jordan (World Health Organization Regional Office for

A. Al-Omari
Office of Scientific Affairs and Research, King Hussein Cancer Center, Amman, Jordan

Translational Research Program, King Hussein Cancer Center, Amman, Jordan

M. Al-Hussaini (✉)
Department of Pathology and Laboratory Medicine, King Hussein Cancer Center, Amman, Jordan

Institutional Review Board (IRB), King Hussein Cancer Center, Amman, Jordan
e-mail: mhussaini@khcc.jo

H. Silverman (ed.), *Research Ethics in the Arab Region*, Research Ethics Forum 5,
https://doi.org/10.1007/978-3-319-65266-5_21

the Eastern Mediterranean 2006; Conesa et al. 2009). However, the average expenditure on R&D was 0.43% of GDP in 2008, which is modest compared with international levels, which is approximately 2–3% (The Global Economy 2015).

Research Governance

Laws and Regulations

Research is governed by the Jordanian Clinical Studies Law (CSL), drafted in 2001 and released in its permanent version in 2011 (Jordan Food and Drug Administration 2001, 2011). The law was primarily extracted from ICH guidelines as well as from U.S. Food and Drug Administration (FDA) and the European Medicines Agency (EMA) regulations. It was enacted to regulate and provide oversight over the expanding number of clinical studies conducted in Jordan. The passage of the CSL has been viewed as a milestone in supporting research, allowing Jordan to be perceived as having an encouraging environment for conducting pharmaceutical-sponsored clinical studies (Shahrouri 2009).

The CSL states that only local organizations licensed by the Minister of Health are allowed to conduct clinical studies, and these organizations include public and private hospitals, universities and academic institutions, scientific research institutions (e.g., Clinical Research Organizations (CROs)), and pharmaceutical companies. However, global pharmaceutical companies and CROs can conduct clinical trials in Jordan through collaboration with a locally licensed clinical site. Licensed organizations and institutions must possess the technical capabilities to provide emergent and intensive care as well as the required laboratory testing. There are currently 17 licensed organizations, seven of which are CROs. Each licensed organization must establish, according to the law and in compliance with the ICH-GCP (good clinical practice) guideline, an IRB of at least five members of both genders with relevant background and experience, including a legal advisor and a representative from the community. The responsibilities and authority of the institutional review boards (IRBs) are to assure the authenticity of the scientific merits of the study, the qualifications of the study team, the voluntary participation of research subjects and the approval and monitoring of the study.

Protection of Subjects in the CSL

Participants in clinical trials are generally well protected by the Jordanian law. For instance, Article 5-a in the CSL states that a voluntary informed consent must be obtained for all human subjects, and that participants should be evaluated for suitability before being admitted to the clinical study. The same Article also states that the collected bio-samples cannot be used for purposes other than what is stated in the study protocol. Members of the clinical research team should have proper education and experience (Article 9-a). The licensed organization(s) and the medical team(s) conducting the study must adhere to the approved clinical protocol as well as to the ethical standards in the Declaration of Helsinki (Article 11). Other unique aspects of the CSL include the requirement to have insurance for research-related injuries and a system of fines and punishments for noncompliance with the law (Article 17).

However, key issues including a favorable benefit–risk balance, fair selection of trial subjects, and protection of minors and vulnerable groups are missing from the law. Also, the CSL does not cover all aspects of the consent procedure and documents, the absence of which may jeopardize the rights, wellbeing, and privacy of the trial participants. A major criticism of the law is the primary focus on BA/BE studies in healthy volunteers. In addition, the CSL in its present form solely covers drug-related clinical studies and needs to be extended to cover other types of research involving humans, such as medical devices, surgical interventions, and social behavioral research. Commentators have recommended amendments to the law or the formulation of guidelines to address these topics (Ramahi and Silverman 2009).

National Authorities

Jordan Food and Drug Administration (JFDA)

In 2003, the Jordan Food and Drug Administration (JFDA) was established as a stand-alone and independent entity to regulate and supervise medicinal products and medical devices in compliance with the effective Drug and Pharmacy Law for the year 2001. To accomplish its mission, it is divided into various directorates. The Drug Directorate deals with regulating and oversight of all drugs synthesized or imported for utilization in Jordan. Within the Drug Directorate, the Clinical Studies Division (CSD) oversees the conduct of clinical trials in Jordan, through the Clinical Studies Committee (CSC), as mandated by the CSL.

Clinical Studies Committee (CSC)

The CSC is constituted of 12 members chaired by the head of JFDA. The membership is for a 2-year renewable term after the approval of the Minister of Health. Membership also includes the director of Drug Directorate, the head of CSD, a pharmacist from the Drug Directorate, two physicians, director of pharmacy at the Royal Medical Services, and five individuals representing universities and private sector who are specialized in the field of pharmacokinetics, analytical pharmacy, biostatistics, clinical pharmacy and pharmacology.

The main responsibilities of the CSC include the review and evaluation of applications for clinical sites and IRB licensing, inspection of licensed sites periodically, evaluation of clinical protocols and follow up on clinical studies, as well as organizing training and educational seminars and workshops (Alnazer 2014). The JFDA also licenses laboratories performing testing on biospecimens for clinical studies.

To maintain oversight of participants of clinical trials across Jordan, the JFDA established in 2005 an online database with guidelines for BA/BE studies, to ensure the safety and protection of the trial participants. Research participants should be 18–50 years old, and they are not permitted to participate in more than one BA/BE study within 80 days. To date; however, there is no national clinical registry system

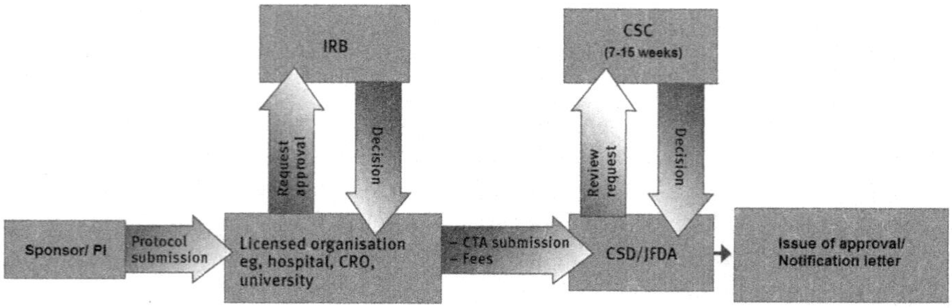

Fig. 1 An overview of the review process for approval of clinical trials in Jordan (adapted from Aroiuri et al. 2015)

in Jordan and information on clinical trials in Jordan is not publicly available. At the moment, JFDA is working on implementing a public local registry for clinical trials. The CSD requests all Phase I–IV clinical trials to be registered before application submission in international or regional registries.

Landscape of RECs in Jordan

There are 22 registered and approved IRBs in Jordan in the various hospitals, institutions and CROs (personal communication with JFDA). Of these, three IRBs hold a Federal Wide Assurance (FWA), which includes KHCC, Ministry of Health and Jordan University of Science and Technology. Aspects of function and responsibilities of the IRBs are detailed in another chapter.

Procedure for Approval of Clinical Trials

Ethics approval of clinical trials is performed both at the institutional and national levels. In accordance with Article 10 in the CSL, clinical trials on medicinal products require an authorization from the CSC based on a favorable opinion from the local IRB. Figure 1 provides an overview of the procedure for submission and evaluation of the clinical trials at JFDA (Aroiuri et al. 2015). Although seemingly lengthy, the ethics review process is usually efficient, as it takes around 4–8 weeks for the approval at the local IRB with a similar period required for the CSC at the JFDA (Alnazer 2014).

Status of Research in Jordan

Since the pharmaceutical industry in Jordan is predominantly devoted to the manufacturing of generics, it is understandable that the majority of CTAs in Jordan represent BA/BE studies (around 92%). Between 2005 and 2013, there were a total of

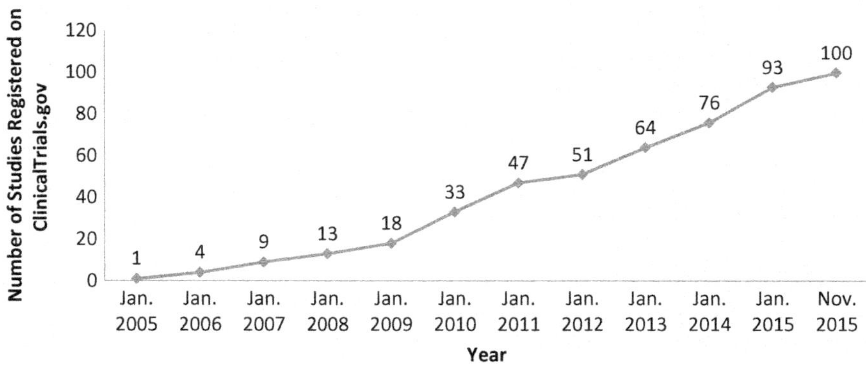

Fig. 2 Evolution of clinical trials in the Jordanian market since 2005 as registered on clinicaltrials.gov

1,471 BA/BEs, 47 Phase I, 17 Phase II, 42 Phase III, and 29 Phase IV CTAs (Aroiuri A et al. 2015). For the same time period only six CTAs were rejected; five applications for safety issues and one application for unsatisfactory preclinical data. The large percentage of accepted trials can be attributed to the fact that almost all multicenter clinical trials initiated in Jordan have already been approved and started overseas. When classified according to the disease category, of the 135 CTAs submitted during the same period for phase I–IV studies, 29% of the applications were for cardiovascular diseases, followed by 16% for oncology, 12% for neuropsychiatric, 11% for diabetes and metabolic diseases, and 9% for blood/immunology/inflammation. The applications for other disease categories were less than 6% (0–6%) (Aroiuri A et al. 2015).

Most CTAs submitted to JFDA were funded by the pharmaceutical industry, with very little contribution by other stakeholders, including academia. Modest expenditure on research from Jordanian academic institutions limits capacity for clinical research. Since the CSL only regulates clinical studies on medicinal products, other types of clinical research conducted at hospitals and universities go unregistered and unreported to the authorities.

Based on data from the WHO International Clinical Trials Registry Platform (ICTRP), only 111 studies (7%) were registered in primary clinical registries. Data from clinicaltrials.gov demonstrates that Jordan shows a modest increase in the number of clinical trials (phase I–IV). The number has increased from 2 studies in 2002 peaking in 2010 with 24 clinical trials, 22% of which are oncology trials. Phase III trials account for the majority of the approved studies (Shafout 2014). This indicates that the information obtained from these registries represents only a small fraction of the trials actually conducted in Jordan, which holds true for the region in general. As of November 2015, 100 clinical trials were registered on clinicaltrials.gov (U.S. National Institutes of Health 2015). Considering that Jordan entered the clinical trial market in the early 2000s, the number of clinical trials in the past 10 years has grown substantially. Figure 2 shows the growth and evolution of clinical trials in the Jordanian market since 2005. Of the 100 registered trials on clinicaltrials.gov, 69 are interventional and 31 non-interventional studies (registered since 2002), out of which 60% are completed (U.S. National Institutes of Health 2015).

Conclusions and Recommendations

The existence of the CSL and a functioning JFDA affords Jordan with a well-regulated system that allows the country to advance within the world of clinical research. A number of factors make Jordan a rich soil for excellent clinical research. First, the geography of the Kingdom that facilitates efficient access for monitoring and audit visits when needed. Second, there are specialized facilities that includes technologically advanced and highly certified hospitals and research facilities. Also, there are many potential expert key leaders, as the country has an estimated number of 25,000 physicians, most of whom are board-certified in the US and western European countries. With proper training and orientation to a clinical research culture, these physicians would be qualified to lead and advance clinical research environment in Jordan.

Understanding the challenges that impede clinical research is essential to advance research in Jordan. These challenges can be addressed at three overlapping levels: the country level, the institutional level and the investigator level.

Country Level

The following factors impact negatively on the conduct of research in Jordan:

1. Jordan is relatively stable and secure, however, regional conflicts and political instability (Arab Spring) have negatively conveyed Jordan among other countries in the Arab region as a less desirable place for conducting clinical studies.
2. Although the CSL was instrumental in providing a legal structure to the performance of research, the law as currently written uses vague statements that are open to individual interpretations and are not tailored to meet the requirements of new research paradigms. National policies and regulatory frameworks will need to be updated to address, the following items: the requirements of investigator-initiated trials, genetic research, tissue banks, material transfers, and research using medical devices. Clear guidelines on any of these topics is lacking in the current regulatory framework.
3. Academic institutions in Jordan are mostly teaching institutions and devote modest monies on research, which limits the capacity for clinical research. Therefore, there is a need in Jordan to encourage and support academic clinical research, by increasing budget allocations dedicated for this purpose.

4. Lack of awareness: Educational campaigns for the public and training workshops targeting professionals involved in clinical studies will improve the overall awareness and capacity within the community.

Institutional Level

Institutions need to allocate resources to advance and promote a clinical research culture. Academic faculty need research protected time, since balancing between heavy clinical loads and research activity demands represent a main challenge. Also needed is a faculty incentive plan that provides financial rewards and recognition for staff who wants to pursue research. These steps can help prevent the current brain drain in which the more experienced, foreign-trained clinical investigators are migrating to GCC countries, EU, and the US.

Investigator Level

Knowledge gaps in research methodology due to inadequate time in the curricula of medical schools devoted to research methods and statistics is a major challenge for investigators, especially for the junior faculty. High level communications with top academic officials is needed to include research methodology and statistics in the curricula of medical schools. Also, building networks of investigators and scientists within and between institutions and with other sponsors of research should be a fundamental objective to improve the clinical research environment. Moreover, most investigators seeking promotion opt for an easy-way to publication by conducting retrospective and observational studies rather than the more impactful but lengthy and complicated interventional clinical trials. The rewarding and recognition system should incentivize the conduct of important research to enable more meaningful clinical research with potential to translate into improved patient care.

References

Alnazer, M. 2014. Jordan's advancement into the clinical market and it regulatory framework. *Journal for Clinical Studies* 6: 16–18.

Aroiuri, A., S. Al-Mahrouq, M. Al-Ghazawl, and D. Russmann. 2015. The evolving clinical research environment in Jordan. *Regulatory Rapporteur* 12: 16–21.

Conesa, S., Yadav, P. and Bader, R. 2009. Analysis of the Pharmaceutical Supply Chain in Jordan. A study funded by The World Bank under the MeTA initiative. Jordan.(www.medicinestransparency.org/fileadmin/uploads/Documents/countries/Supply_Chain_Reports/MeTA_Jordan_Supply_Chain_Report.pdf) accessed 23 Nov 2015.

Jordan Food & Drug Administration. 2001. Clinical research law. Available at: http://www.jfda.jo/EN/Laws/LawInfo.aspx?id=507. Accessed 11 Feb 2007.

Jordan Food and Drug Administration. 2011. Law No. 2 of clinical studies for the year 2011. Available at: http://www.jfda.jo/Default.aspx.

Ramahi, I., and H. Silverman. 2009. Clinical research law in Jordan: An ethical analysis. *Developing World Bioethics* 9 (1): 26–33. https://doi.org/10.1111/j.1471-8847.2007.00221.x.

Shahrouri, R. 2009. Jordan first. *Journal for Clinical Studies*, November, 22.

The Global Economy. 2015. Available at: http://www.theglobaleconomy.com/Jordan/Research_and_development/

The World Bank. 2015. Jordan: Available at: http://www.worldbank.org/en/country/jordan

U.S. National Institutes of Health. 2015. Clinical Trials.Gov. http://clinicaltrials.gov/

World Health Organization Regional Office for the Eastern Mediterranean. 2006. Research and capacity building in trade in health services in the Eastern Mediterranean Region, WHO-EM/PHP/036/E. Retrieved at: http://gis.emro.who.int/HealthSystemObservatory/PDF/Trade And Health Services/Research and capacity building- final.pdf

Research Ethics Governance in the Arab Region – Saudi Arabia

Ghiath Alahmad and Henry Silverman

Health Care System

Saudi Arabia is a monarchical state that has largely been dependent on an oil-based economy, although there have been recent efforts to diversify it economy. The government, which controls most major economic activities, has focused on expanding its healthcare, education, nuclear, construction, and tourism industries (Almalki et al. 2011).

The Ministry of Health (MOH) is considered the lead Government agency responsible for the management, planning, financing and regulating of the health care sector. Health expenditure in Saudi Arabia was reported at 4.68% of the GDP in 2014, according to the World Bank collection of development indicators (Trading Ecoomics 2017). There has been a growing role and increased participation from the private sector in the provision of health care services. The MOH also undertakes the overall supervision and follow-up of health care related activities carried out by the private sector. Therefore, the health care system in Saudi Arabia can be classified as a national health care system (NHS) in which the government provides health care services through a number of government agencies (Almalki et al. 2011; Wikipedia 2017). In addition to the MOH and the private sector, there are also other providers: the Ministry of Defense and Aviation (MODA), the Ministry of Interior (MOI), and the Saudi Arabian National Guard (SANG) finance and deliver primary, secondary and tertiary care to specific enrolled security and armed forces

G. Alahmad (✉)
King Abdullah International Medical Research Center (KAIMRC), King Saud bin Abdulaziz University For Health Sciences (KSAU-HS), King Abdulaziz Medical City, Ministry of National Guard – Health Affairs, P.O. Box 22490, Riyadh 11426, Saudi Arabia
e-mail: ghiathalahmad@hotmail.com

H. Silverman
University of Maryland, Baltimore, MD, USA
e-mail: hsilverm@medicine.umaryland.edu

H. Silverman (ed.), *Research Ethics in the Arab Region*, Research Ethics Forum 5,
https://doi.org/10.1007/978-3-319-65266-5_22

populations. In addition to these agencies, the Ministry of Education provides immediate primary health care to students and the Ministry of Labor and Social Affairs operates institutions for the mentally retarded and custodial homes for orphans (Wikipedia 2017).

Currently, there is a maldistribution of health care services and health professionals within the country that has caused specific populations to experience long waiting lists for many health care services and facilities. Additionally, disadvantaged groups such as the elderly, adolescents and people with special needs such as disability, particularly in rural areas lack access to health care services. Finally, many people living in border and remote areas do not have the ability to access health care facilities. Optimizing the accessibility of health care services requires equity in the distribution of health care facilities throughout the nation and equity of access to health professionals, including transport to services and providers (Almalki et al. 2011). Although the 2016 health care budget was decreased compared with that of 2015, industry players are confident of changes to enhance efficiency and promote better allocation of resources (Oxford Business Group 2017). Furthermore, a fast-growing population coupled with a high incidence of lifestyle-related illnesses such as diabetes and obesity are expected to be the main drivers of new demand for quality health care in the medium to long term.

Of all of the countries in the Gulf Cooperation Council, (GCC), Saudi Arabia maintains the largest pharmaceutical market share as it imports 80% of drugs from other countries; the remaining market share comes from the local pharmaceutical industry. Demand for pharmaceuticals is currently witnessing robust growth in Saudi Arabia, mainly due to increasing prevalence of lifestyle diseases, strong brand loyalty for multinational drugs, and improved healthcare infrastructure. Furthermore, increasing per capita income, growing healthcare infrastructure and increasing penetration of health insurance companies in the country is fuelling growth of the pharmaceuticals market in Saudi Arabia (Future Market Insights 2017).

Research Governance

National Regulations

In 2010, The Law of Ethics of Research on Living Creatures (The Law) was enacted and approved by Royal Decree No. M / 59 on 14/09/1431 Hijri (24/08/2010). The Law establishes guidelines for research involving human subjects according to professional ethics without contradicting Islamic concepts. After the enactment of this law, The Implementing Regulations of the Law of Ethics of Research on Living Things was issued, which explains many of the points in the articles of the Law and provide instructions for its implementation (National Committee of Bioethics (NCBE) 2015). The Law and the Implementing Regulations together form one unit. These legal instruments is reviewed in the chapter by Ghiath Alahmad. Moreover, an ethical analysis of this Law in the same chapter concludes that The Law encodes the seven ethical requirements for research according to the framework developed by Emanuel and colleagues (Emanuel et al. 2000).

On 7 August 2015, the Saudi Food and Drug Authority (SFDA) issued 'Regulations & Requirements for Conducting Clinical Trials on Drugs (Saudi Food and Drug Authority 2015). This guidance is directed towards researchers, sponsors, and contract research organizations (CRO) who need to adhere to the regulations of Research Ethics Code on Living Creatures and good clinical practice (GCP) in accordance with the ICH-E6 guideline. Sponsors include a) governmental research institutions who fund their own investigators and b) private sponsors, e.g., pharmaceutical companies and private research centers. All clinical trials involving drugs must be registered with the SFDA Drug Sector's Clinical Trials Department by the researcher, sponsor or CRO through the Saudi Clinical Trials Registry. Phases II and III trials require approval from the SFDA, Phase IV trials only require approval from an institutional review board and notification to the SFDA (ct.drug@sfda.gov.sa) within 20 working days after obtaining local IRB approval. The guidance also covers the requirements for clinical trial amendments, transporting biological samples and investigator qualifications.

National Authorities

National Ethics Committee

The National Committee of Medical & Bioethics (NCBE) is the main ethics committee in Saudi Arabia. It was established by enactment of the Royal Decree on 18/5/1422H, and is managed by the King Abdulaziz City for Science and Technology (KACST) in Riyadh (King Abdulaziz City for Science and Technology (KACST) 2013). The NCBE provides national oversight to research involving human subjects, exercising its control through its administrative branch called the Research Ethics Monitoring Office. This Office registers and oversees the work of the local institutional research ethics committees (RECs) and ensures that they comply with relevant laws and reviews complaints submitted by the researchers or research participants (Alahmad 2017; Bawazir et al. 2014). The NCBE and the Saudi Law of Ethics of Research on Human Creatures and its implementing regulations are reviewed in the chapter by Ghiath Alahmad.

Drug Regulatory Authority

Since 2010, the Saudi Food and Drug Administration (SFDA) has regulated the conduct of clinical trials in Saudi Arabia (MCT-CRO 2017). Prior to 2009, there were no formal regulations for clinical trials in Saudi Arabia. The Clinical Trial Administration unit was established in 2009 to provide assessment of all clinical trial applications from sponsors and CROs to conduct clinical trials in Saudi Arabia (Bawazir et al. 2014). The SFDA issued in April 2013 the final version of the Clinical Trials Requirements/Guidelines (Saudi Food and Drug Authority 2013).

The Clinical Trial Administration unit evaluates all phase I, II, III and IV clinical protocols as well as trial amendments occurring during or after the submission of the study application (Bawazir et al. 2014). The clinical trial authorization process consists of sequential submission of the clinical trial documents; first to the local

RECs for approval and then followed by the Clinical Trial Administration unit, which then reviews the study protocol, informed consent, investigator brochure, and the prior REC approval.

The Clinical Trial Administration unit has three departments: Clinical Trials Evaluation Department, the Saudi Clinical Trials Registry department (SCTR), and the Good Clinical Practice Department (Bawazir et al. 2014). **The Clinical Trials Evaluation Department conducts** reviews of all types of clinical trial applications, amendments and adverse events generated from the conduct of clinical trials. **The Saudi Clinical Trials Registry** (SCTR) provides an online system for registration of clinical trials conducted in Saudi Arabia. Mandatory registration of all clinical trials is required as of 2013, and hence, the goal of the SCTR is to ensure that every clinical trial conducted in Saudi Arabia is prospectively registered "before the enrollment of the first participant" with full disclosure of the trial data/information all through the entire registry system. **The Good Clinical Practice Department** is responsible for (a) accreditation of CROs and (b) clinical trial inspection program. **The SFDA Inspection Program** verifies that the data generated from each trial have been documented and reported in compliance with the protocol, Good Clinical Practice guidelines, and the sponsor's procedures and regulatory requirement(s) (Bawazir et al. 2014).

Research Ethics Committees (RECs)

The NCBE issued regulations in 2010 (updated 2015) that provide guidance regarding the structure and function of RECs (National Committee of Bioethics (NCBE) 2015). The principal investigator must obtain approval of the trial protocol from the REC Committee prior to submission to the SFDA. The REC should review the proposed clinical trial within a reasonable time and document its views in writing, clearly identifying the trial and the documents reviewed. The REC is also responsible for conducting continuing review of each ongoing trial at intervals appropriate to the degree of risk to subjects, but at least once per year.

The REC should consist of a reasonable number of members, who collectively have the qualifications and experience to review and evaluate the science, medical aspects, and ethics of the proposed trial. It is recommended that the REC should include:

- At least five members.
- At least one member whose primary area of interest is in a nonscientific area.
- At least one member who is independent of the institution/trial site.

Each local research ethics committee should be registered, evaluated and approved by the Monitoring Research Ethics Office at the NCBE. As of January 2017 there were 45 registered ethics committee in different areas in Saudi Arabia.

Status of Research

The number of clinical trials performed in Saudi Arabia as of early 2017 was 242 (source database: www.clinicaltrials.gov - Feb 2017). The distribution of clinical trials per phases was Phase I (27), Phase II (57), Phase III (108), and Phase IV (71). Figure 1 shows the details of clinical trials according to its phases for years 2002–2017.

Ali and colleagues in their review of clinical trials performed in Saudi Arabia concluded that the number of trials is not adequate for a country the size of Saudi Arabia and that many academic institutions only register one trial per year. Barriers to clinical trial conduct include difficulty in the recruitment of study participants and inadequacy in financial resources (Ali et al. 2017). Further, Saudi Arabia contributed only 0.20% of global clinical trials, although this figure is higher than other countries in the region (Ali et al. 2017). Furthermore, according to Saudi Arabia's 2016 fiscal budget, there is a decline of 34% in health and social development budget as compare to 2015, which may adversely affect clinical trials activity of government academic institutions in the Kingdom (Ali et al. 2017).

Jamjoom and colleagues reviewed the "fate" of registered clinical trials performed in Saudi Arabia and observed that when investigators from Saudi Arabia were predominantly responsible for the conduct of the clinical trial compared when they acted merely as collaborators with investigators from other countries, journal publication was less likely (Jamjoom et al. 2015).

Year	Phase 1	Phase 2	Phase 3	Phase 4	Total
2002	0	1	0	1	2
2003	0	0	0	0	0
2004	0	0	0	0	0
2005	1	1	8	6	16
2006	0	2	2	4	8
2007	1	2	7	0	10
2008	0	2	9	3	14
2009	2 (1/2)*	3 (1/2)	10	9	21
2010	3 (1/2)	6 (1/2 + 2/3)	10 (2/3)	9	26
2011	3 (1/2)	5 (1/2 + 2/3)	12 (2/3)	4	22
2012	1	5 (2/3 + 2/3)	12 (2/3 + 2/3)	4	20
2013	2 (1/2)	4 (1/2)	11	7	23
2014	3 (1/2 + 1/2)	12 (1/2 + 1/2)	13	10	36
2015	3 (1/2 + 1/2)	7 (1/2 + 1/2)	9	8	26
2016	2 (1/2 + 1/2)	6 (1/2 + 1/2 + 2/3)	4 (2/3)	7	16
2017	0	0	0	1	1
All years	21	57	108	71	242

Fig. 1 Details of clinical trials according to its phases for years 2002–2017 (*figures in parenthesis refer to a clinical trials that encompassed the indicated two phases)

Conclusion

Saudi Arabia has developed an effective regulatory system for the conduct of clinical trials. That said, several challenges remain and include the following (Bawazir et al. 2014):

- Long ethical approval process at many sites.
- Inadequate financial resources from the national government.
- Inadequate training of members of the research team.
- Adequate procedures for obtaining informed consents are not performed in many cases.
- Inadequate communications between the research investigator and research participants.
- Investigators' poor compliance with clinical trial regulations.
- Difficulties in obtaining informed consent, especially from individuals with illiteracy or from elderly people who are usually surrounded with many family members.
- Difficulty in recruiting the appropriate study sample size.
- Lack of experience in clinical trial conduct.
- Inadequate compliance with Good Clinical Practice (GCP).

Despite these challenges, Saudi Arabia aims to achieve market share levels comparable to that of consumption of developed products, which would enhance annual clinical trial revenues. As such, current plans are in place to promote clinical trials in different areas within Saudi Arabia involving every major research institution. There are plans to involve flexible regulatory processes, especially through allowing a parallel submission process to both the REC and SFDA, rather than sequential process consisting of REC approval prior to submission to SFDA. There are also plans to accredit research sites and CROs within the next five years. Finally, more resources will be devoted to specialized clinical trials training for members of the research team. These enhancements are expected to further attract potential pharmaceutical companies and CROs to help set up clinical trial operations in Saudi Arabia.

References

Alahmad, G. 2017. The Saudi Law of Ethics of Research on Living Creatures and its Implementing Regulations. *Dev World Bioeth* 17(2): 63–69. doi:10.1111/dewb.12114.

Ali, S., M. Alghamdi, A. Alzhrani, and E.B. De Vol. 2017. Magnitude and characteristics of clinical trials in the Kingdom of Saudi Arabia: A cross-sectional analysis. *Contemporary Clinical Trials Communications* 7: 126–129.

Almalki, M., G. Fitzgerald, and M. Clark. 2011. Health care system in Saudi Arabia: an overview. *East Mediterr Health J* 17(10): 784–793.

Bawazir, S., H. Hashan, A. Al Hatareshah, A. Al Ghamdi, and K. Al Shahwan. 2014. Regulating Clinical Trials in Saudi Arabia. *Applied Clinical Research, Clinical Trials & Regulatory Affairs* 1: 2–9.

Emanuel, E.J., D. Wendler, and C. Grady. 2000. What Makes Clinical Research Ethical? *JAMA* 283: 2701–2711.

Future Market Insights. 2017. Saudi Arabia pharmaceutical market: supportive government reforms and rising diseases awareness to fuel revenue growth from branded pharmaceuticals in Saudi Arabia: Industry analysis and opportunity assessment, 2016–2026. Retrieved at: https://www.futuremarketinsights.com/reports/saudi-arabia-pharmaceutical-market.

Jamjoom, A., A. Jamjoom, A. Samman, and A. Gahtani. 2015. Fate of registered clinical trials performed in Sauid Arabia. *Saudi Med J* 36: 1245–1248.

King Abdulaziz City for Science and Technology (KACST). 2013. The *national committee of bioethics*. Retrieved at: http://www.kacst.edu.sa/ar/depts/bioethics/Pages/home.aspx.

MCT-CRO. 2017. *Saudi Arabia*. Retrieved at: http://www.mct-cro.com/regional-reach/cro-saudi-arabia/.

National Committee of Bioethics (NCBE) 2015. *Implementing Regulations of ethics of research on the living Creatures*. Riyadh: King Abdulaziz City of Science and Technology. Retrieved at: http://bioethics.kacst.edu.sa/Document/Regulations/Ethics-Rugl-English.aspx.

Oxford Business Group. 2017. *Health initiatives seek to expand access and improve quality of care in Saudi Arabia*. Retrieved at: http://www.oxfordbusinessgroup.com/overview/hale-and-hearty-initiatives-seek-expand-access-and-improve-quality-care.

Food, Saudi, and Drug Authority. 2013. *Clinical trials requirements/guidelines*. Retrieved at: http://www.sfda.gov.sa/en/drug/Clinical_Trials/Pages/Regulations,-Guidelines-and-Guidance.aspx.

Food, Saudi, and Drug Authority. 2015. *Regulations & requirements for conducting clinical trials on drugs*. Retrieved at: http://www.sfda.gov.sa/en/drug/Clinical_Trials/Pages/Regulations,-Guidelines-and-Guidance.aspx.

Ecoomics, Trading. 2017. *Saudi Arabia health care expenditure*. Retrieved at: https://tradingeconomics.com/saudi-arabia/health-expenditure-total-percent-of-gdp-wb-data.html.

Wikipedia. 2017. *Health care in Saudi Arabia*. Retrieved at: https://en.wikipedia.org/wiki/Health_care_in_Saudi_Arabia.

Research Ethics Governance in the Arab Region: Egypt

Azza Saleh

Health Care System

Healthcare in Egypt consists of both a public and private sector. Public health coverage is offered through the Ministry of Health & Population (MoHP), which operates a series of medical facilities providing free health services. There are two main private insurers: The Health Insurance Organization covers employed persons, students, and widows through premiums deducted from employee salaries and employer payrolls. It operates its own network of medical facilities and contracts with private healthcare providers. The Curative Care Organization operates in specific governorates and contracts with other entities for provision of care. Many mosques operate their own clinics, especially in the large cities. Medical care offered by the public health insurance system is generally of poor quality. Only about 6% of Egyptians who are covered by the Health Insurance Organization utilize its services due to dissatisfaction with the level of care.

Egypt's volatile political environment and numerous changes to the country's leadership in recent years have made it difficult for the MoHP and related entities to push new policies through the government to improve care. However, the size of the population is perhaps the sector's biggest challenge moving forward. That said, there has been several recent successful initiatives and these include: (a) progress made on the health-related Millennium Development Goals; (b) mandatory immunization that eradicated poliomyelitis in Egypt; (c) establishment of an Egyptian national program to combat tuberculosis; (d) development of a national program for prevention and control of Viral Hepatitis B/C; and (e) the near eradication of Bilharziasis. All of the aforementioned initiatives are provided at no cost to all

A. Saleh (✉)
Central Directorate of Research & Health Development, Ministry of Health & Population, Cairo, Egypt

Theodor Bilharz Research Institute, Giza, Egypt
e-mail: azzasaleh@hotmail.com

H. Silverman (ed.), *Research Ethics in the Arab Region*, Research Ethics Forum 5,
https://doi.org/10.1007/978-3-319-65266-5_23

Egyptians, thus uniquely embracing the concept of equity as a guiding principle in healthcare services provision.

Concurrent with these successes, however, there has been an increase of non-communicable diseases, most notably cancer, diabetes, cardiovascular diseases, and chronic respiratory diseases. In response, Egypt has instituted several initiatives – the Children's Cancer Hospital "57357", the National Breast Cancer Screening Programme, the National Hepatitis Campaign, and the National School Feeding Program. A noteworthy establishment is the Regional Centre for Women's Health and Development in Alexandria, with a primary responsibility to focus on research aimed at improving women's health.

Research Governance

Laws and Regulations

Currently, national legislation for the regulation of research and clinical trials in Egypt does not exist. However, a clinical trial law was drafted in 2016 and is awaiting approval by Parliament. Nevertheless, in the absence of such legislation there are several legal policies that address research involving humans. These are as follows:

- The Constitution of 2014 states in Article 60 the following: "The human body is inviolable. Any assault, defilement or mutilation thereof is a crime punishable by Law. Organ trafficking is forbidden, and no medical or scientific experiment may be performed thereon without a documented free consent of the subject according to established principles of the medical field as regulated by law." However, the reference to the clinical trial law in this article remains a draft.
- Law 71/2009: Article 3 of this law regulates the rights of psychiatric patients, while Articles 7 and 8 state the necessity to obtain prior approval from the Research Ethics Committee (RECs) before exposing psychiatric patients to any clinical research. If approval is granted, full explanation of the trial must be provided to the patient. The law also forbids conducting trials involving patients subject to mandatory admission and treatment.
- Law 127/1955 states in Articles 59 and 65 that no foreign pharmaceutical product may enter the country unless it is approved and registered by the Ministry of Health.
- The Egyptian Medical Code of Conduct ("Profession Ethics Regulation"), issued by Ministerial Decree 238/ 2003, provides a set of instructions issued to doctors assigned to clinical trials on humans. These obligations, however, are non-binding and they neither include detailed regulatory procedures nor mention the rights of persons participating in such trials.

In the absence of comprehensive, unified legislation, RECs usually reference international standards (Sleem et al. 2010b). These includes the CIOMS, the Declaration of Helsinki, the International Organization of Medical Sciences (IOMS), and one committee uses the Belmont Report as an international guideline (Sleem et al. 2010b).

National Authorities

Central Directorate for Research & Health Development

The Central Directorate for Research and Health Development in the MoHP is the main organizational body that regulates the conduct of research and RECs throughout Egypt. The CDRHD organizes training courses in the areas of research ethics, good clinical practice, research methodology and biostatistics to build the capacities of health researchers to conduct clinical trials in Egypt. The CDRHD currently monitors clinical trials through annual progress reports submitted to it by the entities conducting the trials.

The CDRHD issued the following ministerial degrees that are aimed at regulating clinical trials in Egypt:

- Ministerial Decree No. (535) of 2012 requires the registration of all Contract Research Organizations (CROs) in Egypt and establishes an inspection process to regularly monitor their activities and their ability to supervise and monitor clinical trials. The total number of CROs registered in the MoHP are now 11, the last one registered in January 2017.
- Ministerial Decree No. (595) of 2012 requires RECs established at the different MoHP ministries, institutions, and scientific organizations to register at the CDRHD. This registration system started in 2017.
- Ministerial Decree No. (235) of 2016 developed standards for establishing and registering clinical research centers.
- Ministerial Decree No (613) of 2016 established a database registry system at the CDRHD for registering all types of research studies approved by RECs in Egypt. The entities required to register their studies include pharmaceutical companies and CROs, universities and research institutions, Ministry of Health departments, and individual master and PhD candidates.
- Ministerial Decree No. (614) of 2016 mandates inspections of ongoing clinical trials at the study sites and any other institution involved with the clinical trial.

Central Scientific and Research Ethics Committee

In 2005, the Egyptian Ministry of Health and Population (MoHP) established a Central Scientific and Research Ethics Committee (CSREC) in the office of the Central Directorate for Research & Health Development (RHD). The Ministerial

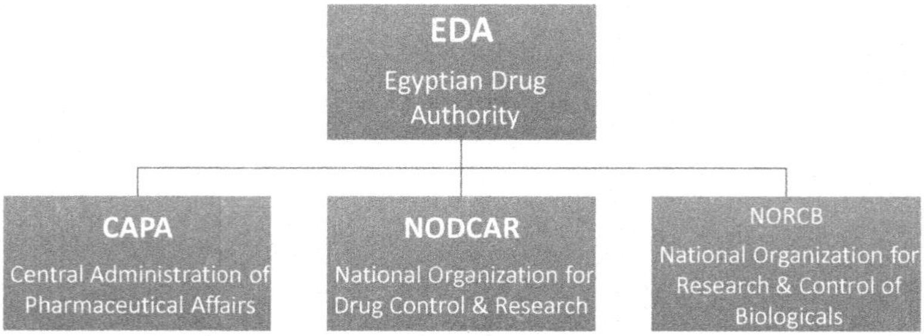

Fig. 1 Organizational structure of the Egyptian Drug Authority

Decree number 95 of 2005 prohibits the conduct of clinical trials before obtaining the approval of the CSREC. This ministerial REC also reviews all Master and Doctorate theses conducted in the governmental hospitals. The Ministerial REC developed its own Standard Operating Procedures (SOPs), as well as guidelines that Egyptian researchers need to follow in their submissions to the REC.

Drug Regulatory Authority

The Egyptian Drug Authority (EDA) is the pharmaceutical regulatory body of the Egyptian Ministry of Health that ensures the safety and quality of medicines, biologicals, medical devices, cosmetics, dietary supplements and pesticides. The EDA has three sub-organizations that work cooperatively and synergistically to assure the achievement of the EDA mission (http://www.eda.mohealth.gov.eg/Articles.aspx?id=4). These include the Central Administration of Pharmaceutical Affairs (CAPA); the National Organization for Drug Control & Research (NODCAR), and the National Organization For research & Control of Biologicals (NORCB) (Fig. 1).

CAPA is a regulatory body that includes four departments as follows:

- Registration Department.
- Licensing and Pharmacists' services Department.
- Inspection and Control Department.
- Importation and Exportation Department.

CAPA gives permission for trial drug importation after it receives the MoHP's CSREC study approval.

NODCAR represents the empowered National Quality Control authority for locally marketed manufactured and imported pharmaceutical products.

NORCB ensures the safety, quality and efficacy of all imported and domestic biologicals in compliance with WHO standards. The Ministry established the NORCB as an official institution to regulate biologicals in close coordination with CAPA. All issued approvals are concurrently communicated to CAPA, MoHP committees as well as to the study sponsor or principal investigator.

Landscape of RECs in Egypt

While the MOH promotes the establishment of research ethics committees (RECs) at the institutional level, no national mandate exists that clearly defines the authority of and the scope of functions of RECs and there is no regulatory body that oversees and regulates the functions of RECs. Instead, all RECs working in Egypt report to their institutional officials, indicating that their mandate comes from a high authority that legitimizes their existence to their peers.

The number of RECs operating in Egypt is more than 50. By searching the OHRP database, 55 RECs are or have been registered as of 2015 (Office for Human Research Protections OHRP 2016). While the establishment of RECs in Egypt has recently increased, the quality and consistency of ethical review remains unclear. Regarding the weaknesses, many RECs do not have adequate financial resources or adequate administrative support personnel. Many of the RECs agree that ongoing challenges include the absence of national ethics guidelines and regularly training of their members, both of which affects their performances. Membership consists mostly of physicians, while lay representation was found to be only 13.7% (Sleem et al. 2010b). The lack of a diversified membership might hinder an objective discussion of the protocol being reviewed and might bias the process towards the interests of researchers versus the interests of research participants.

An Egyptian Network of Research Ethics Committees (ENREC) was established in 2008 to enhance communications between the different RECs in Egypt. As such, it facilitates the exchange of knowledge and the dissemination of teaching materials aiming at optimizing committee functioning. It also helps investigators and their research staff submit their proposals to their respective RECs.

Procedure for Approval of Research and Clinical Trials

Clinical studies in Egypt are regulated by the Central Directorate for Researches and Health Development and operates closely with the Central Scientific and Research Ethics Committee (CSREC) that approves all research.

To begin a clinical trial, a sponsor submits an application to the CSREC and to the REC at the relevant institution where the trial will be conducted, usually a university hospital. Approving clinical trials is a straightforward but lengthy process, as the approval process is sequential: the approval of the department comes first, followed by approval by the institutional REC and finally the CSREC. Each approval serves as a prerequisite for proceeding with the next approval. When exportation of biological samples is involved, the study protocol is submitted concurrently to the national security office within the Ministry of Health for approval.

Status of Research in Egypt

In February 2016 there were 57 active international drug trials in Egypt. Compared to March 2015 and August 2014, based on the same source and using the same methodology, this number represents a slight decrease. Even though the aforementioned timespan is too short to be able to predict future trends, the number seems to have stabilized at around 60 in the past few years.

Even if substantially lower compared to other middle-income economies such as South Africa, China, India and several Latin American countries, the number of active international drug trials suggests that Egypt remains among the favorite destinations for Trans National Corporations (TNCs) to outsource some of their testing. Looking in particular at the two TNCs that run most international drug trials in Egypt at the time of this writing – the Swiss companies Novartis and Roche – one can see that the Arab spring events of early 2011 and its subsequent political unrest did not have a chilling effect on the number of active international drug trials.

Transnational Corporations in Egypt

In February 2016, 21 international pharmaceutical and biotech companies were sponsoring active drug trials in Egypt. The two Swiss giants Novartis and Roche carry out the lion's share of trials. Together, these companies are responsible for almost half of the international drug trials taking place in the country (15 trials or 26% for Novartis, and 13 trials or 23% for Roche). These proportions have remained constant over the past 2 years.

Over half of all international active drug studies in Egypt are cancer trials, followed behind by infectious diseases (10%) and metabolic disorders (10%).

The vast majority (70%) of active international drug trials in Egypt are Phase III trials, with the proportion remaining constant throughout the study period. This finding is not really surprising as the Phase III trials are the ones requiring a larger (statistically significant) number of participants demonstrating efficacy and safety of the treatment, which would thus facilitate obtaining marketing approval.

Conclusions and Recommendations

A fundamental flaw in the Egyptian system of clinical trials is the absence of a comprehensive unified legislation. This means that there is no clear guidance to those bodies charged with conducting or overseeing clinical trials, leaving room for much variability in the conduct of research.

Most of the challenges to the conduct of research relate to the lack of guidance on a national level in terms of standardized research ethics guidelines, lack of standards for operations for research ethics committees, and lack of an accreditation mechanism for RECs. In the absence of accreditation, there is a self-assessment tool that was developed by experts in the Arab region and has been translated in Arabic (Sleem et al. 2010a).

Also needed is the establishment of monitoring and oversight mechanisms for clinical trials, although the Central Directorate for Research and Health Development in the MOH has laid the groundwork to establish a robust oversight system.

References

Office for Human Research Protections OHRP. 2016. Registration of an Institutional Review Board (IRB). Available at: http://www.hhs.gov/ohrp/assurances/

Sleem, H., R. Adelhai, I. Al-Abdallat, M. Al-Naif, H. Gabr, E.T. Kehil, et al. 2010a. Development of an accessible self-assessment tool for research ethics committees in developing countries. *Journal of Empirical Research on Human Research Ethics* 6: 85–96.

Sleem, H., S. El-Kamary, and H.J. Silverman. 2010b. Identifying structures, processes, resources and needs of research ethics committees in Egypt. *BMC Medical Ethics* 11: 12.

Research Ethics Governance in the Arab Region: Lebanon

May M. Al Kassar and Bilal Azakir

Introduction

Lebanon is a low to middle income country situated within the Middle East and the North African region. The country experienced a civil war from 1975 to 1990 and witnessed intermittent disturbances afterwards. Lebanon is usually viewed as an attractive site to conduct clinical trials due to a very short startup time and the availability of many competent physicians (Kumar 2014).

Health Care System

Lebanon has a modern set-up in terms of hospitals' infrastructure and advancements in medical education and in technology, which have enabled Lebanese hospitals to compete with other countries in the region. It is estimated that there are 3.54 doctors per 1,000 people, which is more than double the average in the Arab region. Lebanon spends 8.3% of its GDP on health services (Ammar 2009).

However, the Lebanese health sector is highly fragmented and pluralistic. Widely dominated by the private sector, a total of 163 hospitals contract with the Ministry of Public Health (MoPH), out of which only 28 are public hospitals, representing 16.6% of the total capacity of hospitals in Lebanon (MoPH 2014). Thus, the health care system mainly depends on the highly developed and equipped private hospitals, including a total of 12,648 beds (Private Hospitals Syndicate 2011) distributed

M.M. Al Kassar (✉)
Human Research Protection Program, Weill Cornell Medicine in Qatar, Ar-Rayyan, Qatar

American University of Beirut, Beirut, Lebanon
e-mail: Mak2095@qatar-med.cornell.edu

B. Azakir
Beirut Arab University, Beirut, Lebanon

H. Silverman (ed.), *Research Ethics in the Arab Region*, Research Ethics Forum 5,
https://doi.org/10.1007/978-3-319-65266-5_24

between 80 and 400 beds per hospital. The public sector does not provide more than 10% of Lebanese hospitals capacity; while the Lebanese population health care service is covered by private (social and private insurance) and public providers, (i.e., MoPH and NGOs).

Research Governance

Research Ethics Regulations/Guidelines

Regulations specific for research ethics in Lebanon do not exist, although there are several laws that include multiple provisions pertaining to the conduct of clinical research (UNESCO 2011). The code of medical ethics, law no. 288, for example, was introduced in 1994 and further amended in 2012 under law no. 240 (Code of Medical Ethics 1994). This law, in general, regulates medical practice of physicians in Lebanon and promotes patients' rights.

Article no. 30 of this law includes regulations pertaining to human experiments and clinical research. For example, research requires approval of a hospital ethics committee; informed consent should be obtained from research participants or parents or legal representative for the participation of minors or incapacitated persons; experimental drugs are to be registered at the MoPH; and research participants should receive drugs free of charge. The article also recommends the necessity of establishing an ethics committee at each medical center to follow-up on clinical research.

The Pharmacy Practice law no. 367 (11/8/1994) states in article 55 that only teaching hospitals in Lebanon are allowed to conduct clinical research involving medications. The Ministry further clarified this article by a decree no. 569/2 (December 4, 1996) that limited the conduct of clinical research to teaching hospitals or hospitals affiliated with a medical school (Hamra 2014).

The National Lebanese Consultative Committee on Ethics, (Comité Consultatif National Libanais d'Ethique (CCNLE)) was established in 2001 to provide recommendations regarding research ethical issues (Prime Minister decision No. 63/2001). Since then, the committee passed several laws regulating research. For example, Law No. 574 (dated February 11, 2004) emphasized patients' rights and required informed written consent from research participants. Article 11 of this law makes a clear distinction between consent for clinical treatment and that for clinical research. For example, it emphasizes the following: (a) necessity of voluntary participation in clinical research and necessity of having a documented consent, (b) the need for prior approval from an ethics committee that ensures rigorous scientific background of the research and adherence to ethical principles, (c) requirement of parental consent for minor subjects and that of the legal representative for incapacitated subjects, and (d) consent from a trustworthy person appointed by the subject if the latter is in a state that prohibits him/her from expressing his will. The law also underscored that participation in research must not present actual risk to the participant's welfare and should offer a therapeutic benefit (Act on Patients' Rights and Informed

Consent 2004). This specific requirement, however, would seriously restrict the conduct of many clinical trials if the provision of a therapeutic benefit in research is interpreted strictly.

In 2004, Law no. 625 was passed, which regulated genetic testing for clinical and research purposes (Act on Human Genetic Testing 2004). This law emphasized the rights of individuals undergoing genetic testing or screening. It stresses voluntary consent and prohibits exerting any coercion or any undue influence to acquire such testing (Act on Human Genetic Testing 2004).

The Lebanese MoPH noticed the increase in clinical trials due to the increase in the availability of teaching hospitals, the increase number of researchers interested in conducting clinical trials and the interest of sponsors in conducting research in a LMIC such as Lebanon. It wanted to avoid having Lebanon as an "open market" for all types of clinical research due to the absence of laws regulating clinical research. Accordingly, in 2012, the Ministry took several steps to strengthen the ethical and regulatory oversight of clinical trials while waiting for the Parliament to issue a relevant law for research. For example, the Ministry issued memo no. 27 (April 20, 2012) and memo no. 72 (September 14, 2012) that enforced the registration of clinical trials in Lebanon and requested hospitals involved in clinical trials to submit the following documents to the Ministry for each clinical trial: the clinical research protocol, the REC approval, and the principal investigator declaration that the study is done under his/her direct supervision. Additionally, the Ministry established a national committee that would be responsible for suggesting mechanisms for the regulation of clinical trials (Hamra 2014).

In 2014, the MoPH, in consultation with the Council of State and based on the recommendation of the National Lebanese Consultative Committee on Ethics, issued a ministerial decree (1159/1) based on the law (No. 274, dated April 15, 2015) of the pharmacy practice law. Article 2 of this decree emphasized the Good Clinical Practice and ethical principles in Helsinki Declaration for clinical trials carried out by hospitals in Lebanon. Articles 3 and 4 specified the prior need of an approval from the hospital ethics committee and a request for study drug importation at the MoPH following the ministerial decree (2257/2) regulating drugs importation for research use (issued on December 4, 2015).

While the decree 1159/1 laid down the foundation for clinical trials in Lebanon, the roles and functions of RECs remained unclear. As such, in December 2014, the MoPH issued a ministerial decree (2286/1) to regulate RECs in Lebanon. This decree was developed to give guidance to hospitals and universities who have their own RECs on the requirements needed by the Lebanese MoPH to be officially authorized and allowed to review and oversee the ethical aspects of research that involve human subjects. Article 1 of this decree specified that any health institution conducting medical research required approval from an established and registered REC. Hospitals desiring to pursue research but lacked an REC would need to affiliate with a hospital or an institution that has a registered REC. Reliance agreements between the institutions would need to be submitted to the committee at MOPH for approval.

Article 2 of Decree 2286/1 specified that research had to comply with the following requirements: (a) proposed research requires a scientific basis and clear objectives; (b) use of an investigational product requires prior demonstration of safety; (c) the potential benefits of research must outweigh the risks; (d) informed consent needs to be secured from research subjects after adequate disclosure of the study procedures, the objectives of the research, and any risks or discomfort that might arise from participation; (e) subjects have the right to withdraw from a research study at any stage; (f) minor subjects and others who lack the capacity to consent should not be recruited to research without permission from their legal guardians and the dissent of these subjects need to be respected; (g) confidentiality of research data needs to be safeguarded and privacy needs to be respected; (h) funding is required to cover all expenses of research treatments and procedures; and (i) insurance is required to cover treatment of study adverse events and indemnification for research injury.

This decree also regulated the operations of RECs. It specified that the role of RECs was to ensure that research adheres to principles highlighted by the ministry that aim to protect the rights and welfare of research participants. RECs are required to submit registration and provide other documents demonstrating having met minimum required criteria. These included: standard operating procedures, a statement clarifying its responsibilities and funding sources; the membership roster and the appointment period, the specialty and expertise of members and their conditions of appointments; the policies and guidelines to be followed by the REC in its review; the mechanism of conducting meetings; the mechanism for its decisions and the requirements of quorum; and lastly, the mechanism of disseminating their decisions. A committee at the MoPH was established to review the registration documents.

REC membership required the following representation: (a) three physicians from the institution and one unaffiliated physician i, (b) a social worker and a member with legal expertise, and (c) three community members from the same geographic area where the institution resides. The membership appointments may be executed for 4 years and the committee has to elect a chair and a treasurer. All records of meeting minutes and determinations are required to be kept on file. The committee may request consultants to join its meeting for expert opinions, yet consultants should not be given voting rights. The decision of the committee needs to be taken by voting with no voting rights for the researcher or the study sponsor or right to appeal the REC decision in order to avoid conflict of interest.

Following the decree (2286/1), the MoPH issued an amendment (Decree No. 141/1 December 27, 2016). Article 10 mandated all hospitals and centers that aim to conduct clinical studies and research involving human subjects to comply with decree No. 141/1. Hospitals and centers need to apply to MoPH to recognize officially their REC prior to January 2017; the Ministry will not agree to any clinical study after this date.

Hereby is a list of universities and hospitals that have submitted applications for recognition of ethics committees for clinical trials affiliate and applications that have been studied and approved (Table 1).

Table 1 List of Universities and Hospitals REC submitted, studied or approved by the MoPH (April, 2017)

Submitted RECs	Studied RECs	Approved RECs
1. Saint Joseph University/ Hotel-Dieu Hospital	1. Saint Joseph University/ Hotel-Dieu Hospital	1. Saint Joseph University/ Hotel-Dieu Hospital
2. Rafik Hariri University Hospital	2. Rafik Hariri University Hospital	2. Rafik Hariri University Hospital
3. Lebanese American University/Rizk Hospital	3. Lebanese American University/Rizk Hospital	3. Lebanese American University/Rizk Hospital
4. Hammoud University Hospital	4. Hammoud University Hospital	4. Hammoud University Hospital
5. Balamand/University of St. George University Hospital	5. Balamand/University of St. George University Hospital	5. Balamand/University of St. George University Hospital
6. Bellevue Medical Center and University Hospital	6. Bellevue Medical Center and University Hospital	6. Bellevue Medical Center and University Hospital
7. Nini Hospital	7. Nini Hospital	7. Ain and Zain Hospital
8. Clemenceau Hospital	8. Clemenceau Hospital	8. Makassed General Hospital
9. Mount Lebanon Hospital	9. Mount Lebanon Hospital	9. Jeitwi University Hospital
10. Ain and Zain Hospital	10. Ain and Zain Hospital	10. Beirut Arab University
11. Makassed General Hospital	11. Makassed General Hospital	11. American University of Beirut
12. Jeitwi University Hospital	12.Jeitwi University Hospital	12. Cross Hospital for Lam Land Mental and Psychological
13. Heart of Jesus Hospital	15. Beirut Arab University	
14. Beirut Arab University	16.American University of Beirut	
15. American University of Beirut	17. Permanent Care center	
16. Permanent Care center	18. Our Lady of Succour University Hospital	
17. Our Lady of Succour University Hospital	19. Cross Hospital for Lam Land mental and psychological	
18. Cross Hospital for Lam Land mental and psychological		
19. Middle East Health Center		

RECs were also charged with verifying the qualifications of researchers and the presence of proper infrastructure at the institution where the clinical research will be conducted; approving research studies in accordance with established standards, such as the ICH-GCP; and reviewing research protocols in compliance with WHO standards and operational guidance for ethics review of human related research (World Health Organization 2011).

While these decrees regulate clinical research in Lebanon, it does not have the force of law that can impose punishment due to non-compliance. In addition, establishing a system of oversight for RECs was not addressed by these decrees; and provisions specifying safeguards for vulnerable groups, such as pregnant women, prisoners and refugees, were lacking. Moreover, all existing decrees were drafted to govern biomedical clinical research with no attention to social and behavioral research. As such, there are no rules governing observational research or studies that incur no more than minimal risk.

Although all the above regulatory decrees emphasized the requirement of informed consent, specific listing of required elements to be present in the consent document is absent. Consequently, informed consent documents may consist of few sentences to several pages. Also, a study by Ghandour and colleagues evaluated the consenting practice involving Lebanese university students when they were asked to participate in an online research survey related to sexuality and sexual practices among youth (Ghandour et al. 2013). Students gave consent to the survey without being informed about the topic and the content of the survey. The study showed that 65% of students provided their consent within the first 30 s, whereas 90% of them provided their consent in less than the minimum expected time (Ghandour et al. 2013). In view of this one study and the lack of regulations detailing the required elements of informed consent, follow up studies are warranted to determine the perceptions pertaining to informed consents and the extent of disclosure in the consent forms.

National Authorities

Ministry of Public Health

The vision of the MoPH is "to build an integrated, people centered, health system that promotes and sustains the highest attainable health status of the population, through ensuring a universal health coverage, while addressing the social determinants of health" (MOPH website 2017). The MoPH is in charge of providing proposals for laws and decrees. It has a wide scope of responsibilities that include issuing certifications for medical professions and health facilities; initiating quality control activities and many other services that may have implications on research. Nevertheless, there is no identified department that handles specific matters related to regulating research or overseeing research.

The MoPH also serves as drug regulatory authority. It is responsible, for instance, for drug industry management and control, medicinal imports and exports, drug registration and control, inspectional activities and controlling fraud in the pharmaceutical industry.

Presently, Lebanon lacks a national body that provides oversight of RECs. The requirement of REC registration was introduced in 2014; yet there is no entity established to ensure compliance of RECs to ethical standards and oversee their operations due to lack of logistics and staff members at the MoPH. Therefore, oversight of RECs is lacking and hence, the practice of existing RECs is not uniform. It is rather a self- selected operation based on the preference of each institution.

For example, several RECs have adopted the US regulations as a base for their functions, whereas others follow the ICH-GCP guidelines. Such variations can lead to different ethical assessments by the RECs for the same research studies.

Landscape of RECs in Lebanon

RECs in Lebanon had largely operated without any defined framework until the MoPH issued its decree in 2014 (see above), which was mandated by its 2016 decree.

Examples of operating RECs in Lebanon are as follows:

1. The Rafik Hariri University Hospital (RHUH) is a public institution that offers medical services to Lebanese citizens. Research at RHUH is very attractive to sponsors due to its providing services to a unique population, as it is the only public tertiary care center in Beirut. The REC operates in a manner consistent with ICH GCP guidelines and its membership complies with the membership requirements of 2014 Ministerial decree. RHUH physicians usually attend training sessions organized by local and global CROs (Rafik Hariri University Hospital website, 2015)
2. The American University of Beirut (AUB) is an institution of higher education, chartered in New York State in 1863. The institution has a Federal Wide Assurance (FWA) with the Office of Human Research Protection (OHRP) in the US Department of Health and Human Services (DHHS). The REC at AUB was established in 1996 and operates in a manner consistent with 45.CFR.46 regulations and FDA regulations for clinical investigations (American University of Beirut Website, 2015).
3. The Lebanese American University (LAU) is a private higher education institution. The university has a Federal Wide Assurance (FWA) with OHRP. The membership of the REC is constituted in accordance with the US Code of Federal Regulation 45CFR 46.107, 21CFR 56.107, and Good Clinical Practice ICH Section 3. The responsibility of this committee is to review research projects involving human subjects conducted at LAU and the University Medical Center – Rizk Hospital (UMCRH) (Lebanese American University website, 2015).
4. The Faculty of Medicine at the University of Saint Joseph was created in 1888. Its ethics committee was established at Hotel Dieu de France hospital (HDF) in 1998. The committee consists of members from HDF and external members. The Chair of the Board of Directors at HDF (Hotel Dieu de France website, 2015) appoints the members.
5. Beirut Arab University is a private institution for higher education founded in 1960. The REC was established in 2012 and has adopted international guidelines including Nuremberg code, Helsinki, and Belmont declaration and follows "Ethical Principles and Guidelines for the Protection of Human Subjects of Research" for its human research protection program (Beirut Arab University Website 2017)

Status of Research in Lebanon

Lebanon has been one of the leaders in the conduct of clinical trials since 1990. The number of studies with an open status at clinicaltrials.gov in April 2017 exceeded that of many countries in the Arab region, including Kuwait, Qatar, UAE and Jordan and surpassed only by Egypt and Saudi Arab Kingdom (Clinicaltrial.gov website, 2017). The number of clinical trials conducted in Lebanon has increased steadily from 40 in 2007, 54 in 2008, 68 in 2009, 103 in 2010, 123 trials in 2011, 153 in 2012 to 187 in 2013 (Younes 2014). According to clinicaltrials.gov, in April 2017, there were 323 clinical trials registered in Lebanon (Table 2). Since July 2014, approximately 200 clinical trials were registered at MoPH, mostly Phase III, although all research is open to all different phases of clinical trials.

Many of the clinical trials sites have the highest recruitment worldwide, and in many instances, Lebanon is considered by many sponsors a "rescue" site for ongoing clinical trials due to several advantages (Younes 2014). For example, many sites demonstrate a high recruitment rate, which is probably due to a strong trust relationship between patients and physicians. There is also a lack of health insurance coverage for many individuals and hence lack of access to high quality medical care, which contributes to a desire for individuals to participate in clinical trials. That being said, these characteristics present potential concerns in regards to therapeutic misconception and undue inducement, respectively.

Procedure for Approval of Research and Clinical Trials

In contrast to other countries that operate with a central or national ethics committee that grants ethics approval, in Lebanon there are no requirements for a review or approval for clinical trial protocols by the MoPH. However, the MoPH retains the right to reject, hold, or terminate any clinical trial that does not follow the preceding laws and decrees.

The usual timeline for lunching a clinical trial in Lebanon ranges from 2 to 4 months. This timeline includes approval by local ethics committees and obtaining the drug import license. The Ministry of Public Health is the authority regulating the process of obtaining the import license of drugs. When the drug is already a

Table 2 Status of clinical trials registered in Lebanon according to clinicaltrial.gov in 2017

Status of clinical trial	Number
Completed	170
Recruiting	80
Active not recruiting	27
Terminated	21
Unknown	19
Withdrawn	3
Not yet recruiting	2
Approved for marketing	1

registered product, obtaining an import license goes through the usual process without requiring any additional requirements. However, when the drug is an investigational product, approval from the MOPH is required (Kumar 2014). The process of obtaining import license is estimated to be 2 months (Younes 2014).

Conclusion and Recommendations

In Lebanon, deficiencies exist in terms of having sufficient laws addressing basic aspects of human subjects' protection. Potential liability of institutions and researchers for complying with ethical standards falls in a grey area due to the absence of a specialized body that sets rules and regulations and oversees the conduct of research. As such, we propose the following:

1. More detailed regulations that standardize the ethical practice of research across the country. As opposed to general international regulations, country specific regulations would take into consideration the local context and the Arab culture and norms. Once laws are established, different institutions may develop their own standard operating procedures that are specific to their institutions, while still in compliance with national regulations.
2. Establishment of a national regulatory oversight body: A national entity is needed to provide oversight of research. Such an entity would assure compliance of institutions and provide oversight to RECs. An essential component of its mandate would be monitoring REC operations and the conduct of research.
3. Setting of national research priorities: Assessing research studies at a central level before going through the process of ethical review at the site of implementation would ensure that research is in alignment with national priorities. This evaluation will help filter research studies based on the country needs and priorities, and restrict implementation of high risk clinical trials to specific sites.
4. Registering clinical trials to track all clinical trials being performed in the country serves to manage research studies and monitor data safety. A central bureau tasked to register clinical trials would provide for the public disclosure of active research in order to capitalize on expanding benefits to a bigger proportion of our communities. MoPH is ready to launch a national registry for clinical trials in Lebanon in collaboration with and following the WHO standards.
5. Organizing and regulating the work of CROs and pharmaceutical companies: The number of CROs is increasing in Lebanon, which represents a natural phenomenon since the market of research is expanding. A major drawback with these CROs is the current lack of regulations that ensure their accountability. Regulating these entities, the mode of their operation and setting requirements for the qualifications of their personnel are key factors to ensure good quality research. Developing and updating laws to regulate importing, storing, distributing and transporting investigational drugs are an absolute necessity.

Although the steps outlined above will require a huge amount of time, effort and resources, such a journey is needed to enhance the protection of the rights and welfare of our people.

References

Ammar, W. 2009. Health beyond politics. WHO and Ministry of Public Health in Lebanon.

Ghandour, L., R. Yasmine, and F. El-Kak. 2013. Giving consent without getting informed: A cross-cultural issue in research ethics. *Journal of Empirical Research on Human Research Ethics* 8 (3): 12–21. https://doi.org/10.1525/jer.2013.8.3.12.

Hamra, R. 2014. Role of the ministry of public health in clinical research in Lebanon: History, present situation, and plans for the future. *Human & Health* 28: 8–9.

Kumar, A.S. 2014. Lebanon watch. *Journal for Clinical Studies* 5 (6): 28–29.

UNESCO. 2011. Ethics and law in biomedicine and genetics. An overview of the national regulations in the Arab States. Accessed at: http://unesdoc.unesco.org/images/0021/002152/215207E.pdf

World Health Organization. 2011. *Standards and operational guidance for ethics review of health-related research with human participants*. Available at: http://www.who.int/ethics/research/en/.

Younes, A. 2014. Conducting clinical studies in Lebanon. *Journal for Clinical Studies* 6 (2): 36–38.

Health Research, Regulations and Ethics in the United Arab Emirates

Satish Chandrasekhar Nair, Farida Al Marzooqi, and Aisha Al Khamiri

Introduction

The Gulf Cooperation Countries (GCC) represents a political and economic union of six Arab states bordering the Persian Gulf, consisting of the United Arab Emirates, Bahrain, Qatar, Kuwait, Oman and Saudi Arabia. The GCC ranks high in economic growth and has a modern infrastructure, associated with a small population size. Conversely, the other countries in the Arab region have relatively undeveloped infrastructure associated with a larger population living in economic poverty. The GCC accounts for less than 10% of the population in the Arab region (Nair et al. 2013; The World Bank 2016).

The United Arab Emirates, a member country of the GCC, is a confederation of seven emirates, Abu Dhabi is the largest emirate and is the capital. The other emirates, in descending order of size, includes Dubai, Sharjah, Ras Al Khaima, Fujairah and Umm Al Qwain. The UAE has a population of 9.2 million, consisting of predominantly expatriates who represent multiple different nationalities, languages and cultures. UAE nationals account for 19% of the total population (Nair et al. 2013; The World Bank 2016). The per capita income is among the top 10 countries of the world (The World Bank 2016). Economic prosperity followed the discovery of oil and natural gas almost 45 years ago. Despite the spike in the number of publications in recent years addressing public health and the business of healthcare (The World Bank 2016; Colliers International 2013; Loney et al. 2013), a systematic review of

S.C. Nair (✉)
Departments of Academic Affairs and Internal Medicine Residency Program, Tawam Hospital in Affiliation with Johns Hopkins Medicine USA, P.O. Box 15258, Al Ain, UAE
e-mail: schandra@seha.ae; satchi2000@outlook.com

F. Al Marzooqi • A. Al Khamiri
Internal Medicine Resident, Tawam Hospital, Abu Dhabi, UAE

H. Silverman (ed.), *Research Ethics in the Arab Region*, Research Ethics Forum 5,
https://doi.org/10.1007/978-3-319-65266-5_25

health regulations, research infrastructure, and ethics regulations has been long overdue. Herein, we aim to close the gap through this review.

Healthcare System

Healthcare services is regulated by the Ministry of Health (MOH), which also operates more than one-third of hospitals in the country (Colliers International 2013). Depending on the emirate, the operational functions of the MOH are delegated to the local health regulators, such as the Health Authority Abu Dhabi (HAAD), Dubai Health Authority (DHA), the Sharjah Health Authority (SHA), the Ajman Health Authority (Ajman), Umm Al Qwain Healthcare, Ras Al Khaima Municipality – Public Health and Environment and the Fujairah Municipality- Public Health and Environment (Colliers International 2013).

According to the World Bank, health expenditure has escalated from 2.6% in 1995 to 3.6% in 2016 as a percentage of total Gross Domestic Product (GDP) (The World Bank 2016). The distribution of public and private hospitals is uneven. The majority of the hospitals (63%, 66/104) are private-owned and the remainder are public hospitals (37%, 38/104), although more than three-quarters of the total beds are in the public hospitals (Colliers International 2013). However, by 2008 the National Health Council established a more efficient system of coordination between the different health care providers across the country, including the private sectors (Koornneef et al. 2012). The government has continuously strived to ensure that healthcare facilities are equipped with technologically-advanced equipment for the diagnosis and treatment of diseases to sustain the optimum quality of health and wellbeing of the population. The health authorities verify the qualification, experience, competence and licensing of the healthcare providers to meet the expectations of high quality healthcare service delivery (Colliers International 2013; U.S.-U.A.E. Business Council 2016). Key performance indicators, to assure effectiveness and efficiency in delivering healthcare services, are continuously measured by the regulators (Colliers International 2013; U.S.-U.A.E. Business Council 2016).

Affiliation with western managed healthcare organizations, such as Mayo Clinic, Cleveland Clinic, Johns Hopkins Medicine International, Bumrungrad International and University of Vienna, to name a few, was initiated in 2005 to transform healthcare to modern practices (Colliers International 2013; U.S.-U.A.E. Business Council 2016). Effective 2007, health insurance coverage was made mandatory in the emirate of Abu Dhabi and recently enforced in Dubai (Colliers International 2013; U.S.-U.A.E. Business Council 2016). The Daman insurance provider is the leading insurance company in the country in addition to various others such as Abu Dhabi National Insurance Company and Saudi Arabian Cooperative Insurance Company. Malaffi hospital information system provides exchange of health information across the various public hospitals (U.S.-U.A.E. Business Council 2016). The federal medical liability law governs the practice of healthcare in the UAE. The law (Law number 10, 2008) was recently modified (Law number 4, 2016) to accommodate stringent patient safety measures and to enhance medical practice accountability (Hajat et al. 2012).

Disease Spectrum

The healthcare market continues to grow in the UAE, primarily due to the growing demand from urbanization, an increasing population, and an increase in chronic diseases previously uncommon to the region (Al Sarraj et al. 2015; Hajat et al. 2012). Cultural and genetic differences within the local populations offer unique opportunities for medical research. Genetic and congenital defects are high given the high rate of consanguinity and lack of prenatal genetic screening (Hamamy n.d.; El-Hajj Fuleihan 2009; Al-Rawi and Al-Tajir 2012). Inherited hematological disorders, including sickle cell anemia and thalassemia, have mandated pre-marriage screening by the government (Hamamy n.d.; El-Hajj Fuleihan 2009; Al-Rawi and Al-Tajir 2012). Hypovitaminosis D, in spite of the abundant sunshine, is among the highest in the world (Hamamy n.d.; El-Hajj Fuleihan 2009; Al-Rawi and Al-Tajir 2012). Nearly one-quarter of the population is obese, adding high risk for hyperlipidemia, hypertension, diabetes and coronary heart disease (Aljefree and Ahmed 2015). The three major non-communicable diseases such as cardiovascular disease, cancer and diabetes contribute to the vast majority of deaths in the country. Not surprising, the UAE has the second highest prevalence of diabetes in the world (18.7%) compared to the global average of 6.4% (Sreedharan et al. 2015). The Government's Vision 2021 lists cardiovascular diseases, diabetes, child obesity and

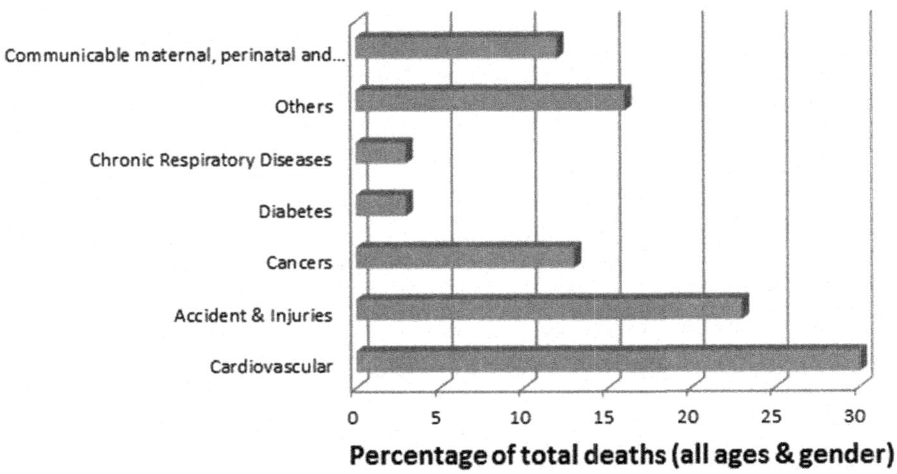

Fig. 1 The three major non-communicable diseases, cardiovascular disease, cancer and diabetes, contribute to the vast majority of deaths in the UAE (Adapted from http://www.who.int/nmh/countries/are_en.pdf?ua=1)

cancer as among the top 5 health priorities (UAE Vision 2021, Fig. 1). The high prevalence of genetic and metabolic diseases make the UAE an ideal location for the conduct of clinical research.

Research Governance

The surge in clinical research and clinical trial activities in the UAE in the past few years has encouraged the need to develop an effective regulatory framework. Health research governance in the UAE, summarized in Fig. 2, can be classified into six categories: (1) regulations and guidelines, (2) national authorities; (3) research ethics committees; (4) financial transparency, (5) compliance audits, and (6) training.

Regulations and Guidelines

The UAE Medical Liability Law No. 10 (2016) (8) prohibits medical research involving human participants unless a license is obtained from one of the following bodies, as per their jurisdiction:

- Dubai Health Authority
- Dubai Healthcare City Authority

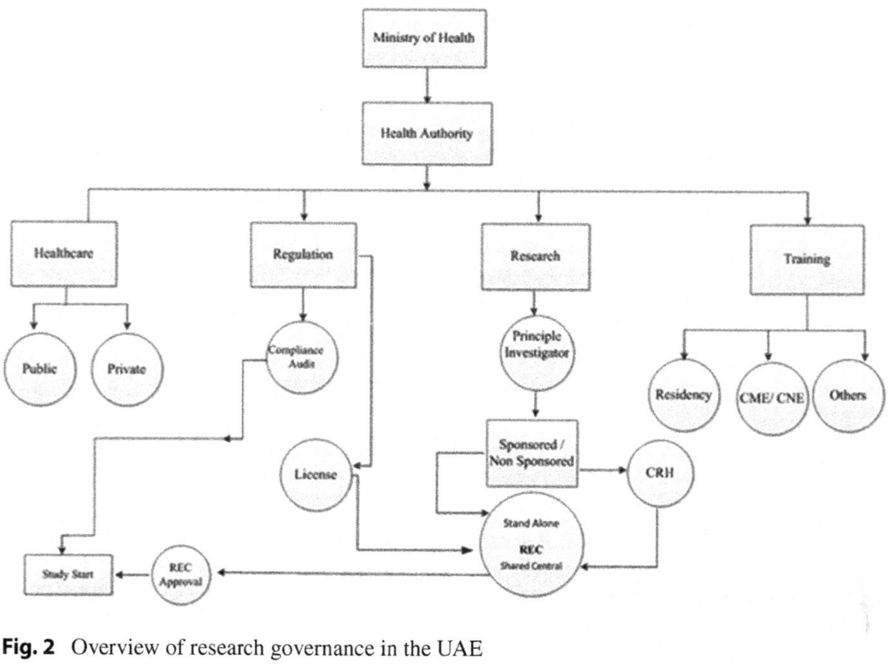

Fig. 2 Overview of research governance in the UAE

- Ministry of Health
- Abu Dhabi Health Authority
- Public Universities

The MOH requires that the International Conference on Harmonization and Good Clinical Practice (ICH-GCP) guidelines to be followed for all types of human research in the UAE (Ibrahim et al. 2006).

National Authorities

Similar to the health sector, health research is governed by the MOH and the delegated health authorities in each emirate (Nair et al. 2013), of which the Dubai Health Authority and the Health Authority of Abu Dhabi (HAAD) are considered important regulatory authorities for the different centres where research will be performed (Kumar 2015)

Every clinical trial involving a new investigational drug requires to be registered with the MOH for drug importation procedures. The MOH in the UAE requires a provisional approval by a research ethics committee before granting approval for drug importation. Study sponsors, such as pharmaceutical sponsors, are required to adhere to specific labelling, licensing, and expiration and shipping requirements (Nair et al. 2013; Nair and Ibrahim 2015a). The overall approval time for investigational new drug importation, from the initial submission of the protocol to the research ethics committee to the first patient enrolment takes nearly 3 months (Nair et al. 2013; Nair and Ibrahim 2015a).

Dubai Health Authority

The Dubai Health Authority's Medical Research Committee (MRC) acts as the research ethics committee at Dubai Health Authority. The primary objective of the MRC is to protect the mental and physical welfare, rights, dignity and safety of participants in research, to facilitate ethical research through efficient and effective review processes, to promote ethical standards of human research, and to review research in accordance with the DHA code of ethics and the ICH-GCP guidelines, ensuring that all such investigations conform to ethical principles including those described in the Declaration of Helsinki (Kumar 2015).

Health Authority Abu Dhabi (HAAD)

HAAD has established research policies, standards, and the governance structure to oversee regulation of human subjects research in Abu Dhabi (HAAD). The Abu Dhabi Health Research Council (HRC) is the governing body established by HAAD to supervise health research. HAAD-licensed health care facilities must receive HAAD authorization to conduct human subjects research. Authorization requires:

- Approval from a Research Ethics Committee.
- Report of research to HAAD annually (or upon request).

- An application for Authorization to Conduct Human Subjects Research.

The Mission of HAAD's Medical Research Section is to promote world-class research that improves health and quality of life for all people in the Emirate of Abu Dhabi, while ensuring the conduct of ethical research and the protection of the rights and welfare of human subjects. The Medical Research Section facilitates the work of the Abu Dhabi Health Research Council, the Abu Dhabi Research Ethics Committee (ADREC), and the Scientific Peer Review Committees (PRCs). The Medical Research Section helps to develop the Abu Dhabi Health Research Strategy, define research ethics policies and standards, create research funding/grant administration procedures, apply evaluation methods, and measure key performance indicators of Abu Dhabi's progress in health research (Kumar 2015).

In the UAE, the Clinical Research Organizations (CROs) foster a bridge between the pharmaceutical sponsor, investigator and the study site (Nair et al. 2013; Nair and Ibrahim 2015a). The CROs are not required to be licensed in the UAE, however in the emirate of Abu Dhabi, Tawam hospital has made it mandatory for CROs and sponsors to be registered. Similarly, all sponsored studies are required to have third-party insurance coverage for participants to protect them from the study related hazards (Nair et al. 2013; Nair and Ibrahim 2015a).

Research Ethics Committees

The MOH prescribes Standard Operating Procedures (SOP) in accordance with the ICH-GCP standards for the research ethics committees (REC) in the UAE (Ibrahim et al. 2006). Accordingly, each REC provides research ethical review, approval, and study oversight in accordance with the GCP (Nair and Ibrahim 2015a). A recent nationwide study examined the structure, function and operations of the RECs (Abdulrahman and Nair 2017). A total of 21 individual RECs distributed in the different emirates in the UAE (including a central REC in the Al Ain region of Abu Dhabi) provide ethics oversight over all the health facilities and academic institutions in the UAE (Abdulrahman and Nair 2017). Almost all RECs (90%) follow ICH-GCP guidelines, 67% have been in operation for more than 5 years, and proposals are reviewed for scientific and ethical merit within 8 weeks from protocol submission (Abdulrahman and Nair 2017). The remainder 10% of the RECs that do not follow ICG-GCP guidelines are housed in academic institutions and are involved in basic science research. None of the RECs provide financial compensation for their members to review a research protocol (Abdulrahman and Nair 2017).

A clinical research hub (CRH) is engineered within the hospitals and academic health centers in the emirate of Abu Dhabi (Tawam hospital), accredited by the Joint Commission. The CRH serves as an interface between the investigators and the central RECs (one central REC for the Al Ain Medical District) to promote ethical research. The Al Ain Medical District Human Research Ethics Committee is the only central committee in the eastern region of Abu Dhabi. The Mafraq REC caters to the western region of the emirate of Abu Dhabi. – The CRH facilitates verification of investigator credentials, feasibility of the research proposal, funding transparency, conflicts of interest, ethics training and compliance with local, national laws and international guidelines including Joint Commission. The CRH model has been hugely successful to ensure regulatory oversight and patient protection compliance for research studies, especially for clinical trials that are otherwise left for supervision by the pharmaceutical sponsors (Nair and Ibrahim 2015a; Abdulrahman and Nair 2017).

Each of the RECs in the UAE establish their own specific research policies and standards. For example, the RECs in the emirate of Abu Dhabi are required to be licensed by the HAAD and is renewable annually. RECs are also licensed by the Dubai Health Authority. As such, there is heterogeneity among the RECs in terms of requirements and evaluations, patient information and consent document, and investigator qualifications. The application requirements and processes are also different between these two emirates. Specifically, there are some discrepancies in the approaches of different ethics committees as regards inclusion and exclusion criteria, and some ethics committees require applicants to have certificates in research (e.g. GCP). As such, there is a need for a common regulatory framework to establish harmonization among the RECs in the UAE. The need to formally establishing a central IRB in the UAE has met with resistance among the stakeholders due to the lack of clinical and patient protection expertise in the country.

Financial Transparency

Research in the UAE is funded predominantly by academic grants (61%, non-sponsored studies), pharmaceutical sponsorships (28%, sponsored studies) and the remainder through other vehicles, such as endowments. A clinical study agreement between the study site, investigator, CROs and the sponsor of research is mandatory for studies involving external sponsors. The clinical study agreement is a legal document that ensures the roles and responsibility of all the study stakeholders, verified for both ethical and legal implications in the UAE. Scope, duration, risks, benefits, study budget, terms of payment, number of patient visits, data sharing, data protection, insurance and indemnification for participants as coverage towards study related adverse events are some highlights of the clinical study agreement. As such, sponsors of research studies are therefore required to transfer funds to the institution study site/corporate account. The study site in turn distributes the funds to the investigators as "investigator fees." Similarly, study coordinators, research nurses and other support staff are remunerated for research activities over and beyond normal working hours. Almost one-third of the total study budget as detailed in the clinical study agreement, is allocated for overhead costs by the study sites. Study extensions and amendments also entail a nominal fee, directly credited to the study-site accounts. Government-run, public hospitals, with a variety of specialties, infrastructure and patients are the major beneficiaries of sponsored research funds. A recent report indicates that less than 50% of the research sites and RECs have enforced research funding transparency systems (Abdulrahman and Nair 2017).

Compliance Audit

The health authorities such as the Dubai Health and the Abu Dhabi Health Authority, require mandatory reporting of clinical research activities (Nair et al. 2013, 2016; Nair and Ibrahim 2014, 2015a). Research projects, especially clinical trials that pose more than minimal risk, may be subjected to ethical approval by the REC. Although clinical research and clinical trials are relatively new to the UAE, significant measures have been adopted to protect patient privacy and data confidentiality (Nair and Ibrahim 2015b). This is particularly important given the national law to protect and preserve patient medical records of UAE nationals for their lifetime and the non-nationals for up to 7 years after the last clinic visit (Nair and Ibrahim 2015b). Cultural aspects of research subject privacy and data confidentiality in the UAE has been examined (Nair and Ibrahim 2015b). Assessment of the informed consents compliance against GCP guidelines indicated that elements involving subject understanding of the risks and benefits of research participation both for clinical trials and genetic studies, needed improvement (Nair and Ibrahim 2014, 2015a; Nair et al. 2016). Informed consent readability challenges encountered by the research participants have also been accounted in the UAE (Nair and Ibrahim 2014, 2015a; Nair et al. 2016;).

Training in Research and Research Ethics

The health authorities require Good Clinical Practice training certification for physicians and other health care providers prior to obtaining ethical approval for a research study in the UAE (Ibrahim et al. 2006). Pharmaceutical sponsors have constantly provided GCP training for their investigators and support staff engaged in sponsoring research in the UAE (Sponsor Training n.d.; Sleem et al. 2010). Although there are several providers for GCP and research training in the UAE, a systematic iterated learning model to train health care providers, especially physicians engaged in research is still lacking (Abdulrahman and Nair 2017). The global providers of research training have met with limited success in the UAE because of largely overlooking the impact of regional, cultural and social factors and, constantly changing research and regulations (Kripalani et al. 2006). The emirate of Abu Dhabi piloted a home grown training program to train medical residents (Tawam hospital) in research in 2015 (Al Marzooqi et al. 2016). The program, accredited by the Abu Dhabi health authority, called Abu Dhabi Clinical Research Excellence Development for Innovation and Technology (ACREDIT), addressed the basic to advanced level research needs of medical residents (Al Marzooqi et al.

2016). Major modules of the ACREDIT program include data understanding, research design, protocol development, patient protection, ethics, regulations and statistics. The success of the ACREDIT program among medical residents was measured by the number of research projects started by the resident and research publications in journals with good impact and presentations at international conferences (Abdulrahman and Nair 2017; Al Marzooqi et al. 2016). Participant satisfaction, accreditation body support and social media discussions by the participants about ACREDIT helped to expand the scope of the program to include physicians, pharmacists and others (Abdulrahman and Nair 2017; Al Marzooqi et al. 2016). The recent accreditation inspection by the ACGME-I alluded to the contributions made by ACREDIT to enhance research in Abu Dhabi (Abdulrahman and Nair 2017; Al Marzooqi et al. 2016).

Status of Research in the UAE

Research involving human subjects is relatively new to the UAE. Table 1 shows that less than 0.2% of the global human health research publications is contributed by the UAE. Historically, human research studies in this region have not been properly identified as such, but rather considered quality improvement initiatives until 2005 (Nair and Ibrahim 2015b). Still, basic science and behavioral studies contributed to the bulk of human research in the country until 2011. Since 2012, there has been an increase in the number of human research publications from the UAE (Table 1). The transformation of healthcare in the UAE began with the collaboration with western managed health care providers, introduction of medical insurance, development of the medical residency program and accreditation by the Accreditation Council for Graduate Medical Education-I (Abdulrahman and Nair 2017). Recent initiatives by the government to encourage medical research, including research conducted by medical trainees, has enabled a change from the traditional practice of medicine to evidence-based (Abdulrahman and Nair 2017). Retrospective chart reviews, case reports in addition to a high number of observational studies, are conducted every year in the country (Ibrahim and Nair 2013). Survey and questionnaire studies have aided in the understanding of physician career preferences, satisfaction and burnout among medical residents, and accreditation perceptions (Schiess et al. 2015; El

Table 1 Publications involving human subject research in the UAE

	Human research publication		
	Global (#)	UAE (#)	% of total
1971–1980	113,690	11	0.009675433
1981–1990	545,190	87	0.01595774
1991–2000	1,069,038	955	0.089332652
2001–2010	2,045,668	1983	0.096936551
2011–2016	1,850,113	3515	0.189988395

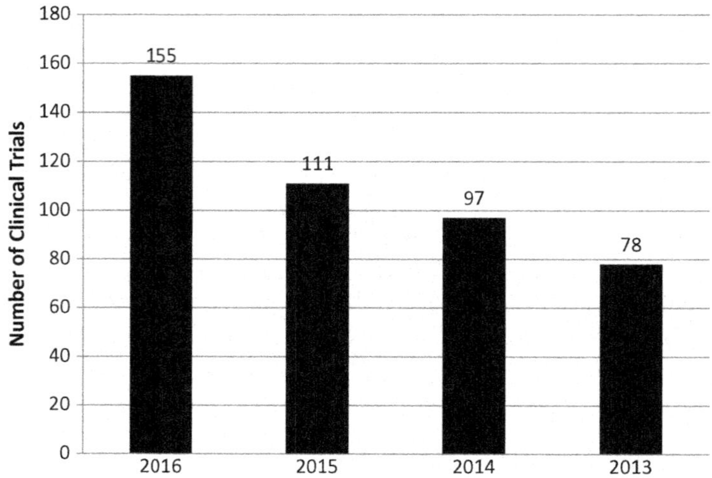

Fig. 3 Number of clinical trials in the UAE

Miedany et al. 2011). Clinical research and patient reported outcomes research is slowly gaining momentum in the UAE (El Miedany et al. 2011).

Saudi Arabia, followed by the UAE, leads the region in the total number of clinical trials conducted per year. Approximately 34% of all registered studies are observational in Saudi Arabia, 37% in the UAE and between 48% and 65% collectively in Bahrain, Oman, Qatar and Kuwait (Nair et al. 2016). In comparison, Asian countries, such as India, China and Japan, have 10–20% of the total studies registered as observational (Nair et al. 2016). Currently, almost 155 clinical trials (Clinical Trials 2017) have been conducted in the UAE (Fig. 3). These predominantly include phase III and Phase IV studies, although a few Phase II studies have also been conducted depending on the subspecialty, type and stage of the disease (Nair et al. 2013). The health authorities do not permit Phase I trials (Nair et al. 2013). Oncology, metabolic diseases, infectious disease top the list of clinical trials in the UAE (Clinical Trials 2017). The increase in clinical trials ranged from 24% in 2014 to 99% increase in 2016, compared to baseline year 2013 (Fig. 3).

Conclusion

Adoption of ICH-GCP guidelines to review and approve research studies, compliance audits and periodic reporting to the regulators reflect the main ethical mechanisms to protect research participants. Verification of investigator credentials, competence and measures to ensure financial transparency are the highlights of the prevalent regulatory system. The success of the research training program, ACREDIT, will be a great step forward to standardize training among all the investigators in the country.

Several gaps, however, need to be addressed in order to establish harmonization among the RECs in the UAE. First, national regulations need to ensure that research is performed based on cultural aspects of the region, rather than just relying on international standards. Second, there is a need for a common regulatory framework for all of the emirates. Finally, a central monitoring system is needed for all of the RECs in the UAE.

Although the UAE is new to the area of human clinical research, adherence to the constantly evolving regulations and the willingness to comply with regulations by the investigators make the UAE unique for developing a robust human research enterprise and should serve as an example for similar countries of the Arab world.

References

Abdulrahman, M., and S. Nair 2017. Overall assessment of human research and ethics committees in The United Arab Emirates. *The Journal of Empirical Research on Human Research Ethics.* In press.

Al Marzooqi, F., and A. Al Khamiri, S.C. Nair 2016. *Medical residency research perceptions: A cross-sectional study from The Abu Dhabi Services Company Residency Centers In The UAE.* Poster session presented at the UAEU Annual Research & Innovation Conference 2016, Al Ain, UAE. Reterived from: http://conferences.uaeu.ac.ae/aric/en/about.shtml

Al Sarraj, Y., S. Nair, A. Al Siraj, and M. AlShayeb. 2015. Characteristics of salivary gland tumours in the United Arab Emirates. *Ecancermedicalscience* 9: 583. https://doi.org/10.3332/ecancer.2015.583.

Aljefree, N., and F. Ahmed. 2015. Prevalence of cardiovascular disease and associated risk factors among adult population in the gulf region: A systematic review. *Advances in Public Health* 2015: 1–23. https://doi.org/10.1155/2015/235101.

Al-Rawi, Y., G. Al-Tajir 2012. MENA region. *ACRP Monitor*, September 2012, 33–37.

Clinical Trials. Retrieved January 23, 2017, from Clinical Trials.gov, http://www.clinicaltrials.gv

Colliers International. 2013. UAE Health Overview. Retrieved January 16, 2017, from http://www.colliers.com/en-gb/unitedarabemirates/services/healthcare

El Miedany, Y., M. El Gaafary, N. El Aroussy, I. Ahmed, S. Youssef, and D. Palmer. 2011. Patient reported outcomes in ankylosing spondylitis: development and validation of a new questionnaire for functional impairment and quality of life assessment. *Clinical and Experimental Rheumatology* 29 (5): 801–810.

El-Hajj Fuleihan, G. 2009. Vitamin D deficiency in the middle east and its health consequences for children and adults. *Clinical Reviews in Bone and Mineral Metabolism* 7 (1): 77–93. https://doi.org/10.1007/s12018-009-9027-9.

Hajat, C., O. Harrison, and Z. Shather. 2012. A profile and approach to chronic disease in Abu Dhabi. *Globalization and Health* 8 (1): 18. https://doi.org/10.1186/1744-8603-8-18.

Hamamy, H. n.d. Consanguineous marriages: Preconception consultation in primaryhealth care settings. *Journal of Community Genetics* 3 (3): 185–192. https://doi.org/10.1007/s12687-011-0072-y.

http://www.tamimi.com/en/magazine/law-update/section-14/november-7/the-new-uae-medical-liability-lawan- analysis.html. Accessed 15 Feb 2017

Ibrahim, H., and S.C. Nair. 2013. Focus on international research strategy and teaching: The FIRST programme. *Perspectives on Medical Education* 3 (2): 129–135. https://doi.org/10.1007/s40037-013-0098-4.

Ibrahim, K., E.A. Eada, and N. Younis. 2006. Guidelines: Ministry of health-drug control-UAE guidance for conducting clinical trials based on drugs/medical products and good. *Clinical Practice* 6: 1–44.

Koornneef, E.J., P.B.M. Robben, M.B. Al Seiari, and Z. Al Siksek. 2012. Health system reform in the Emirate of Abu Dhabi, United Arab Emirates. *Health Policy* 108 (2–3): 115–121. https://doi.org/10.1016/j.healthpol.2012.08.026.

Kripalani, S., J. Bussey-Jones, M.G. Katz, and I. Genao. 2006. A prescription for cultural competence in medical education. *Journal of General Internal Medicine* 21 (10): 1116–1120.

Kumar, A.S. 2015. Clinical research in the United Arab Emirates. *Journal of Clinical Studies* 6 (6): 30–31.

Loney, T., T.-C. Aw, D.G. Handysides, R. Ali, I. Blair, M. Grivna, ... Y. El-Obaid. 2013. An analysis of the health status of the United Arab Emirates: The "big 4" public health issues. *Global Health Action*, 6. doi:https://doi.org/10.3402/gha.v6i0.20100

Nair, S.C., and H. Ibrahim. 2014. Informed consent form challenges for genetic research in a developing Arab country with high risk for genetic disease. *Journal of Genetic Counseling* 24 (2): 294–299. https://doi.org/10.1007/s10897-014-976.

Nair, S., and H. Ibrahim. 2015a. GCP compliance and readability of informed consent forms from an emerging hub for clinical trials. *Perspectives in Clinical Research* 6 (2): 104. https://doi.org/10.4103/2229-3485.154012.

Nair, S.C., and H. Ibrahim. 2015b. Assessing subject privacy and data confidentiality in an emerging region for clinical trials: United Arab Emirates. *Accountability in Research* 22 (4): 205–221. https://doi.org/10.1080/08989621.2014.942452.

Nair, S.C., H. Ibrahim, and D.D. Celentano. 2013. Clinical trials in the middle east and north Africa (MENA) region: Grandstanding or grandeur? *Contemporary Clinical Trials* 36 (2): 704–710. https://doi.org/10.1016/j.cct.2013.05.009.

Nair, S., H. Ibrahim, and O. Askar. 2016. Comparison of good clinical practice compliance and readability ease of the informed consents between observational and interventional clinical studies in the Emirates. *Perspectives in Clinical Research* 7 (3): 123. https://doi.org/10.4103/2229-3485.184815.

Schiess, N., H. Ibrahim, S. Shaban, M.N. Perez, and S.C. Nair. 2015. Career choice and primary care in the United Arab Emirates. *The Journal of Graduate Medical Education* 7 (4): 663–666. https://doi.org/10.4300/JGME-D-14-00780.1.

Sleem, H., S.S. El-Kamary, and H.J. Silverman. 2010. Identifying structures, processes, resources and needs of research ethics committees in Egypt. *BMC Medical Ethics* 11: 12. https://doi.org/10.1186/1472-6939-11-12.

Sponsor Training n.d.. Retrieved January 21, 2017, from PAREXEL academy, http://www.parexel-academy.com/deu/about-us/parexel-academy/

Sreedharan, J., J. Muttappallymyalil, S. al Sharbatti, S. Hassoun, R. Safadi, I. Abderahman, ... A. M. Fouda. 2015. Incidence of type 2 diabetes Mellitus among Emirati residents in Ajman, United Arab Emirates. *Korean Journal of Family Medicine* 36(5): 253. doi:https://doi.org/10.4082/kjfm.2015.36.5.253

The World Bank. 2016. United Arab Emirates. Retrieved January 16, 2017 from *The World Bank*, https://data.worldbank.org/country/united-arab-emirates.

U.S.-U.A.E. Business Council. 2016. *The UAE Healthsector: An Update*. Retrieved January 25, 2017, from http://usuaebusiness.org/wpcontent/uploads/2016/09/Healthcare-Report-Final.pdf

Part V

Responsibilities and Functions of Research Ethics Committees

Establishing Functioning Research Ethics Committees: Introduction

Henry Silverman

Formal ethics review of research has increasingly become a requirement in the Arab region, motivated by the recent passage of national regulations, by the increased funding of research by international sponsors, including pharmaceutical companies, and the prerequisite for ethics review mandated by international journals. Finally, a functioning ethics review system helps to build public confidence and trust in the integrity of the research process. As prior ethics review has become a widely accepted safeguard for the protection of the welfare and rights of research participants, this chapter will review several factors that are instrumental for effective ethics review systems.

First, establishing the legitimacy of research ethics committees (RECs) represents a primary issue insofar as it plays a key role in confirming the authority of RECs to approve, disapprove, delay, and require changes in research. Legitimacy is usually achieved by having a high-ranking institutional official (e.g., President, Vice-President, Dean, Minister of Health) establish the REC and designate the chair and vice-chair and even nominate its members. Such a process declares to the faculty that ethics review is mandatory rather than discretionary, and that the REC is authorized to make decisions regarding the approvability of submitted research. Such authority conferred by legitimacy within the institution also enables the REC to function both as independently and as effectively as possible.

To be sure, the political and cultural environments of the institution will dictate how effectively the REC can exercise its authority. For instance, the REC may be pressured to approve questionable research at the university due to financial or reputational considerations. The culture of the institution is also pivotal with respect to the responsible conduct of researchers regarding the protection of human subjects of research. While an REC-approved protocol may include adequate protections of

H. Silverman (✉)
University of Maryland, Baltimore, MD, USA
e-mail: hsilverm@medicine.umaryland.edu

H. Silverman (ed.), *Research Ethics in the Arab Region*, Research Ethics Forum 5,
https://doi.org/10.1007/978-3-319-65266-5_26

the human subjects, unless the protocol is appropriately implemented by researchers, human subjects cannot be protected. Thus, researchers have the responsibility of complying with their REC-approved protocols.

Second, institutional officials should also ensure the adequacy of resources (human, capital, and financial) for RECs to operate efficiently and effectively. Such resources are justifiable, as leadership in research institutions expect that their RECs will provide a service to the researchers - their actions will facilitate research and ensure that it is being conducted in an ethical manner. Third, defining accountability mechanisms is fundamental in establishing credible ethics review (Hirtle and Sprumont 2000). The accountability of RECs may be achieved by formal or informal mechanisms, or a combination of both. Formal mechanisms are usually accomplished when the ethics review system is integrated in the regulatory framework of the national government and consist of registering RECs or performing audits and inspections. Alternatively, the national government may require RECs to obtain accreditation. An accreditation process, however, will prove to be problematic due to the amount of resources necessary to institute such a mechanism. Instead, a self-assessment activity as described elsewhere may prove to be an acceptable substitute.

Constraints to effective accountability mechanisms include the lack of clear reporting structures, especially in countries where there may be a division of powers between national and regional governments (as occurs in the UAE). The presence of different regulatory bodies that have overlapping functions, e.g., National Ethics Committees and the National Drug Regulatory Authorities (as occurs in Sudan) can lead to situations where the lines of authority are unclear. Absence of a formal regulatory structure will lead to questions as to who should regulate RECs and whether and which governmental agencies should intervene in the regulations of RECs. Finally, even when a regulatory oversight system is established at the national level, the lack of appropriate resources available to the regulatory authorities would undermine their efforts (Hirtle et al. 2000).

In the absence of RECs being integrated into a national regulatory framework, local institutional policies may provide informal solutions, such as requiring RECs to submit annual reports and other documents (e.g., records of their decisions) to the high ranking officials of the institution. Unless rigorously enforced, such mechanisms may make the accountability of RECs somewhat ambiguous.

Other accountability mechanisms include appropriate monitoring and review by the institution and establishment of a quality assurance and improvement program. Establishing a procedure to receive complaints from research participants also helps with establishing accountability of RECs.

Ensuring transparency represents another important aspect of RECs, both for the institution and for the RECs. For example, RECs must be diligent about conflicts of interests at the institutional and investigator levels, which emanate from the prospect of obtaining academic rewards (prestige and reputation) as well as from obtaining financial resources, as e.g., pharmaceutical funding has increasingly become a major source of revenues for the conduct of clinical trials, especially as governmental funding of research remains scant in the Arab region compared with other regions

(UNESCO Institute for Statistics 2015). As members of RECs are part of the institutions, their institutional conflicts of interests may undermine their independence (Campbell et al. 2006). The increasing prevalence of and hence, concern for conflicts of interest in research enhances the necessity for RECs to determine the extent to which financial conflicts of interest threatens the protection of the welfare and rights of research participants (Ghooi 2015; Rockey and Collins 2010). Unfortunately, regulation of conflicts of interests at the institutional levels remains elusive in many institutions in the Arab region (Silverman et al. 2015).

Finally, achieving independence represents another important characteristic for RECs, as a primary task of RECs is to function as a counterbalance to research and financial interests that might be present both at the institutional and investigator levels (Hirtle et al. 2000). The independence of ethics committee members can be compromised by a variety of factors. The person in charge of appointing the committee members as well as the chair of the committee may have a professional responsibility (e.g., obtaining institutional funding) that conflicts with the work of the REC. Additionally, as ethics committees function within their institutions, they might, consciously or unconsciously, not reject protocols from their colleagues, as they share a commitment to their institution to obtain research funding. RECs, however, should not allow the financial interests of researchers and institutions make them lose sight of the rights and welfare of human subjects.

Independence of RECs can be advanced by several mechanisms. First, clear written policies regarding the appointment and replacement of members can lessen arbitrary decisions by institutional officials. Second, institutional officials should be prohibited from serving on the committee either as chair or as a member. Third, RECs' disapproval of research should not be overturned by institutional officials, although their approvals may be questioned at the institutional level. Fourth, the appointment of members without institutional affiliation (e.g., community members) can help provide a neutral balance to REC discussions.

This review of the important characteristics of RECs serves as background for a further examination of the RECs existing in the Arab region. The chapters in this Part will examine the challenges faced by RECs, explore the views of investigators in the Arab region towards RECs, and review the utility of a self-assessment tool for RECs that was developed for LMICs. The section will also review the structures and processes of two RECs in the Arab region, one at Cairo University and the other at the King Hussein Cancer Center. These two RECs have reached a level of sophistication that can serve as models for other RECs in the region. This section will end with Farida Lada describing pragmatic aspects of establishing an REC, including the development of policies and standard operating procedures that should serve as a guide for its functioning.

References

Campbell, E.G., J.S. Weissman, C. Vogeli, B.R. Clarridge, M. Abraham, J.E. Marder, and G. Koski. 2006. Financial relationships between institutional review board members and industry. *The New England Journal of Medicine* 355 (22): 2321–2329. https://doi.org/10.1056/NEJMsa061457.

Ghooi, R.B. 2015. Conflict of interest in clinical research. *Perspectives Clinical Research* 6 (1): 10–14. https://doi.org/10.4103/2229-3485.148794.

Hirtle, M.T.L., and D. Sprumont. 2000. A comparative analysis of research ethics review mechanisms and the ICH good clinical practice guideline. *European Journal of Health Law* 7: 267.

Rockey, S.J., and F.S. Collins. 2010. Managing financial conflict of interest in biomedical research. *JAMA* 303 (23): 2400–2402. https://doi.org/10.1001/jama.2010.774.

Silverman, H., H. Sleem, K. Moodley, N. Kumar, S. Naidoo, T. Subramanian, et al. 2015. Results of a self-assessment tool to assess the operational characteristics of research ethics committees in low- and middle-income countries. *Journal of Medical Ethics* 41 (4): 332–337. https://doi.org/10.1136/medethics-2013-101587.

UNESCO Institute for Statistics. 2015. How much does your country invest in R&D?, Retrievable at: http://uis.unesco.org/apps/visualisations/research-and-development-spending/.

Challenges of Research Ethics Committees in the Arab Region

Hany M. Sleem and Henry Silverman

Introduction

In the last decade health research, including international clinical trials, has increased greatly in many regions of the world, including the Arab region. Many international research ethics guidelines mandate that all research involving human subjects be reviewed by a research ethic committee (REC) (Council for International Organizations of Medical Sciences (CIOMS) and World Health Organization (WHO) 2016; World Medical Association 2013). As such, many RECs have been established in the Arab region during the last decade (Office of Human Research Protections (OHRP) 2015).

However, commentators have voiced concerns that many RECs in low and middle income countries (LMICs) might not be able to promote high standards of human subject protection due to several challenges that they face. To better address the quality of RECs, it is paramount to understand the specific challenges that RECs encounter so that policy makers (e.g., Ministry of Health and top officials at academic institutions) can better support these committees. Accordingly, the purpose of this chapter is to review the existing literature on the needs and challenges of RECs.

Most of our data are from several studies performed in Egypt (Abdel-Aal et al. 2013; Matar and Silverman 2013; Silverman et al. 2015; Sleem et al. 2010a), as well as studies performed in Africa (Milford et al. 2006; Moodley and Myer 2007; Silaigwana and Wassenaar 2015). These studies show that the challenges RECs face include inadequate or absence of national laws for the regulation of research, lack

H.M. Sleem (✉)
Egyptian Network of Research Ethics Committees (ENREC), Cairo, Egypt

National Hepatology and Tropical Medicine Research Institute (NHTMRI), Cairo, Egypt
e-mail: hanysleem@hotmail.com

H. Silverman
University of Maryland, Baltimore, MD, USA
e-mail: hsilverm@medicine.umaryland.edu

H. Silverman (ed.), *Research Ethics in the Arab Region*, Research Ethics Forum 5,
https://doi.org/10.1007/978-3-319-65266-5_27

of institutional support, inadequate financial, material and human resources, lack of adequately trained REC members, insufficient diversity of membership, lack of independence, and inadequate internal and external quality improvement efforts (Hyder et al. 2004; Kass et al. 2003).

Inadequate or Absence of National Laws Regulating Health Research

Several studies have demonstrated that RECs harbor concerns regarding the inadequacy or absence of national ethics regulations, as it might be difficult to adapt international guidelines to the local context. Also, without regulations at the national level, it might be challenging to promote the importance of requiring ethics review and also communicate and justify the authority of RECs. Finally, although international guidelines suggest structures of RECs and processes for their review functions, without guidance from national regulations variability in operations will exist between the different RECs within the same country, which may lead to variability in the protection of research participants (Younis 2015).

Extent of Institutional Support

Institutional commitment and support of RECs is crucial for affirming the legitimacy and functioning of RECs. Such legitimization helps with establishing the authority of the RECs to approve and disapprove research; promotes investigator compliance with the decisions of RECs; and enhances the independence of RECs from institutional pressures. The following indices serve as indicators of institutional commitment:

- REC is established under a high-ranking authority
- The institution regularly evaluates the operations of the REC
- The institution requires that those involved in research receive training in research ethics in order to submit protocols to the REC
- Institution requires a conflict of interest policy for members of the research staff
- REC is given its own budget
- REC has its own administrative staff and access to capital resources

One study that involved 64 RECs from Egypt, India, and South Africa showed that institutional support was lacking for many RECs, as only 25% of the RECs were established under a high ranking official, less than 40% had the availability of a budget, 69% had access to an administrative staff, and approximately 70% had access to capital resources, such as computer, fax machines, availability of a meeting room (Silverman et al. 2015). Other studies have shown similar results (Milford et al. 2006; Moodley and Myer 2007).

Inadequate Member Training

The extent of adequately trained members is variable amongst RECs. All of the studies reviewed for this chapter uniformly reported that the majority of committee members need more ethics training. Sleem and colleagues showed that almost three-quarters (72.6%) of the members from all the 12 RECs they surveyed indicated they received some training in ethics, although the specification of the extent of such training was not elicited (Sleem et al. 2010a). Chairs from all of the RECs indicated that they had received some prior ethics training. Eleven RECs indicated that it had at least two members with training in ethics. One REC indicated that none of its members had received any training in research ethics. Another study showed that only 40% of all members received ethics training prior to joining their committees, while just over half had received training after assuming their position on the committees (Milford et al. 2006).

In another study, 54% of REC members had received training in research ethics or Good Clinical Practice (Moodley and Myer 2007). A survey of REC chairs in Egypt found that 12 out of 13 RECS felt that lack of ethics training hampered effective functioning of their committees (Matar and Silverman 2013). A report detailing the operations of an Egyptian REC also concluded that more training was required to improve the functioning of the REC (Abdel-Aal et al. 2013). Finally, Silverman and colleagues reported in their study that only 45% of the RECs provided continuing education in ethics for their members (Silverman et al. 2015).

In general, a large majority of RECs have insufficient training of their members. Inadequate training of REC members can compromise the quality, efficiency and consistency of ethical reviews. Most new committee members lack special training and experience in research ethics, although they typically have significant expertise in their primary specialities.

We recommend that REC members have formal training on research ethics, research methodology, design aspects of clinical trial and Good Clinical Practice (GCP). RECs should document the type of training that their membership receives and terms of appointment should be conditioned on such training. Additionally, there should be a requirement for continuous education, as research ethics guidelines are being continually updated as science continues to advance.

Successful RECs usually begins the process of training for new members upon appointment to the committee. As such, it might be helpful to provide members with orientation books, internet sites and online courses in research ethics and GCP. Many eLearning modules are available online. One recommendation is that researchers should complete human subjects protection training through an online program that is verified by a certificate.

Member Composition

Studies have demonstrated a lack of member diversity among many committees. Specifically, there is inadequate representation of women, non-scientists, and community members. One study showed that only 50% of the RECs surveyed had adequate gender balance (defined as having gender representation between 40% and 60% of the total membership) (Silverman et al.2015). Studies have also shown a predominance of physicians and scientists on the committee. For example, Sleem and colleagues showed that of the RECs they surveyed in 2008, about 90% of members of the RECs in Egypt were physicians and scientists (Sleem et al. 2010a). Another study in Africa demonstrated that among the surveyed RECs, a majority of the members (56%) were scientists or clinicians and community representatives accounted for only 8% of membership (Moodley and Myer 2007). Such memberships skewed toward physicians and scientists may bias decisions towards the interests of researchers against that of research participants. An inadequate number of members from the community may lead to unsatisfactory representation of the community's attitudes and values.

Lack of Independence

Achieving independence represents another challenge for RECs. Such independence assures that RECs operate free from the potential financial interests of their institutions that might conflict with its independent review of research. Independence of RECs can be advanced by the development of clear written policies regarding the appointment of members, prohibiting institutional officials from serving on the committee either as chair or as a member, not allowing institutional officials to overturn RECs' disapprovals of research, and appointing members without institutional affiliation (e.g., community members), as they can help provide a neutral balance to REC discussions.

Accountability Mechanisms

Many RECs lack accountability mechanisms at the national level and institutional levels. RECs need to be held accountable for their practices and actions to ensure public confidence with their review functions. Accountability can be achieved by the national government in a variety of mechanisms. For example, the Saudi law of research ethics mandates that every REC member pass an online research ethics exam available at the website of the national committee of bioethics. RECs cannot be approved by the national committee unless all members have passed this online exam. In Egypt, according to Ministerial Decree (No. 595 of 2012), all RECs must register with the Egyptian MOH and one of their submitted documents include the training plan that is established for members of the RECs. At the institutional level, accountability can be achieved by instituting a quality assurance and improvement program and establishing a procedure for participants' complaints

Transparency

In regards to transparency, although a large percentage of RECs in Egypt have written Standard Operating Procedures, many lack a conflict of interest policy (Silverman et al. 2015). Furthermore, RECs tend to operate without knowledge of how other RECs operate in their country. One method to achieve better transparency between intra-country RECs is the establishment of a network of RECs. To address this issue, the Egyptian Network of Research Ethics Committees (ENREC) was established in 2008 (Egyptian Network of Research Ethics Committees (ENREC) 2015). Such a network allows an optimum degree of visibility and interaction between RECs, thus facilitating and rendering more uniform the operating procedures between RECs. The ENREC network facilitates communications between the RECs' members in Egypt through the exchange of knowledge and the dissemination of teaching materials aiming at optimizing RECs functioning.

Evaluation of REC Performance

Evaluating the effectiveness of RECs remains challenging, particularly as there are no gold standards to measure the quality of REC reviews or the impact of RECs on research practices. Governmental or private auditing and accreditation initiatives have been put in place recently to formally evaluate RECs. These efforts include various external review mechanisms based on standards drawn from existing regulatory requirements. Examples of such accreditation efforts include the Strategic Initiative for Developing Capacity in Ethical Review (SIDCER), which endorses a two-step process for RECs in LMICs: a self-assessment performed by the REC followed by an external review by SIDCER (Strategic Initiative for Developing Capacity in Ethical Review (SIDCER) 2015). The Association for the Accreditation of Human Research Protection Programs (AAHRPP), a private organization based in the USA, evaluates an institution's human research protection program, including the institution's REC. AAHRPP has predominantly been focused on RECs in the USA, but has also extended its program to RECs in LMICs (Association for the Accreditation of Human Research Protection Programs (AAHRPP) 2015).

Accreditation contributes to maintenance of public trust and respect from international and national bodies, as well as sponsors and research organizations. However, a comprehensive auditing or accreditation mechanism remains unlikely for many LMICs due to the large investment of human and financial resources needed for such efforts. Also, many LMICs do not have a legal or regulatory framework for clinical research and therefore, an external review mechanism based on national standards may be problematic for these countries. However, a self-assessment process provides an intermediate step to help RECs evaluate their performance against a standard and demonstrates their legitimacy to their stakeholders. We previously developed a self-assessment tool for RECs from LMICs based on international standards for RECs (Sleem et al. 2010 b). Such a self-assessment process also serves as a quality improvement activity for RECs. As this self-assessment tool is scored (maximum point total is 200), data obtained from more than 60 RECs from LMICs can be used as a benchmarking indicator for RECs (Silverman et al. 2015).

Conclusion

The functioning of RECs are impeded by several challenges that include the lack of an enabling legal framework at the national level, inadequate institutional support that includes appropriate human and capital resources, insufficient training of members to review studies, inadequate membership diversity, lack of transparency and accountability mechanisms, absence of internal quality improvement programs, and lack of assessment mechanisms.

We recommend that national governments and institutional officials invest in capacity-enhancing programs to maximize the efficiency and effectiveness of their ethics programs, which includes functioning RECs, so that the protection of rights and welfare of research participants can be optimized. We also recommend that the national regulatory bodies establish minimum registration criteria for all of the RECs in their respective countries. This would represent a needed first step at determining whether important characteristics of RECs (e.g., member composition and training, interval of periodic review) exist in the country, which would make subsequent attempts at establishing robust accreditation standards more feasible. Such a registration system has been established in Egypt, where the Ministry of Health has partnered with ENREC to help with their efforts at registering identified RECs in Egypt.

References

Abdel-Aal, W., E.A. Ghaffar, and O. El Shabrawy. 2013. Review of the Medical Research Ethics Committee (MREC), National Research Center of Egypt, 2003–2011. *Current Medical Research and Opinion* 29 (10): 1411–1417. https://doi.org/10.1185/03007995.2013.815158.

Association for the Accreditation of Human Research Protection Programs (AAHRPP). 2015. Available at: http://www.aahrpp.org

Council for International Organizations of Medical Sciences (CIOMS), and World Health Organization (WHO). 2016. *International ethical guidelines for health-related research involving humans*. Geneva: CIOMS.

Egyptian Network of Research Ethics Committees (ENREC). 2015. Available at: www.enrec.org.

Hyder, A.A., S.A. Wali, A.N. Khan, N.B. Teoh, N.E. Kass, and L. Dawson. 2004. Ethical review of health research: A perspective from developing country researchers. *Journal of Medical Ethics* 38: 68–72.

Kass, N., L. Dawson, and N.I. Loyo-Berrios. 2003. Ethical oversight of research in developing countries. *IRB: Ethics & Human Research* 25: 1–10.

Matar, A., and H. Silverman. 2013. Perspectives of Egyptian research ethics committees regarding their effective functioning. *Journal of Empirical Research on Human Research Ethics* 8 (1): 32–44. https://doi.org/10.1525/jer.2013.8.1.32.

Milford, C., D. Wassenaar, and C. Slack. 2006. Resources and needs of research ethics committees in Africa: Preparations for HIV vaccine trials. *IRB: Ethics & Human Research* 28: 1–9.

Moodley, K., and L. Myer. 2007. Health research ethics committees in South Africa 12 years into democracy. *BMC Medical Ethics* 8: 1. https://doi.org/10.1186/1472-6939-8-1.

Office of Human Research Protections (OHRP). 2015. IRBs and assurances. Available at: http://www.hhs.gov/ohrp/assurances/index.html.

Silaigwana, B., and D. Wassenaar. 2015. Biomedical research ethics committees in sub-Saharan Africa: A collective review of their structure, functioning, and outcomes. *Journal of Empirical Research on Human Research Ethics* 10 (2): 169–184. https://doi.org/10.1177/1556264615575511.

Silverman, H., H. Sleem, K. Moodley, N. Kumar, S. Naidoo, T. Subramanian,. .. M. Moni 2015. Results of a self-assessment tool to assess the operational characteristics of research ethics committees in low- and middle-income countries. *Journal of Medical Ethics* 41(4): 332–337. doi:10.1136/medethics-2013-101587.

Sleem, H., S. El-Kamary, and H.J. Silverman. 2010a. Identifying structures, processes, resources and needs of research ethics committees in Egypt. *BMC Medical Ethics* 11: 12.

Sleem, H., R.A. Abdelhai, I. Al-Abdallat, M. Al-Naif, H.M. Gabr, E. T. Kehil, . .. H. Silverman. 2010b. Development of an accessible self-assessment tool for research ethics committees in developing countries. *Journal of Empirical Research Human Reseach Ethics* 5(3): 85–96; quiz 97–88. doi:10.1525/jer.2010.5.3.85.

Strategic Initiative for Developing Capacity in Ethical Review (SIDCER). 2015. SIDCER recognition programme: Available at: http://www.who.int/sidcer/en/

World Medical Association. 2013. Declaration of Helsinki. Available at: http://www.wma.net/en/30publications/10policies/b3/

Younis, I.M. 2015. Overview of research committees status in Egypt: Challenges aspirations and current situation. *Accountability in Research* 22 (4): 222–236. https://doi.org/10.1080/08989621.2014.956869.

Challenges to Research Ethics Regulations: Academic Researchers' Voices in the Arab World

Jihad Makhoul and Rima Nakkash

Introduction

The Arab region has recently witnessed widespread financial support for collaborative research involving human subjects (Chin et al. 2011; Neitzke 2012; UNESCO 2009) and accordingly, this has been met with an increase in the number of academic institutions that conduct research (Sleem et al. 2010). However, this increase has not been coupled with a similar rise in the number of research ethics committees (RECs) and many of those in place lack sufficient functionality (Silverman et al. 2014). Another concern emanates from the lack of a culturally sensitive framework to guide oversight, as regulations and guidelines in the region have been adopted from western or international standards (Sleem et al. 2010). As such, this recent surge in funding and the corresponding conduct of health research has fueled a growing interest in the development of research ethics instruments in non–western settings.

Studies focused on the views of researchers themselves can be helpful in understanding aspects of research ethics in the local context, but such studies have been scarce. Investigating academic researchers' views regarding conducting research and their subsequent experiences with applying ethics regulations largely adopted from western countries but applied in non-western countries of the world is an emerging field. A comprehensive search employing a number of academic electronic databases yielded eleven publications from the low- and middle-income countries compared to the large number on the same topic from high-income countries in the west. The studies identified used quantitative research approaches, while a few used qualitative methods to investigate researchers' knowledge, attitudes, perceptions, and practices pertaining to research ethics and research ethics committees.

J. Makhoul (✉) • R. Nakkash
Department of Health Promotion and Community Health, Faculty of Health Sciences, American University of Beirut, Beirut, Lebanon
e-mail: jm04@aub.edu.lb

H. Silverman (ed.), *Research Ethics in the Arab Region*, Research Ethics Forum 5,
https://doi.org/10.1007/978-3-319-65266-5_28

The vast majority of these studies come from Africa, such as Uganda (Ibingira and Ochieng 2010), Kenya (Lairumbi et al. 2012), South Africa (Mamotte and Wassenaar 2009), Ethiopia (Addissie et al. 2014), Sudan (Elsayed and Kass 2007) and Egypt (El-Dessouky et al. 2011; Kandeel et al. 2011). They focus on perspectives of researchers as well as doctoral students in health research institutions, universities, and hospitals. These studies report on concerns regarding the informed consent process (Addissie et al. 2014; Hyder et al. 2004; Newton and Appiah-Poku 2007; Rivera et al. 2007), the impact of requirements of research ethics committees (RECs) on their research activities (Ibingira and Ochieng 2010; Mamotte and Wassenaar 2009, El-Dessouky et al. 2011; Elsayed and Kass 2007; Hyder et al. 2004; Ibingira and Ochieng 2010; Kandeel et al. 2011; Mamotte and Wassenaar 2009; Rivera et al. 2007) and the importance of training in research ethics for involved stakeholders (El-Dessouky et al. 2011).

Only four of these studies report on work done specifically in Arab countries and they include Egypt (El-Dessouky et al. 2011; Kandeel et al. 2011), Sudan (Elsayed and Kass 2007), and Jordan (Bin Tareef 2009). These studies highlight similar concerns regarding the absence of frameworks that define and govern the functions of RECs and the lack of national ethics guidelines to guide research (Elsayed and Kass 2007; Bin Tareef 2009). In the two Egyptian studies (El-Dessouky et al. 2011; Kandeel et al. 2011), investigators acknowledge the importance of RECs, but they also describe them as burdensome on the research process in terms of delays and bureaucratic red tape, lack of REC members' familiarity with the methodology used in the protocols and with the process of obtaining informed consent.

While these studies investigating research ethics practices in non-western settings (Hyder et al. 2004; Newton and Appiah-Poku 2007; Rivera et al. 2007) bring to light important issues, several of these reports aggregate their data from different countries and hence, refer their findings as being related to the 'developing world'. Such classification, as we will point out below, fails to acknowledge the socio-cultural specificities and the sociopolitical variations between the countries. These socio-cultural and sociopolitical factors pertaining to the research study sites are important factors to take into consideration as they contribute to how research is conducted.

This chapter will contribute to the emerging body of knowledge about the challenges researchers face in the conduct of research, and how those challenges are often linked to the contexts where research takes place. We aim to discuss the underlying reasons for these challenges and irregularities; a discussion that will also point out routes of interventions at national and academic levels that will lead to enhancements in research quality.

Background

Research in the Arab region is in its infancy (Waast 2010), and not always regulated by national research ethics committees or ethics guidelines enforced by law (Alahmad et al. 2012). Furthermore, not all countries have highly functioning RECs, and given that experience with research ethics is in its infancy, there are gaps in the knowledge base of researchers and regulators regarding research ethics, as well as imperfections in the application of research ethics principles to the conduct of research (Abdur Rab et al. 2008).

In order to understand the experiences of researchers in conducting research and specifically, how they apply research ethics in the Arab region, we interviewed academic researchers who conduct research involving human subjects in two different countries, Qatar representing the high income oil producing Gulf countries and Lebanon, a middle income country, which has social and economic features similar to a number of other countries in the Middle East (Makhoul et al. 2014). A sample of 52 researchers in biomedical and social behavioral sciences were recruited (23 in Qatar and 29 in Lebanon) and subsequently participated in in-depth interviews. Of these 52 participants, 15 from Lebanon and 11 from Qatar have biomedical research backgrounds, while 14 from Lebanon and 23 from Qatar have social behavioral backgrounds. The open-ended interview questions inquired about their perspectives and experiences of conducting research in their respective fields and about the challenges they encounter in conducting their research with particular focus on research ethics. The questions also asked about clearance procedures, capacity for research, and suggestions to improve research conduct.

Results

Research Ethics Training

Findings reveal that despite complaints voiced by the participants regarding the procedures necessary for ethics approval, they reported that the presence of a functional REC in the university had a positive influence on them as academic researchers. Requiring faculty to complete training courses on research ethics sensitizes them to ethics related terminology and concepts. The Collaborative Institutional Training Initiative (CITI) is the most recurring form of online training that the participants reported to have taken, perhaps because the majority of the universities in Qatar and Lebanon are connected to North American universities and the Qatari national regulations have required it as stipulated in "Policies, regulations, and guidelines for research involving human subjects" (Qatar Supreme Council of Health 2009).

In addition to having research ethics training as required by their institutions, the majority of the participants also commented on sources of obtaining research ethics skills. These include gaining experience through their graduate or postgraduate studies, serving as an REC member, attending conferences in their disciplines, learning from peers, and reading on their own. A few reported learning about research ethics through continuing education workshops, seminars and conferences. Approximately one third of the participants in Lebanon received formal training in research ethics and the rest acquired such capacity through experience, some referring to it as "on the job training". Meanwhile, almost all the *non-Qatari* participants in Qatar reported a more involved research portfolio of 6–25 years in several countries including the Arab region, North America, Europe, and Southeast Asia.

While all the participants from private universities in Qatar reported having had training in ethical research conduct, only half of the interviewed public university participants reported such training.

National and Institutional Environment

A supportive institutional environment is necessary for enhancing ethical research, providing opportunities for capacity building, and requiring research training for academic faculty. This was evident in the narratives of participants from the universities that have RECs and who are well versed in research ethics terminology and report that their research teams (research assistants, colleagues, field workers and data collectors) have similar competences. In Qatar, the state‘s determination to improve research capacity has led to mandatory research guidelines outlined by the Qatari Supreme Council for Health, which requires ethics review of research projects, including those conducted by students. The internal and external research collaborations also contribute to learning about ethical research conduct.

In contrast, the Lebanese participants complained about the poor research ethics training of their co-researchers. This again could be attributed to the absence of a system that supports ethical research conduct at a national level, as reflected by the lack of research ethics regulations in Lebanon, in contrast to those that exist in Qatar.

Challenges for Researchers in Both Countries

The challenges with conducting ethical research reported by the participants pertain to *institutional, individual, and cultural* factors. Insitutionally, they reported delays in approvals and lack of effective communication between themselves and the RECs. At an individual level, challenges include inadequate research ethics training and inadequate time and funding for research, all of which one could argue are related to lack of institutional support for research initiatives.

To exacerbate the situation, participants in both countries describe the environments they work in as a "non-research culture", as both the general public and institutional officials are neither responsive to nor interested in research. Both academic and non-academic institutions that are considered research sites, such as schools and hospitals, are similarly seen as "not research-oriented", although Qatar has witnessed a surge in research with the establishment of the satellite western university campuses.

Regarding culture, there are requirements that are not culturally sensitive, for example, those involved with obtaining and documenting informed consent. By approaching informed consent processes with a "one size fits all" approach, researchers risk oversimplifying the process and treating groups and communities as homogenous. Using Del Pozo's and Fins' words, this is similar to extrapolating western standards inappropriately to the Arab world (Del Pozo and Fins 2008). For example, in a predominantly Muslim country, religion sets the values for ethical conduct, in general, and research ethics, in particular. Hence, Islamic ethics guidelines for research and what constitutes men and women's rights are derived from the principles of Islamic law, Shari'a (Afifi 2007a). For example, Islamic law values women as 'a cornerstone of the family' and it is the man in the family who has the responsibility to ensure her welfare. This means that for women to participate in research, their husbands or family must approve their participation (Afifi 2007b).

A similar concern pertains to REC requirements for informed consent that emphasize individual autonomy and the signing of consent forms, which the participants described as imported requirements from the West and therefore, not applicable in the Arab culture. One participant stated:

> *I think our comprehension, autonomy, decision-making and research are very different from the West so when we come and bring these principles and apply them here they don't make sense. I think we need to adapt them to make more sense and to be more contextual.* (Medical doctor, Lebanon)

The use of consent forms that require signatures was seen as being inappropriate in non-research cultures, where people are not interested in research and are afraid of signing forms.

Another culture-related challenge involves the use of written consent forms in social contexts where there is a fear of written information (Del Pozo and Fins 2008). This relates to the differences in the ways that information is shared in 'high context' and 'low context' societies (Hofstede and Hofstede 2010). In *high context* societies, information sharing is evident in the social environment and is publicly known. High context societies is a feature of collectivist societies, such as those of the Arab world where information sharing largely takes place through oral rather than written routes, and through family and informal networks rather than written documents. In the Arab world, decisions are taken based on and with feedback from extended family members or the elderly (Joseph 1994).

This variation in decision making processes between societies with different social contexts is also apparent in other non-western settings. For example, African philosophies and perspectives inform ways of 'seeing and doing' based on an African value system. In reference to that, Chilisa discusses the notion of an Afrocentric paradigm, which is a culturally specific worldview that draws on African philosophical assumptions and guides the research process, viewing human beings in relation to others, emphasizing the value of religiosity, consensus building, kindness, respect and care (Chilisa 2009). This communal culture informs African traditional medicine wherein patients make medical decisions and give consent in consultation with both the members of their community and the traditional doctor. This means that the final consent in their decision-making process rests on the consensus reached in consultation with the group rather than by individuals alone (Osuji 2014).

This situation regarding decision making is similar in most Asian cultures, where the family is highly valued and individuals' decisions about informed consent are influenced by family as well. From an East Asian Confucian virtue perspective, the family has a moral obligation to protect the interests of its members who are ill or interested in participating in research (Yu 2015). In case of health related matters for example, the patient does not have an individual right to include or exclude family decision making. Instead, this Confucian perspective emphasizes human relations with others of significance in social relations (familial and non-familial relations) (Choi 2015). The Chinese consider that society is centered around the self in its connections to different people with different types and degrees of relationships (Yu 2015). Therefore, a shared decisional authority is enjoyed by both individuals and their families and individuals engage on decision making processes taking into consideration the impact of their decision on others' welfare and wellbeing (Fan 2015). The examples mentioned above are in contrast with how consent issues are dealt with in European or American societies, which are more individualistic and value personal independence over duty to in-groups (Oyserman et al. 2002).

REC Related Challenges

In their description of the role of RECs in their context, our participants used the terms "cooperative", "fast in responses", "available for counseling, monitoring and training" and "setting best practices and standards". Advantages to REC review included safeguarding human subjects from harm, enhancing research credibility, and improving the likelihood of publishing in international journals.

Despite these reported advantages, there were also complaints about RECs' practices that overshadowed the perceived advantages. For example, the participants in Lebanon spoke about the effects of REC reviews on their research, using terms such as "police", "radar", "adds burden", and "overdoing their job". REC regulations were described as "inconsistent" and their processes as "mechanical" and "rigid".

> *The attitude with which it's done and the approach is very important and when they are acting like a police that can stop you and can hurt you, it's not nice. [But] when it's a collaborative constructive process, it can be very good.* (Medical doctor, Lebanon)

Other recurring challenges reported included delays in REC responses, and consequent slowing down of the research process, using terms, such as "hindering", "delaying" and "limiting". The perceived reasons reported behind these delays are mainly due to inexperienced reviewers, understaffing, and requiring multiple submissions to the RECs of collaborating universities and institutions, which result in duplication and often conflicting REC requirements:

> *I think one of the challenges here is that we have to submit, like for....especially for me, I have to submit for you know.... Hamad Medical Corporation, Qatar University, Weill*

Cornell, umm.....So as you can see, it is a lot of work.... you still have to go through all that duplication process to submit to each institution. (Public health researcher, Qatar)

A study investigating research ethics committees in Egypt (Silverman et al. 2013) concurs with some of the findings reported here regarding challenges. Problems cited in this study included RECs acting as hindrances to optimal functioning of research, with inadequate research ethics training of reviewers and the shortage of human resources for the RECs (which results in delays), all of which have implications on the quality of reviews and the review process.

Our participants also reported ambiguity of the review processes, rigid requirements, and confusion regarding the reasons for the required changes to their protocols. These issues signaled weak communications between the participants and their RECs. Examples of the terms they used include "mismatch", "disconnect", "aggressive", "tension" and "weird".

There are [requirements] that the REC office rightfully requests....There are others which are weird and others that are acceptable. (Human resources researcher, Lebanon)

An analysis of the university websites in both Lebanon and Qatar (Makhoul et al. 2016) indicates a grim shortage of relevant and updated information on REC policies, review processes and forms, which may contribute to this ambiguity and confusion regarding the review process.

The participants also expressed dissatisfaction with the use of REC consent forms that adversely affect the recruitment of research participants into their studies because of their content and the signature requirement. As a result of the above, researchers reported often opting to follow alternative methods for consent, such as oral consent or shorter versions of the same forms, which indicates clear deviations from ethics guidelines, as stipulated by their RECs.

The social science participants expressed concerns regarding the use of biomedical research standards to review social behavioral research. Participants described the RECs' changes and requirement as "funny" or "frustrating" and not applicable to social research approaches. Sometimes, the participants reported they would have to change their research protocols to speed up the review processes.

....It is an issue not just here, it is an issue in North America too, having a medical model for ethics in research and applying it to research in say social sciences where it is not the same ....And there is something called research chill....where people are changing the kind of research they do or they're not doing empirical research because they are afraid it is not gonna get passed by the REC. (Linguistics researcher, Qatar)

Finally, the absence of much needed outreach activities for researchers or on-going educational programs to build their research capacity to meet the REC requirements recurred in both sites, although more so in Lebanon.

Honestly, the REC is not doing anything; they're not doing workshops, nor approaching the investigators....their [the REC's] role shouldn't be like a tower that is disconnected of the masses, and only punishes, it is sad.... (Food Sciences researcher, Lebanon)

One thing that I would like to see from the REC is at least one year seminar to let us know: the researchers, the newcomers to the university, to get acquainted with procedures of getting ethics approval....that will be a good idea. (Nutrition researcher, Qatar)

Conclusions

Challenges to responsible ethical conduct for the protection of participants in research in the Arab region emanate from scarcity in national regulations, sub-optimal research ethics capacity, and cultural insensitivity. The underlying reasons for the challenges that have been discussed point to a number of remedies at national and institutional (academic) levels that will lead to an enhancement in the ethical conduct of research. At the national level, a political commitment to ethical research should require the development of research ethics regulations that include the requirement that all universities establish RECs on their campuses. Ethics guidelines should accommodate the complexities of the non-western multi-cultural research sites. For example, the large extent of variability in consent issues between the Arab region and the West is unsurprising given the nature of the social contexts in the Arab region; and as a result, culturally sensitive consent seeking processes and forms should be developed. Finally, national governments should develop regulatory and oversight mechanisms for research.

At the institutional level, academic institutions should improve effective communication between RECs and researchers, both through on-line and interpersonal channels, and encourage dialogue among them to reduce barriers and improve trust. There is also the need for institutions to develop local guidelines governing recruitment processes that respect prevailing cultural values, yet protect all individuals. Research universities should invest in human resources to enhance REC functioning and also work towards strengthening continuing education that include both online and face to face in-house training for both researchers and REC members.

References

Abdur Rab, M., A. Abou-Zeid, M. Afzal, and H.J. Silverman. 2008. Ethical practices for health research in the Eastern Mediterranean Region of the World Health Organization: A retrospective data analysis. *PloS One* 3: e2094.

Addissie, A., G. Davey, M.J. Newport, T. Addissie, H. MacGregor, Y. Feleke, and B. Farsides. 2014. A mixed-methods study on perceptions towards use of rapid ethical assessment to improve informed consent processes for health research in a low-income setting. *BMC Medical Ethics* 15: 35.–6939-15-35. https://doi.org/10.1186/1472-6939-15-35.

Afifi, R.Y. 2007a. Biomedical research ethics: An Islamic view–Part I. *International Journal of Surgery* 5 (5): 292–296.

———. 2007b. Biomedical research ethics: An Islamic view part II. *International Journal of Surgery* 5 (6): 381–383.

Alahmad, G., M. Al-Jumah, and K. Dierickx. 2012. Review of national research ethics regulations and guidelines in Middle Eastern Arab countries. *BMC Medical Ethics* 13: 34. http://doi.org/10.1186/1472-6939-13-34.

Bin Tareef, A. 2009. Scientific research in Jordanian higher education institutions: An evaluation of the status and obstacles. *Journal of Instructional Psychology* 36 (2): 158.

Chilisa, B. 2009. Indigenous African-centered ethics: Contesting and complementing dominant models. In *The handbook of social research ethics*, ed. D.M. Mertens and P.E. Ginsberg, 407–426. Thousand Oaks: Sage.

Chin, L.J., H. Rifai-Bashjawish, K. Kleinert, A. Saltman, C.S. Leu, and R. Klitzman. 2011. HIV/AIDS research conducted in the developing world and sponsored by the developed world: Reporting of research ethics committee review in two countries. *Journal of Empirical Research on Human Research Ethics: JERHRE* 6 (3): 83–91. https://doi.org/10.1525/jer.2011.6.3.83.

Choi, K. 2015. The ideal of autonomy and its misuse. In *Family-oriented informed consent: East Asian and American perspective*, ed. C. Fan, 83–91. New York: Springer.

Del Pozo, P.R., and J.J. Fins. 2008. Islam and informed consent: Notes from Doha. *Cambridge Quarterly of Healthcare Ethics* 17 (03): 273–279.

El-Dessouky, H.F., A.M. Abdel-Aziz, C. Ibrahim, M. Moni, R. Abul Fadl, and H. Silverman. 2011. Knowledge, awareness, and attitudes about research ethics among dental faculty in the middle east: A pilot study. *International Journal of Dentistry* 2011: 694759. https://doi.org/10.1155/2011/694759.

Elsayed, D.E.M., and N.E. Kass. 2007. Assessment of the ethical review process in Sudan. *Developing World Bioethics* 7 (3): 143–148.

Fan, R. 2015. *Family-oriented informed consent: East Asian and American perspectives*. New York: Springer.

Hofstede, G., and G. Hofstede. 2010. *Culture and organizations: Software of the mind: Intercultural cooperation and its importance for survival*. 3rd ed. New York: McGraw Hill.

Hyder, A.A., S.A. Wali, A.N. Khan, N.B. Teoh, N.E. Kass, and L. Dawson. 2004. Ethical review of health research: A perspective from developing country researchers. *Journal of Medical Ethics* 30 (1): 68–72.

Ibingira, C., and J. Ochieng. 2010. Attitudes and perceptions about the research and ethics committee in Kampala, Uganda. *The International Journal of Medicine* 3 (2): 347–351. Available at: http://intermedjournal.page.tl/Home-TIJM.htm.

Joseph, S. 1994. Brother/sister relationships: Connectivity, love, and power in the reproduction of patriarchy in Lebanon. *American Ethnologist* 21 (1): 50–73.

Kandeel, N., A. El-Nemer, N.M. Ali, H. Kassem, M. El-Setouhy, M.E. Elgharieb, and H.J. Silverman. 2011. A multicenter study of the awareness and attitudes of Egyptian faculty towards research ethics: A pilot study. *Journal of Empirical Research on Human Research Ethics : JERHRE* 6 (4): 99–108. https://doi.org/10.1525/jer.2011.6.4.99.

Lairumbi, G.M., M. Parker, R. Fitzpatrick, and M.C. English. 2012. Forms of benefit sharing in global health research undertaken in resource poor settings: A qualitative study of stakeholders' views in Kenya. *Philosophy, Ethics, and Humanities in Medicine* 7: 7.

Makhoul, J., L. El-Alti, Y. Qutteina, C. Nasrallah, C. Sakr, R. Nakkash, and K. Alali. 2014. "Protecting" or "policing": Academic researchers' view of RECs in an arab context. *Journal of Empirical Research on Human Research Ethics: JERHRE* 9 (5): 25–35. https://doi.org/10.1177/1556264614553170.

Makhoul, J., Y. Qutteina, L. El-Alti, M. Baroud, and C. Nasrallah 2016. Human subjects research in the Arab world: What do university websites say? Unpublished report. American University of Beirut.

Mamotte, N., and D. Wassenaar. 2009. Ethics review in a developing country: A survey of South African social scientists' experiences. *Journal of Empirical Research on Human Research Ethics: JERHRE* 4 (4): 69–78. https://doi.org/10.1525/jer.2009.4.4.69.

Neitzke, A.B. 2012. Globalizing research ethics: Justice & biomedical research in developing countries. *Perspectives on Global Development and Technology* 11 (1): 145–153.

Newton, S.K., and J. Appiah-Poku. 2007. The perspectives of researchers on obtaining informed consent in developing countries. *Developing World Bioethics* 7 (1): 19–24.

Osuji, P.I. 2014. *African traditional medicine: Autonomy and informed consent*. New York: Springer.

Oyserman, D., H.M. Coon, and M. Kemmelmeier. 2002. Rethinking individualism and collectivism: Evaluation of theoretical assumptions and meta-analyses. *Psychological Bulletin* 128 (1): 3.

Qatar Supreme Council of Health. 2009. *Policies, regulations, and guidelines for research involving human (publication no. 1)*. Qatar: State of Qatar. Available at: http://www.moph.qa/app/media/24.

Rivera, R., D. Borasky, R. Rice, F. Carayon, and E. Wong. 2007. Informed consent: An international researchers' perspective. *American Journal of Public Health* 97 (1): 25.

Silverman, H., H. Edwards, A. Shamoo, and A. Matar. 2013. Enhancing research ethics capacity in the Middle East: Experience and challenges of a Fogarty-sponsored training program. *Journal of Empirical Research on Human Research Ethics* 8 (5): 40–51.

Silverman, H., H. Sleem, K. Moodley, N. Kumar, S. Naidoo, T. Subramanian, and M. Moni. 2014. Results of a self-assessment tool to assess the operational characteristics of research ethics committees in low- and middle-income countries. *Journal of Medical Ethics* 41 (4): 332–339. https://doi.org/10.1136/medethics-2013-101587.

Sleem, H., S.S. El-Kamary, and H.J. Silverman. 2010. Identifying structures, processes, resources and needs of research ethics committees in Egypt. *BMC Medical Ethics* 11: 12.–6939-11-12. https://doi.org/10.1186/1472-6939-11-12.

UNESCO 2009. Mapping research systems in developing countries. Available at: unesdoc.unesco.org/images/0018/001833/183365e.pdf.

Waast, R. 2010. Research in Arab countries (North Africa and West Asia). *Science Technology & Society* 15 (2): 187–231.

Yu, K. 2015. The Confucian alternative to the individual-oriented model of informed consent: Family and beyond. In *Family-oriented informed consent: East Asian and American perspectives*, ed. C. Fan, 93–106. New York: Springer.

Assessment of Research Ethics Committees

Henry Silverman

The establishment of research ethics committees (RECs) in the Arab Region has increased during the last decade in response to the increased research that has occurred in this region. However, the extent of their functioning remains unknown. Accordingly, there has been a growing interest in establishing mechanisms to assess RECs' operations, policies, and procedures. Although assessing RECs' structures and processes of operations do not indicate functioning, they can serve as surrogate measures of functionality.

Assessment efforts have included REC registration coupled with audits that assess REC compliance with established national regulations regarding research. In South Africa, the National Health Research Ethics Council (NHREC) has a registration process and in 2012 it conducted its first audit of all 33 registered RECs to assess their compliance with the Department of Health's Research Ethics Guidelines (National Health Research Ethics Council (NHREC) 2016).

Similar activities are being performed in the Arab Region. For example, Jordan's Law of Clinical Studies requires RECs to register with the Jordan Food and Drug Administration to ensure that they are meeting requirements related to members' diversity and qualifications; regular audits are not performed (Jordan Food and Drug Administration 2011). Similar registration efforts exist in Saudi Arabia and Egypt (see Appendix III).

Additionally, there have been initiatives to formally evaluate RECs via an accreditation process that includes an external review mechanism based on standards drawn from international regulatory requirements, but adapted to existing national standards of the country where the institution resides. Such an effort has been instituted by the Association for the Accreditation of Human Research Protection Programs (AAHRPP) (Association for the Accreditation of Human

H. Silverman (✉)
University of Maryland, Baltimore, MD, USA
e-mail: hsilverm@medicine.umaryland.edu

H. Silverman (ed.), *Research Ethics in the Arab Region*, Research Ethics Forum 5,
https://doi.org/10.1007/978-3-319-65266-5_29

Research Protection Programs (AAHRPP) 2015). This private U.S. organization evaluates an institution's Human Research Protection Program (HRPP), including its IRB(s)/REC(s); accreditation is voluntary. Currently, AAHRPP has conducted reviews of HRPPs and its associated RECs from several institutions in the Arab region.

The Strategic Initiative for Developing Capacity in Ethical Review (SIDCER) implements a two-step process for accreditation (Strategic Initiative for Developing Capacity in Ethical Review (Strategic Initiative for Developing Capacity in Ethical Review (SIDCER) 2015). The first step involves an institution's self-assessment of its program followed by an on-site review by SIDCER.

Since only a few countries have a legal or regulatory framework for clinical research, an accreditation process consisting of an external review mechanism based on national standards is problematic for many countries in the Arab region. In addition, an accreditation mechanism remains problematic for many countries due to the large investment of human and financial resources needed to prepare for such efforts.

Alternatively, RECs can conduct a self-assessment to evaluate their operating characteristics against international standards and demonstrate to their stakeholders the legitimacy of their review mechanisms. Recently, a working group comprised of experts in the Arab region developed an accessible self-assessment tool for RECs based on international standards (Sleem et al. 2010). The self-assessment tool is shown in Appendix III. The tool is divided into the following categories:

- Institutional Commitment
- Policies and procedures of the REC
- Membership composition and educational training
- Submission processes
- Aspects of Minutes Procedures
- Procedures for Protocol review
- Criteria for Informed Consent review
- Processes regarding Communicating a Decision
- Processes for Continuing Review
- REC Resources.

The 'institutional commitment' domain consists of the following items:

- The REC is established under a high-ranking authority;
- Institution regularly evaluates the operations of the REC;
- Institution requires investigators to have training in research ethics in order to submit protocols to the REC;
- Institution requires a conflict of interest policy for members of the research staff;
- The institution provides the following resources:
  - Budget
  - Administrative staff
  - Capital resources

As part of the self-assessment tool, points (1, 2, or 5 points) are assigned to each of the items within each category. A maximum point score of 5 is assigned to those items believed to represent significant aspects of RECs' operations. For example, five points are given to items concerned with the educational efforts of the REC, presence of conflict of interest policies, and extent of the diversity of member composition. In contrast, only one point is given to each of the review criteria. The maximum achievable point total is 200 points. Major limitations of the use of a self-assessment tool involve the objectivity and accuracy with which an REC would have in completing such a tool. Such limitations, however, are inherent in any quality improvement measure.

To assess the feasibility of this self-assessment tool, we performed a study in which we recruited 64 chairs of RECs from three different countries (Egypt, South Africa, and India) to complete this tool (Silverman et al. 2015). The aggregate mean score was 137.4 ± 35.8 and the median score was 145. As a group, RECs achieved more than 80 % of the maximum scores for the following domains:

- Submission processes and documents received
- Aspects of meeting minutes
- Criteria for informed consent

RECs achieved less than 80% of the maximum scores for the following domains:

- Institutional commitment
- Policies and procedures of the REC
- Membership composition and training
- Policies and procedures for protocol review
- Processes regarding communicating a decision letter
- Criteria for continuing review

More than 85% of the REC chairs thought that the tool gave useful information and more than 85% completed the survey in less than 1 hour.

While it is difficult to interpret the meaning of any absolute score obtained on a self-assessment tool, such a tool can provide helpful information to RECs in several ways. First, it can serve as a quality improvement mechanism by identifying standards that need improvement. Second, RECs can compare their scores against the mean scores obtained in the above mentioned study as a benchmark for how well they are operating compared to other RECs in the other regions of the world. Accordingly, chairs can use such data to lobby for more human and capital resources. Finally, the process of self-assessment can raise awareness regarding the strengths and challenges at the level of their individual REC.

References

Association for the Accreditation of Human Research Protection Programs (AAHRPP). 2015. Available at: http://www.aahrpp.org.

Jordan Food and Drug Administration. 2011. Law no. 2 of clinical studies for the year 2011. Available at: http://www.jfda.jo/Default.aspx.

National Health Research Ethics Council (NHREC). 2016. Registration of ethics committees. Available at: http://www.nhrec.org.za/index.php/registration-of-ethics-committees.

Silverman, H., H. Sleem, K. Moodley, N. Kumar, S. Naidoo, T. Subramanian, … M. Moni. 2015. Results of a self-assessment tool to assess the operational characteristics of research ethics committees in low- and middle-income countries. *Journal of Medical Ethics*, 41(4): 332–337. doi:https://doi.org/10.1136/medethics-2013-101587.

Sleem H, R. Adelhai, I. Al-Abdallat, M. Al-Naif, H. Gabr, E.T. Kehil,… H. Silverman. 2010. Development of an accessible self-assessment tool for research ethics committees in developing countries. *Journal of Empirical Research on Human Research Ethics* 6: 85–96.

Strategic Initiative for Developing Capacity in Ethical Review (SIDCER). 2015. SIDCER recognition programme. Available at: http://www.who.int/sidcer/en/.

Case Study: Research Ethics Committee at Cairo University, Egypt

Noha Asem

Introduction

The Faculty of Medicine at Cairo University in Egypt has a responsibility to ensure that scientifically valid research is conducted according to accepted ethical practices that promote the rights and welfare of research subjects. As such, i**n 2002, the Dean of the Faculty of Medicine established a research ethics committee (REC) to review human subject research conducted by staff at Kasr Al Ainy hospital.** Also, Cairo University obtained an FWA from the United States Office of Human Research Protections (OHRP) and the REC registered at OHRP.

The Cairo REC had encountered many challenges during its inception phase. This included insufficient training for its members, lack of diverse membership, and limited resources. All of these challenges have been documented for other RECs in Egypt (Sleem et al. 2010). In addition, at the time of its establishment, **there was a lack of awareness among the faculty regarding research ethics and the functions of the REC. A survey study that involved medical staff members of Cairo University showed that many of the faculty had limited knowledge regarding research ethics and that only 31.4% (27 of 88) had previously submitted a protocol to REC** (Asem and Silverman 2009)**. Raising awareness about research ethics and the roles of the REC became an important mission that the REC achieved primarily through the conduct of several workshops in research ethics, including a faculty conference in 2013. In addition, REC members made presentations in different departments of the faculty about the roles and responsibilities of the REC.**

Originally, the faculty were not required to submit their researches to the REC. Only internationally sponsored clinical trials were required as per the sponsor's country regulations to seek site specific REC approval. Beginning in

N. Asem (✉)
Faculty of Medicine, Cairo University, Cairo, Egypt
e-mail: noha_asem@yahoo.com

H. Silverman (ed.), *Research Ethics in the Arab Region*, Research Ethics Forum 5,
https://doi.org/10.1007/978-3-319-65266-5_30

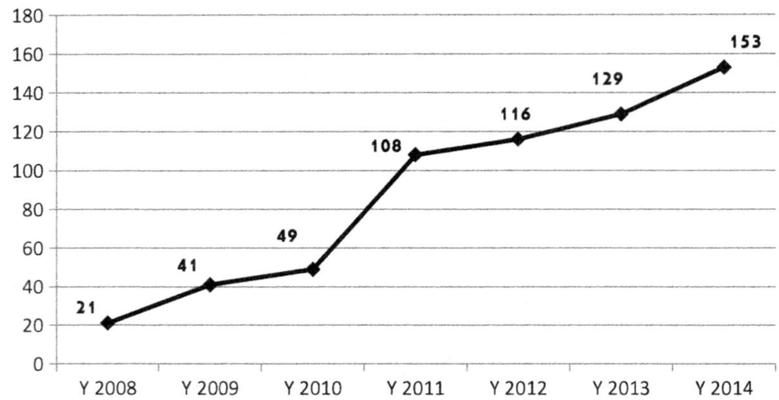

Fig. 1 Numbers of applications to REC from 2008 to 2014

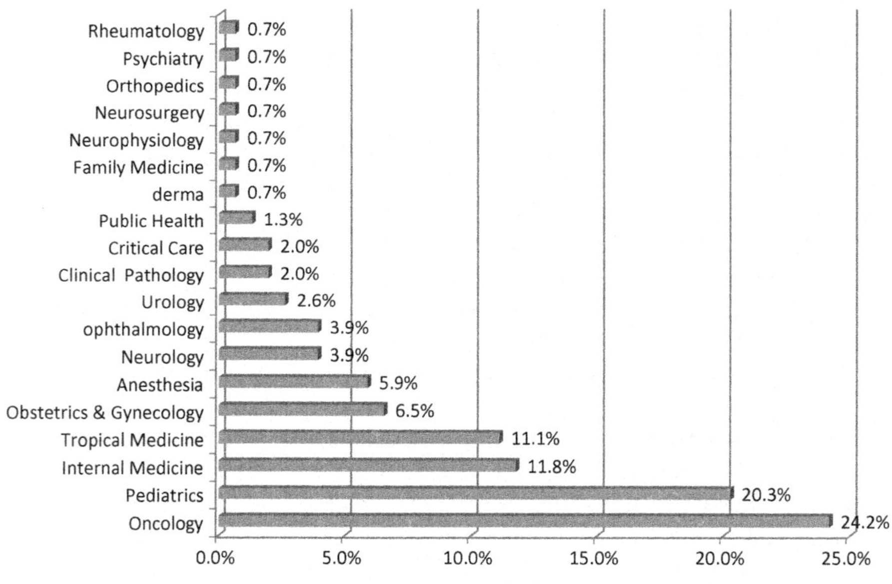

Fig. 2 Applications in 2014 categorized by specialty

2010, the Faculty of Medicine made it mandatory for faculty to submit other types of research for REC approval; these included all master's and doctoral theses that represent high risk interventional studies. This change led to increased applications to the REC, as shown in Figs. 1 and 2. In 2008, 21 applications were submitted, whereas in 2014 the number of applications reached 153 (Fig. 1), representing submissions from 19 departments as shown (Fig. 2).

Governance

The REC is under the governance of the Faculty of Medicine. In 2009, the Vice Dean for Research appointed a senior professor as chair of the REC. Subsequently, the chair made recommendations for who could serve as members, which was presented to the faculty council for approval. The composition of the REC represents a gender-balanced committee comprised of faculty from medicine and other departments. In response to the increased number and diversity of protocol submissions to the REC, an advisory board of 34 staff members from several faculty departments was established. An advisory board member can be invited to review a protocol application and attend certain REC meetings based on the domain of the applied research protocol.

Structure and Operations

Regulations and Guidelines

The REC operates according to Declaration of Helsinki, the WHO Standards and Operational Guidance for Ethics Review of Health-Related Research with Human Participants, the Council for International Organizations of Medical Sciences (CIOMS) and the International Conference of Harmonization, Good Clinical Practice.

Administrative Staff

The increased numbers and complexity of applications to REC raised the need to hire an administrative secretary for the REC office. An REC coordinator has also been assigned since 2010, who has qualifications in research ethics and Good Clinical Practice (GCP).

The main responsibilities of the REC coordinator are as follows:

- Serves as liaison to the research community;
- Conducts initial review of all submissions for completion and identifies regulatory and ethical concerns prior to full board review;
- Gives presentations about the REC to departments at the university;
- Provides consultation to faculty regarding the review process and the technical and ethical requirements for conducting research involving human subjects;
- Helps with designing culturally relevant informed consent forms;
- Works in partnership with the REC chairperson and members to develop and upgrade written guidelines and templates to improve communication and understanding of human research requirements among the faculty;
- Tracks status of submitted and approved studies;
- Records the meeting minutes; and
- Coordinates expedited review of eligible submissions.

Documents

The REC developed several documents and templates to enhance transparency. These include the following: Standard Operating Procedures (SOPs); a standardized REC application form; standardized REC review form; standardized letters for the PI to communicate REC decisions; conflict of interest management plan; confidentiality agreement; continuing review submission form and review form; and amendments submission and review form.

Meetings

The REC meets monthly on Saturdays. A quorum (half of REC membership plus one) is required for a meeting to be held.

Member Training

Four members of the REC received advanced training in research ethics from the Fogarty International Health/NIH -sponsored Middle East Research Ethics Training Initiative (MERETI) that is administered at the University of Maryland University. Other members receive training from the following variety of resources: (1) educational sessions held during REC meetings, (2) online training, including the MERETI, WHO, and CITI programs, and (3) workshops and conferences held at Cairo University. All advisory board members attended a full day workshop in research ethics that was organized by the REC in 2010. Future workshops are planned.

Conflict of Interest Policy

Members are required to reveal their conflict of interests before their first REC meeting. In addition, members are required to declare any professional conflict of interest at the outset of the meeting and if present, do not participate in the subsequent review of that research.

Submissions of Applications

Researchers are requested to complete a standardized REC application form (see Appendix III) accompanied by supporting documents, including their curriculum vitae, study protocol, data collection sheet and informed consent form. All materials must be delivered to the REC office at least 2 weeks before the monthly meeting.

REC ID:

Application for REC Review

Section One: Application Information

Principal Investigator/s:		
Department:		
Title:		
Phone/Pager:		
Fax:		
E-mail address:		
Mailing Address:		

Co Investigators:			
Department:			
Title:			
Phone/Pager:			
Fax:			
E-mail address:			
Mailing Address:			

Title of Project	**Purpose of Project (one or two sentences)**

Estimated duration of total project	
Estimated total number of subjects (including control subjects)	
Age range of subjects	
Sex of subjects	
Where will study be conducted?	
Source of subjects	
Experience of Principal Investigator: Brief summary (also attach a CV)	
What is the total budget of the research?	
Who is the sponsoring agency?	

1-This research project is: (Check all that applies)

1-☐ Single site project
2-☐ Multi-center project
3-☐ National collaborative project
4-☐ International collaborative project

2-What is the type of the research?

1. ☐ Interventional study: Specify the phase: **(1) I** ☐ **(2) II** ☐ **(3) III** ☐ **(4)IV**☐
2. ☐ Observational Descriptive Study (Case report, Case series, Survey)
3. ☐ Observational Analytic study (Cross-sectional, Case-control, Cohort)
4. ☐ Diagnostic test evaluation study
5. ☐ Other: Specify____

REC ID:

3-Does this study include? (Check all that applies)

1. ☐ Placebo
2. ☐ Randomization
3. ☐ Genetic testing
4. ☐ Human Embryo research
5. ☐ Stem cell research
6. ☐ Biological specimens collection
7. ☐ Invasive Techniques

4-Does a Data Safety and Monitoring Board exist for this study?

1. ☐ Yes 2.☐ No

5-Has this study undergone previous scientific review?

1. ☐ Yes 2.☐ No

6-Risks: Indicate what you consider to be the risks to subjects and indicate the precautions to be taken to minimize or eliminate these risks. Justify the need for a placebo control group if one is included in this study. Where appropriate, describe the data monitoring procedures that will be employed to ensure the safety of subjects. Use additional sheets as needed.

____

____

____

7-Benefits: Indicate what you consider to be the benefits to subjects and the society. Indicate the procedures to be taken to maximize these Benefits. Use additional sheets as needed.

____

____

____

8-Indicate whether this project involves any of the following subject populations?

1. ☐ Children (Children are defined by local law as anyone under age 18.)
2. ☐ Prisoners
3. ☐ Pregnant women
4. ☐ Cognitively impaired or mentally disabled subjects
5. ☐ Economically or educationally disadvantaged subjects

9-What type of consent will be obtained from research subjects?

☐ Written consent
☐ Oral consent
☐ Will not obtain consent

10-If written consent will not be obtained, explain why.

____

____

____

11-Will subjects receive any compensation for participation in cash or in kind?

1. ☐ Yes 2.☐ No

12-If subjects receive any compensation; please describe amount or kind of compensation

____

____

____

13-Will identifiable, private, or sensitive information be obtained about the subjects or other living individuals?

REC ID:

1. ☐ Yes 2.☐ No

14-Explain how Privacy and Confidentiality of Data and Records will be maintained:

15-Briefly outline in average "300 words" the expected benefits of the proposed research regarding health development in Egypt and the expected progress of medical knowledge and medical care to our community

16-Kindly, provide information regarding any changes in the original study protocol and outline the details of his study in the local Egyptian study site.

PI Signature:

Date:

Type of Submissions

Table 1 shows the major research designs of the submissions to the REC between 2011 and 2014. Interventional studies represent the main type of research submitted to the REC, which has increased yearly since 2011, reflecting the increased number of industry sponsored clinical trials conducted at the Faculty of Medicine. Also, masters and doctoral theses are increasingly involving experimental studies. Table 1 also shows that phase III clinical trials represents the main category of submitted experimental studies; 63.3% in 2011 and 71.1% in 2014. The percentage of Phase II and Phase IV studies range between 10% and 20%, while the number of Phase I studies is no more than 1 or 2 studies per year. Beginning in 2013 and 2014, slightly more than half of the applications to REC represented multicenter studies (data not shown). Also, international collaborative studies represented 50.4% and 49.0% of the total number of submitted proposals for years 2013 and 2014, respectively (data not shown).

Table 1 Clinical designs of researches submitted to the REC 2011–2014

Research category		2011 n	2011 %	2012 n	2012 %	2013 n	2013 %	2014 n	2014 %
Interventional studies		60	55.6	77	66.4	92	71.3	114	74.5
Phase of experimental studies	Phase I	2.0	3.3	1.0	1.3	2.0	2.2	1.0	0.9
	Phase II	10	16.7	16	20.8	17	18.5	20	17.5
	Phase III	38	63.3	51	66.2	62	67.3	81	71.1
	Phase IV	10	16.7	9	11.7	11	12.0	12	10.5
Observational		48	44.4	39	33.6	37	28.7	39	25.5
Total		108	100.0	116	100.0	129	100.0	153	100.0

Table 2 Specific issues included in studies submitted to REC 2011–2014; total n = 108

Research category	2011 n	2011 %	2012 n	2012 %	2013 n	2013 %	2014 n	2014 %
Biological specimens collection	31	28.7	52	44.8	57	44.2	65	42.5
Genetic testing	9	8.3	17	14.7	30	23.3	33	21.6
Stem cell research	1	0.9	6	5.2	2	1.6	2	1.3

Table 2 shows specific research issues involved with many of the submitted proposals. As shown, there has been an increase in number of studies involving biological samples/specimens; 31 applications (28.7%) in 2011, which increased to 65 (42.5%) in 2014. Application involving genetic testing progressively increased from 9 (8.3%) in 2011 to 33 (21.6%) in 2014. The number of submissions for stem cell research has not increased, which reflects the concerns of REC regarding aspects of stem cell research.

Informed Consent

Guidelines emphasize that written consent is required for human subject research with few exceptions, e.g., to waive the documentation of signature or waive any or all of the basic elements of informed consent. Table 3 shows that documentation by a written signature has increased from 77.8% of studies in 2011 to 97.4% in 2014. The increase in documentation by written consent is mainly attributed to the increased number of interventional studies. Very few studies are performed in which a waiver of consent is granted.

Table 3 Types of informed consent in research submitted to REC 2011–2014

	2011		2012		2013		2014	
	n	%	n	%	n	%	n	%
Written	84	77.8	106	91.4	118	91.5	149	97.4
Verbal	20	18.5	8	6.9	5	3.9	4	2.6
Waiver	4	3.7	2	1.7	6	4.7	0	0.0
Total	108	100.0	116	100.0	129	100.0	153	100.0

Table 4 REC decisions: 2011–2014

	2011		2012		2013		2014	
	n	%	n	%	n	%	n	%
Unconditional approval	63	58.3	62	53.4	66	51.2	83	54.2
Conditional approval	34	31.5	44	37.9	51	39.5	61	39.9
Deferral	9	8.3	8	6.9	9	7.0	7	4.6
Disapproval	2	1.9	2	1.7	3	2.3	2	1.3
Total	108	100	116	100	129	100	153	100

Decisions of the REC

One of the four following decisions is made after protocol review:

1. Unconditional approval;
2. Conditional approval with clarifications or modifications;
3. Deferral due to insufficient information to make a decision
4. Disapproval when a proposal lacks sufficient social values or present major safety concerns that does not appear to be remedial.

Table 4 shows the REC decisions from 2011 to 2014. It shows that the most common decisions are unconditional approval (above 50%) followed by conditional approval. Deferral decisions are less frequent (less than 10%). Common reasons for deferrals include: unacceptable study design, insufficient supportive documents or published papers related to the safety of study intervention, or insufficient preclinical data, pharmacological or pharmacokinetics of a study drug. Disapproval decisions are the least common decision given for the submitted studies (less than 3%). Most common reasons for disapproval includes an unfavorable assessment of the risk benefit ratio and the prospect of risky adverse events.

Monitoring of REC Approved Studies

The REC monitors approved studies through continuing review, which is required on a yearly basis for most protocols and more frequently for high risk protocols with potential major safety concerns. Monitoring is also achieved by mandatory reporting requirements that includes safety reports, progress reports, protocol deviations, end-of-study notification, and clinical study reports. Local serious adverse events must be reported within 24 h to the REC. The auditing role of the REC is still limited to individual cases where protocol deviations are reported or complaints are received from research participants.

Special Considerations

International Research

There has been an increased number of international studies submitted to the REC during the past few years. Concerns regarding these studies are mainly related to research design issues and the nature and extent of post-trial benefits. Specifically, the most common concerns are as follows: relevance of the research to the health needs of the local population; applicability of the research design to the local cultural context, especially among socially or economically disadvantaged people; presence of insurance coverage; presence of Data Safety and Monitoring Board (DSMB), including national and international clinical trials; informed consent that is sensitive to the local setting; post-trial benefits to research participants and to the local population.

Stem Cell Research

Standard practice in clinical stem cell research necessitates specific regulations to ensure the biological safety of the infused stem cells, including consideration of long range side effects and minimizing exposure to unknown risks. As such, there are additional regulatory requirements for stem cell research that uses ex-vivo expanded stem cells that regulates methods of stem cell preparation in the laboratory. For example, stem cells for human use must be collected and expanded ex vivo in dedicated facilities, with filtered laminar flow of environmental air and controlled access in compliance with Good Manufacturing Practice (GMP) rules. Oversight and regular auditing of these processes are necessary ("ISSCR Guidelines for the Clinical Translation of Stem Cells" 2009).

Based on REC responsibility in ensuring safety and welfare of patients who participate in stem cell studies, while promoting ethical research in the institute, the REC requires the following actions to be implemented before clinical stem cell researches can proceed:

- Examining the available stem cell laboratory for compliance with the facility requirements of stem cell research regulations and recommending the required improvements if any.

- Establishing the critical preparatory requirements for cells to be infused into patients including sampling, culture and growth factor, cell infusion, in vivo cell tracking and follow up issues.
- Establishing the necessary quality control and biosafety measures to be implemented and monitored.
- Establishing the frequency and requirements for regulatory audit of stem cell clinical studies.
- Establishing an institutional policy and procedures that ensure and enforce the above measures.

Research Involving Storage/Exportation of Biological Samples

There was an increase in number of studies submitted to REC that involved collection of biological samples/specimens (Table 2). There are compelling scientific reasons for the collection, export, storage and reuse of human biological samples for research purposes (Tindana et al. 2014). However, the practice of exporting and sharing human biological samples from Africa and the Arab region have raised concerns about appropriate mechanisms to safeguard the interests of sample donors and their communities (Zhang et al. 2010). Specific issues involve safeguarding confidentiality, benefit-sharing, and informed consent, particularly for future use of stored samples. Obtaining appropriate consent for sample export and reuse that allows research participants to put limits for using of their stored samples in future research is the most frequent concern. Finally, approval is required from the Egyptian National Security Agency before exportation of any biological material outside the country.

Informed Consent

Inform consent forms for international researches have usually led to the use of lengthy and complex consent documents, especially after translation into the Arabic language. A large proportion of the narrative in such consent forms are usually due to the input of legal language required by sponsors. Such language is complex and makes comprehension problematic for many potential research participants, thus presenting difficulties for the consent process.

This issue was discussed in several REC meetings and accordingly, a site specific consent form template was developed (see Appendix IV). It provides a guide to the essential components of the consent form, as well as site specific contact information for research participants. When an applied consent document is more than five pages, the principal investigator may be required to submit a consent form that provides potential research participants with the most essential and site specific information they need to know in a simpler more reader friendly form in the beginning of the ICF. Subsequently, the full consent document is presented.

استمارة الموافقة على المشاركة في البحث

عنوان البحث

الباحثون: استاذ دكتور جامعة

استاذ دكتور جامعه

استاذ دكتور جامعه

الغرض من الدراسة:

الإجراءات / الأعمال المطلوبة من المشارك:

الفترة الزمنية المطلوبة للمشاركة:

المخاطر:

.

الفوائد للمشارك والمجتمع:

حماية خصوصية المشارك و سرية البيانات:

المشاركة تطوعية:

تكاليف المشاركة في البحث: :

التعويض:

Version……, Date……….

الحق في الانسحاب:

البدائل المتاحة في حالة عدم الرغبة في المشاركة:

(لا يحرمك التوقيع على نموذج الموافقة هذا أى من حقوقك القانونية بأى حال كما لا يعفي الباحثين أو الراعى أو المؤسسة المشاركة من مسئولياتهم المهنية او القانونية)

- لمعرفة المزيد عن هذه الدراسة يمكنك الاتصال بالدكتور-------------- ت: ------------- 02

أو الاتصال بالدكتور-------------- ت: ------------- 02

- فى حالة حدوث متاعب صحية نتيجة المشاركة فى الدراسة يمكنك الاتصال بالدكتور------------ ت:---------- -02

أو الاتصال بالدكتور-------------- ت: ------------- 02

أو التوجه الي --.

- فى حالة وجود شكوى، يرجى الاتصال بمكتب لجنة مراجعة اخلاقيات البحوث تليفون رقم.....................

إذا كنت توافق على الاشتراك فى هذه الدراسة، قم بالإشارة فى المكان المناسب فى الجزء التالى:

_____: لقد تم شرح كل المعلومات الواردة فى هذه الاتفاقية.

_____: لقد قرأت وفهمت المعلومات الواردة فى هذه الاتفاقية.

اسم المشارك: ______________________ توقيعه: ______________________

شاهد علي إجراءات الموافقة : ______________________ توقيعه: ______________________

توقيع مسئول الدراسة: ______________________________________

التاريخ: ____________________

لا تعتمد إلا إذا كان خاتم لجنة مراجعة اخلاقيات البحوث عليها .

سارية من : / / 201 إلى / / 201

تسلم نسخة للمشارك وتحفظ النسخة الأصلية مع الباحث فى ملف المشارك

Version……, Date……….

Challenges Facing the Cairo University REC

The following represent challenges to the REC at Cairo University:

Lack of National Regulations for Research Ethics

To date, there are no national regulations for research ethics in Egypt to provide specific guidance to RECs in its review of research that is responsive to the local context. However, a draft law for guiding clinical research has been drafted and waiting for the parliament to discuss, make any necessary changes, and grant approval.

Resources

A lack of human and physical resources represents a common challenge, as mentioned before and identified for other RECs in Egypt (Sleem et al. 2010)**. Initially, the REC had no dedicated office space, supplies, computer or other IT facilities. In 2008,** the Dean and Vice Dean for Research and Postgraduate Studies provided additional meeting space and office equipment **in 2010.**

Current efforts are directed to the development of a complete management information system. This has been a priority for the REC's plan of improvement in response to the increased numbers and complexity of applications. On the other hand, continuous updating and capacity building among all members of REC to keep the pace with advancements of research is important for continuous capacity building.

Awareness and Knowledge of Researchers Regarding Issues in Research Ethics

Concerns have been expressed about the awareness and knowledge of researchers regarding issues in research ethics. For example, a study conducted among 135 medical researchers from Cairo University in 2008 showed that they desired more training on the principles of research ethics and writing a proper informed consent (Asem and Silverman 2009). Another study performed in south Egypt showed that the academic medical staff had deficient knowledge about research ethics and that they desired more research ethics training (Shabrawy et al. 2014). Template submission forms for researchers applying to REC were developed to overcome some of their knowledge-based challenges. Also, the REC has organized several faculty annual conferences aimed at raising awareness and knowledge regarding research ethics among staff and students.

Monitoring and Auditing Role

Parties responsible for the oversight of multi-centre clinical trials include researchers, institutions, sponsors of research, and RECs. It remains controversial regarding best practices for a monitoring role for RECs (Pickworth 2000). Currently, REC monitoring is limited to specific studies and occurs only after being notified of adverse events and protocol violations. Extension of the monitoring role of REC beyond the mere receipt of reports will require additional human and capital resources.

Next Steps

The REC is taking steps towards expanding its role in raising awareness and building capacity among the staff and students at Kasr Al-Ainy. Intense efforts are also planned to enhance the service it provides to researchers, e.g., faster turnaround times of ethical review. Finally, strengthening the REC's information system as well as automation of several of its functions will be more cost-effective.

References

Asem, N., and H.J. Silverman. 2009. *Perspectives of faculty at Cairo University towards research ethics and informed consent*. Abstract Presentation at PRIM&R, Nashville, Tenn.

ISSCR Guidelines for the Clinical Translation of Stem Cells. 2009. *Current Protocols Stem Cell Biology*., Appendix 1, Appendix 1B. https://doi.org/10.1002/9780470151808.sca01bs9.

Pickworth, E. 2000. Should local research ethics committees monitor research they have approved? *Journal of Medical Ethics* 26 (5): 330–333.

Shabrawy, E., T. Hifnawy, and H. Reda. 2014. Applying ethical guidelines in clinical researches among Academic Medical Staff: An experience from South Egypt. *British Journal of Medicine and Medical Research* 4 (10): 2014–2024.

Sleem, H., S. El-Kamary, and H.J. Silverman. 2010. Identifying structures, processes, resources and needs of research ethics committees in Egypt. *BMC Medical Ethics* 11: 12.

Tindana, P., C.S. Molyneux, S. Bull, and M. Parker. 2014. Ethical issues in the export, storage and reuse of human biological samples in biomedical research: perspectives of key stakeholders in Ghana and Kenya. *BMC Medical Ethics* 15: 76. https://doi.org/10.1186/1472-6939-15-76.

Zhang, X., K. Matsui, B. Krohmal, A.A. Zeid, V. Muthuswamy, Y.M. Koo, … R.K. Lie. 2010. Attitudes towards transfers of human tissue samples across borders: an international survey of researchers and policy makers in five countries. *BMC Medical Ethics* 11: 16. doi:https://doi.org/10.1186/1472-6939-11-16.

Case Study: Research Ethics Committee at King Hussein Cancer Center, Jordan

Maysa Al-Hussaini

Introduction

The King Hussein Cancer Center (KHCC) established its Institutional Review Board (KHCC-IRB) in 2003. It aims at protecting the rights and welfare of human research participants during the conduct of research. In addition to the regulations in the Jordanian Clinical Studies Law (Jordan Food & Drug Administration 2011), the KHCC-IRB functions in accordance with international standards, which includes the Belmont report, the Declaration of Helsinki, and the International Conference of Harmonization-Good Clinical Practice (ICH-GCP). KHCC acquired an FWA since 2003 and its IRB is also registered with OHRP.

Governance, Structure, and Operations

The governance, structure, and operations (including policies and procedures that regulate the functions of the KHCC-IRB) are defined in the IRB manual that was developed and approved by KHCC in 2003. It was reviewed and updated in 2008 and is regularly up-dated when necessary. This latest update included an ethical framework for biobank research, as a new biobank (KHCCBIO) was established in 2012. The manual is currently undergoing another update in preparation for an impending accreditation by the Association for the Accreditation of Human Research Protection Programs (AAHRPP).

M. Al-Hussaini (✉)
Department of Pathology and Laboratory Medicine, King Hussein Cancer Center, Amman, Jordan

Institutional Review Board (IRB), King Hussein Cancer Center, Amman, Jordan
e-mail: mhussaini@khcc.jo

H. Silverman (ed.), *Research Ethics in the Arab Region*, Research Ethics Forum 5,
https://doi.org/10.1007/978-3-319-65266-5_31

Governance

The Director General (DG)/Chief Executive Officer (CEO) of KHCC appoints the IRB Chair, who in turn nominates the IRB members. The IRB Chair reports directly to the DG/CEO. An IRB coordinator manages the daily operations, who acts as a liaison between the IRB Chair and members on one hand, and researchers and other research stakeholders at KHCC on the other hand. The IRB coordinator is a full time employee at KHCC and administratively is part of the Office of Research and Scientific Affairs (OSAR).

Member Composition

The KHCC-IRB is composed of 24 members consisting of a Chair and a Deputy Chair, as well as regular and alternate members. Each regular member has a matching alternate member with equivalent qualifications. If a regular member cannot attend a meeting, the corresponding alternate assumes his/her role with full voting privileges. The term of membership is 2 years and is renewable. Members are appointed based on recommendation from the IRB Chair to the DG/CEO.

The KHCC-IRB is composed of a mixture of physicians, pharmacists, nurses and scientists, in addition to community representatives and a lawyer. The KHCC-IRB members reflect the diversity of the departments, programs and services available at KHCC. Figure 1 shows the composition of the KHCC-IRB from 2009 to 2013 and shows that the male to female and MD to non-MD ratios have been well balanced (King Hussein Cancer Center – IRB. Five year summary. Annual report 2009–2013).

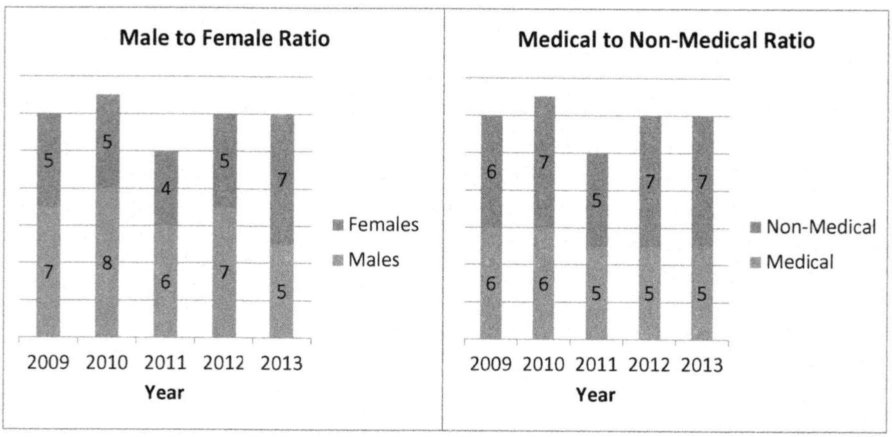

Fig. 1 Composition of the KHCC-IRB (2009–2013)

Operations

Protocol Submission Details

Submitting a study proposal for ethics review and approval at KHCC follows an established process. Investigators are required to use specific submission forms (Appendix V: Form A and Appendix VI (Form B) to facilitate the submission process. Form A is designated for Exempt reviews, while Form B is more detailed and is for Expedited and Full Board reviews. The first two pages of both forms are almost identical. The first page contains the title of proposal, the IRB accession number and a list of all documents that should be submitted. The second page contains details of the research team composition including the Principal Investigator (PI) and co-investigators (Co-Is), who should all sign the form's hard copy. Soft and hard copies (with signatures) are requested for all submissions.

Templates of informed consent forms (ICF) are available in Arabic and English languages (Appendix VII). They serve to guide researchers on the essential elements that should be included in any ICF. If appropriate, there is a form which investigators should submit if they are requesting a waiver of consent. Additionally, there are forms for continuing reviews, modification of approved proposals, end of study reports, reporting of adverse events, disclosure of conflict of interest (COI), and for a confidentiality agreement. All forms are readily available and easily accessible on the IRB webpage at KHCC's intranet. For interventional studies, including PI-initiated studies, a full study protocol must be submitted as well. Once all submission requirements are completed, a unique IRB accession number is assigned.

Numbers and Types of Studies

The number of studies submitted for review at KHCC-IRB have ranged from 71 to 96 studies per year (King Hussein Cancer Center – IRB. Five year summary. Annual report 2009–2013). The top 5 submitting departments are medical oncology, surgery, pediatrics, nursing and pathology. The use of pre-existing data, including archived pathology material, is the most common type of research category; in 2014, 42 of 80 (52.5%) submitted studies represented this category. Questionnaire/survey studies represent the next most frequent type of studies (n = 27, 33.75%), whereas only two (2.5%) phase-3 clinical studies were submitted in 2014.

Types of IRB Review

Each study is assigned a review type, which includes exempt, expedited, or full board review. These review types are determined by the study's level of risk and the type of study population, especially when including a vulnerable population, e.g., children, mentally incapacitated, etc.

Exempt review is the most common type, accounting for 81.0% of reviewed studies in 2014. Research is classified as being exempt when the level of risk is no more than minimal risk, does not involve vulnerable populations, and falls under one of the categories for Exempt review listed in Form-A, e.g., the secondary use of pre-existing biospecimens, or de-identified laboratory samples and survey/interview type of research. The review is completed by the IRB Chair, his/her designee, or an assigned IRB member.

Expedited review represents the least common type of review, accounting for 9% of studies submitted in 2014. Expedited review occurs when the protocol's risk is no more than minimal risk and falls under one of the listed categories in Form-B. The IRB Chair or his/her designee plus another IRB member review the proposal and associated documents.

Studies judged to have more than minimal risk require Full-Board review. This is the second most common type of review, accounting for 11% of all studies reviewed in 2014.

The most common initial decision granted to submitted studies is "Approval with clarifications". On average, one to two studies are rejected/year, which have been mostly due to the lack of adequate experience by the PI to conduct the study or when the study population is determined non-suitable to participate in the study. Examples include high-risk populations, such as bone marrow transplant patients or patients in ICU settings.

Turnaround Time

The turnaround time (TAT), from the day of assignment of an accession number to the time of final approval, is monitored for all submissions. The median TAT for the Exempt review is 2 days (range 2–6 days), for expedited review is 31 days (range 22–35 days), and for Full-Board review is 68 days (range 63–106 days); see Fig. 2 (TAT by the type of submission). A recent increase in the TAT has occurred with the intra-mural grants program, representing KHCC investigator-initiated studies/clinical trials. These studies first undergo a scientific review by the Research Council (RC) followed by IRB review. An IRB decision can override that of the RC. A Notice of Award is issued only after IRB approval.

Meeting Details

The tentative meeting dates of the IRB are scheduled at the beginning of each calendar year and posted on the IRB webpage at KHCC's intranet. The committee meets no less than once per month. At least 5 days prior to each meeting, all members receive the minutes of the previous meeting, the agenda, which lists all approved studies by Exempt, Expedited or Full-Board reviews, all updates on previously approved studies, and adverse event reports.

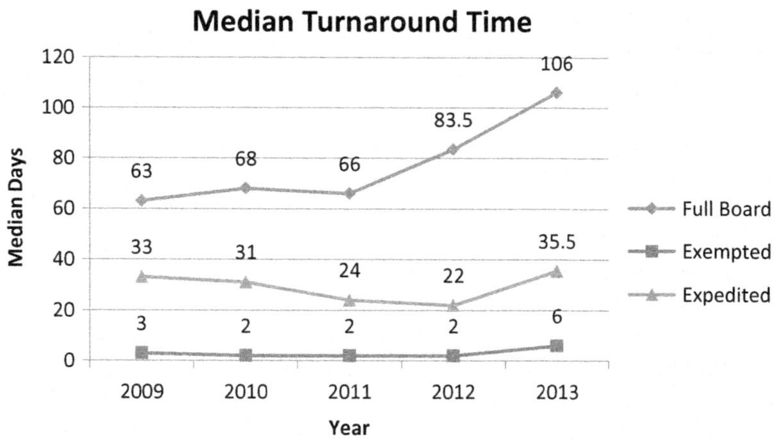

Fig. 2 Median turnaround time for IRB approval by the category of submission, 2009–2013 King Hussein Cancer Center – IRB. Five year summary. Annual report 2009–2013

The meeting begins with approval of the minutes, followed by reviewing the items on the agenda. The bulk of the time is spent on new business, which includes administrative issues (if applicable) and new studies. Examples of administrative issues include: updating the IRB Manual to reflect changing practices, e.g. the need to have a witness signature on the consent form in interventional studies, mandating the signature of the Chief Medical Officer when the Chair of the Department is the PI or Co-I, and discussing new paradigm of research (e.g., the use of stem cells in research).

On average, the full board of the IRB reviews one to two studies per month. All study documents are sent in advance to three regular IRB members and their alternates who serve as the primary reviewers for the protocol. These documents are sent no less than 2 weeks before a scheduled meeting. The IRB members use a specific "IRB Member Review Form" for their review. A checklist for the essential elements that should be present in the Informed Consent Form (ICF), which is available both in English and Arabic languages, is sent with the ICF for the IRB members involved in the primary review as well as the community representative(s). At the meeting, the assigned reviewers, both regular and alternate, provide their assessment of the scientific and ethical merits of the study. This is followed by a discussion among the other attending members. The ICF, when available, is reviewed and discussed meticulously with special attention to the comments by the community representative(s).

Voting takes place at the end of the discussion and one of the following determinations is given: approval, approval with clarifications, deferral until further modifications, or rejection decisions. All attending regular members, as well as alternates for their respective non-attending regular members, have the right to vote or abstain. A decision is determined by a majority of the voting members, which requires 50% of the members plus 1 additional vote. Proposals given a determination of approved or approved with clarifications can later be signed by the IRB-Chair, upon satisfying the clarifications (if applicable). Deferral decisions, however, are brought back to a full board IBB meeting for further discussions. Occasionally, the IRB invites the PI to respond to the comments. At least two-third of the members must be present to maintain the quorum, which must include the Chair or Deputy, and the community representative. On average, the meeting time ranges between 1.06 and 1.32 h (King Hussein Cancer Center – IRB. Five year summary. Annual report 2009–2013).

Post-meeting Actions

The IRB coordinator prepares the meeting minutes, which are reviewed by the Chair. Within 1 week of the meeting, an email is sent to the PI with the IRB's determination and recommendations. If the study is approved, then the PI receives a list of the PI's responsibilities, and IRB-approved stamped versions of any study related documents that will be used in the study; e.g., ICF and/or questionnaires. The IRB stamp contains a clear statement of approval ("IRB Approved"), as well as the approval and expiration dates, which is one calendar year from the date of the IRB determination. Only valid copies of stamped documents are allowed to be used with research participants during the active conduct of research. An electronic alert is sent to the PI(s) requesting their attendance at the IRB Office to receive a hard copy of the approval letter and all stamped documents. A letter directed to the Medical Records Department is issued, to grant access to the confidential medical records of the patients, if needed.

Continuing Review

PIs are required to submit continuing review reports at least annually. To achieve this purpose, an automatic email is generated from the IRB database, 11 months from the approval date, addressed to the PI(s), requesting an update on the status of the study. In addition, PI(s) are required to provide other updates, such as "adverse events reports", important changes to the protocol or the ICF, as well as any changes in the composition of the research team.

Annual Reports: Quality Assurance Activity

The IRB submits annual reports at the end of each calendar year compiling the different indicators monitored by the IRB. A 5-year summary report was prepared summarizing and outlining the various indicators from 2009 to 2013 King Hussein Cancer Center – IRB. Five year summary. Annual report 2009–2013. The KHCC IRB is meeting most of the set targets for the following indicators (see also Figs. 1 and 2):

- IRB composition; this includes the IRB member list since the last JFDA approval with any resignations, appointments or change in the status from alternate to regular members, the male to female and MD to non-MD ratios.
- Number of Full-Board meetings held during the year, the percentage of members attending (quorum), and duration of meetings.
- Submitted proposals: this includes the total number of submitted proposals classified by type of review (Exempt, Expedited, Full-Board), the type of sponsorship (none, intra-mural grants, extramural grants and pharmaceutically-sponsored studies), and the submitting departments as determined by the department of the PI.
- Status of the submitted proposals at the end of the year: this is determined as approved, rejected, and withdrawn by the PI and pending approval.
- The turnaround time (TAT) from submission to approval is also monitored for each type of review process which are compared against set targets (the targets are Exempt studies, 7 working days; Expedited, 30 working days and Full-Board, 90 working days).

The annual report also summarizes any educational activities held for the IRB members. One example was a teleconference workshop sponsored by MERETI in 2009. This program included seven teleconference seminars with assignments held over a 3-month period. The annual report also states future goals to be accomplished in the following year. An example of such a goal was the awareness campaign launched in 2013, which targeted patients, visitors, and employees at the KHCC. We also organized a 2-day workshop on the ethics of biobanks to help IRB members understand the various ethical issues that might be encountered, including the types of consent forms used (broad versus specific), and ethical issues regarding re-contact of participants and the return of results and incidental findings.

Recurring Educational Activities

We recently instituted at the IRB meetings regular educational sessions in which IRB members give 10–15 minutes presentation at the beginning of the meetings. New IRB members are requested to complete the NIH course on "Protection of Human Research Participants".

Conflict of Interest Policy

A Conflict of Interest (COI) policy for IRB members was developed in 2009. This policy clearly defines and states the conditions under which a COI exists. Procedures to be taken once a COI is declared includes leaving the IRB meeting during the discussion of the protocol, prohibition to voting and actions taken if quorum is lost due to COI by one of the IRB members.

We conducted a survey in 2009 to measure the satisfaction of the various stakeholders with their interactions with the IRB. Most respondents found the webpage of the IRB at KHCC's intranet useful and contains the information needed to facilitate the submission process and that the IRB generated forms are user-friendly. Respondents felt that the IRB coordinator was helpful with facilitating communications with the IRB. Educational sessions on the submission process, the types of reviews and the IRB function were requested. Accordingly, we organized several teaching sessions to the various groups, which included the Surgical Department, the Pathology Department and Hospice and Palliative Care Program, who are frequent users of the IRB. However, many investigators thought that the approval process was lengthy. Accordingly, the IRB set TAT targets that were conveyed to the investigators and monitored.

Challenges

The KHCC-IRB encounters many challenges, some of which are common to other IRBs in the country and the region and other emerging clinical trial markets. Some of the challenges include the following;

IRB Membership

(a) **Turnover of IRB members**: on average, 20 % of IRB members leave the IRB each year. This has ranged from 8 % in 2012 to 29 % in 2011. Resigning from the IRB is more frequent among non-MDs compared to MDs. The major drawback is the need for continuous recruiting and training of new members.

(b) **Lack of regular training for IRB members**: Reviewing a proposal under an Expedited or Full-Board review categories require special skills. Similar to other functioning IRBs in the emerging clinical trial markets (Lansang and Dennis 2004), there is a lack of dedicated training for IRB members and investigators in research ethics. The Jordanian Food and Drug Administration (JFDA) used to hold a full day symposium for IRB members and investigators on the essentials of research ethics with a focus on the principles of research ethics, the informed consent process and documents, and the role of the IRBs in ensuring ethical research. However, these symposia have been suspended and training of IRB members is only accomplished by briefings provided by the IRB Chair at the beginning of their membership.

(c) **IRB Members' Workload:** Many IRB members find it difficult to accommodate their IRB obligations within their busy schedules. Apart from the IRB coordinator, who is the only full time employee at the IRB Office, all other members, including the Chair and Deputy, do not receive any reduction of their other professional obligations when joining the IRB. As such, it becomes difficult to attract members from the hospital staff to join. Additionally; there is no financial compensation for IRB members.

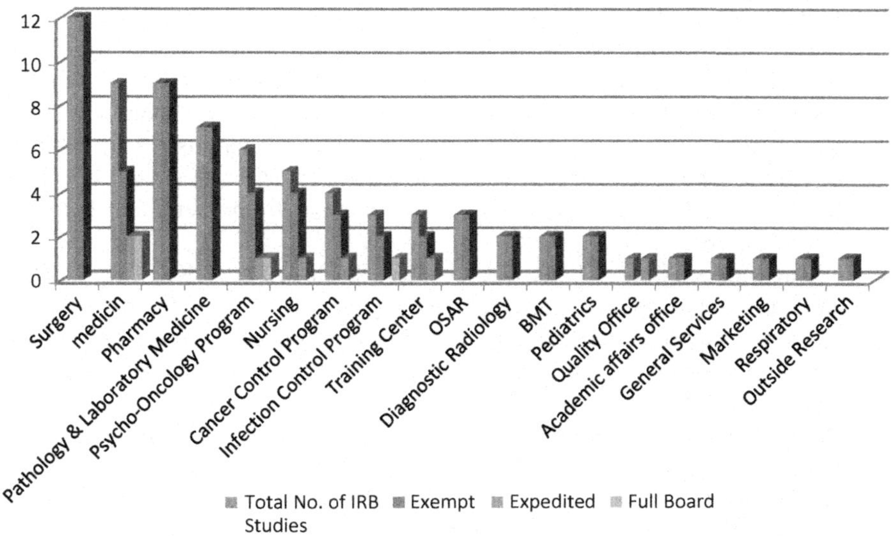

Fig. 3 Studies approved by category of submission from different departments at KHCC 2009–2013 King Hussein Cancer Center – IRB. Five year summary. Annual report 2009–2013

(d) **Diverse Research Portfolio:** KHCC is a comprehensive cancer center that encompasses many departments, programs and services, with varying specialties and sub-specialties. This has resulted in a relatively large and diverse research portfolio. Figure 3 illustrates the number of studies submitted from the various departments in 2009–2013. The IRB has addressed this diverse research portfolio by recruiting members with different scientific backgrounds. In spite of this strategy, members occasionally find it difficult to understand the scientific merits, assess the risk: benefit ratio and the relationship of certain aspects of the protocol to the current standards of practice. As deemed necessary, ad hoc members are invited to help in the review process of complex protocols.

Addressing New Research Paradigms in the Absence of Guidance from a National Law

(a) **Genetic research**: this type of research needs to be reviewed cautiously, as it is associated with several potential risks, including breach of confidentiality, which can lead to social stigma, discrimination, and community harms. Such research may also reveal information about relatives' health status. Potential re-contact of participants regarding genetic results relevant to their health represents another controversial issue. Experience in this type of research is limited at our center for both IRB members and investigators. The first genetic study submitted to KHCC-IRB was related to incidence of BRCA gene mutations in a subset of high risk breast cancer patients diagnosed and managed at

KHCC. This study was discussed at a Full-Board meeting with an initial decision of "deferral until modifications". This included modifying the design of the study from anonymous to coded, with reversal of the code upon receiving the results of the tests, so that patients can become informed and counseled to the next step for themselves and family members. Interim reports were submitted and discussed at IRB meetings every 10th patient. The ICF was amended 3 times to reflect the new IRB recommendations. Opinions from international experts were obtained twice.

(b) **Tissue banks**: A tissue bank was recently established at KHCC (KHCCBIO) and controversial issues related to this type of research involves ownership of the tissue and generated data, transport of tissue samples to other countries, the appropriate limits on the use of tissue samples in future research, and benefit-sharing.

(c) **Data Transfer and Material Transfer**: In a recent study, most patients at the KHCC did not object to the transfer of tissue abroad for research purposes (Al-Hussaini and Abu-Hmaidan 2014). However; in the absence of national regulations on the status of material transfer to regional and international institutions, the IRB and the institution needed to decide on the appropriateness of material transfer on a case-by-case basis. KHCC recently approved a "Data and Material Transfer Agreement" that incorporated the international standards and was approval by the legal representative of the Center. This will alleviate the problem of data and material transfer, while at the same time provide a legal umbrella for the transfer of tissue.

Deficiencies in the Current Clinical Studies Law

The Jordanian Law was the first national effort to regulate the conduct of clinical research Jordan Food & Drug Administration (2001, 2011) and the first document in the Arab countries to reference international guidelines and regulations (Alahmad et al. 2012). However, this Clinical Studies Law has been found to be deficient in several aspects. For example, in comparison to ICH-GCP, it only includes 3 out of 19 essential elements of informed consent. Similar findings were addressed by Ramahi and Silverman, who noted deficiencies in the law, which included the absence of the following requirements for ethical approval: favorable assessment of risks and benefits, the fair selection of subjects, the protection of the rights and welfare of children and other vulnerable subjects participating in research (Ramahi and Silverman 2009). That said, the KHCC-IRB includes all the elements of the ICF as advised by international documents. However, without a national law, there can be variability between different IRBs in Jordan.

Interactions with Investigators

(a) **Tension between researchers and IRB:** The requirement for ethical approval before any study can be performed is now well acknowledged at KHCC, although it took tenacious efforts and support to achieve investigators' compliance. However, many investigators still view the IRB as an additional obstacle for research, and several perceive any comments from the IRB with skepticism. Through their reviews, the IRB members strive to ensure that national/international standards are met, and that research undertaken at the KHCC protects participants' welfare and rights and provides the maximum potential benefits with the minimization of risks. To meet these standards, not infrequently, there are necessary modifications to the ICF, recommendations for additional measures to minimize risks and to ensure protection of the privacy and confidentiality, as well as occasional requests for changes in the design of the study. Investigators, who undoubtedly share these ethical goals, are concerned however, that the IRB imposes impractical demands that impede the ability to conduct research. This doesn't appear to be unique to KHCC. This type of tension is well documented in international literature, although its magnitude might be more exaggerated in this part of the world (Klitzman 2012).

(b) **Confusion with understanding the role of IRB:** Many investigators find it difficult to separate the role of the Research Council, whose primary concern is the scientific review, from that of the IRB, whose primary concern is with ethical review. Continued efforts are made to clarify the separate distinctive roles.

Complexity of Informed Consent Forms (ICF)

Dealing with informed consent in general and informed consent for international research in particular represents one of the most challenging tasks that many IRBs face (Bhutta 2004). The ICF should act as a guide during the consenting process. Surveying the ICFs that the KHCC-IRB received from investigators during the last few years revealed that the documents are translated in a complex, highly- professional medical language that is difficult to comprehend by the average lay person. Ideally, the language of the consent document should be at or below an eighth grade school level. Additionally, the translation is often performed in other Arab countries where the dialect might be different. Several examples are presented in the Table 1. The complexity of the language used in international research is not unique to KHCC, as it has been described across other regions (Hyder et al. 2004). Moreover, not uncommonly the ICF is lengthy. The number of pages in ICFs from international studies submitted to KHCC ranges between 11 and 23 pages, which makes the consenting process problematic for both the research team member and potential research participants.

Table 1 Examples of difficult language used in some of the ICFs and the corrections suggested by KHCC-IRB

التصحيح	الأصلي
عينات دراسة حركة الدواء في الجسم	عينات الحرائك الدوائية
جلسات التسمير	وتجنب استخدام السولاريوم
رئتيك	أنّ رئاك تعرّض للضرر
نقص كرات الدم البيضاء المتعادلة	نقص العدلات
الحزام الناري	الهربس النطاقي
المنتشر	الورم النقيلي
تآكل	وارتشاف العظم

International and Multi-institutional Collaborative Research

In international collaborative research, the foreign investigators would occasionally approach the KHCC-IRB asking whether approval from KHCC was needed if approval was granted from their other IRB(s). A similar problem was described by Hyder et al. who investigated the practices of investigators from low and middle income countries that involved research funded from sponsors from western countries (Hyder et al. 2004). Often, the investigators thought that local IRB approval was not needed once the study was approved by external international IRBs. Also, with multi-institutional PI-initiated research studies, local IRBs might request modifications that differ from the other participating IRBs and the PI might find it difficult to obtain approval on the suggested modifications, an occurrence that can lead to significant delays or inability to perform the research (Ahmed and Nicholson 1996; Menikoff 2010).

Monitoring of Ongoing Studies

Once the IRB approves a proposal, obtaining updates on the status of the study is challenging. In 2013, the IRB sent 71 emails to investigators requesting continuing review reports on their IRB- approved studies. Only 31 (44 %) replied back after the first email. Additionally; proper monitoring of the on-going studies, especially during the process of recruitment, consenting, and conduct of the study, is problematic. Internal audits have been conducted on a few investigator-initiated studies, the findings of which are presented to the IRB and discussed with the PIs. However, systematic monitoring and auditing of all on-going studies has yet to be developed.

Electronic Health Records (EHR)

KHCC is currently in the process of implementing "Vista" EHR system. This is a national E-Health program that aims to link many governmental and military hospitals, allowing sharing the confidential information in the medical records across the different participating premises. Policies governing access to patients' records for research purposes from the participating hospitals have not been developed.

Next Steps

The KHCC has embarked on an ambitious program to enhance its operations. Aspects of this program includes the following:

1. KHCC is in the process of preparing for the AAHRPP accreditation; a process that will enhance the status of KHCC-IRB both nationally and internationally. This process will help us institute the necessary changes to address the several deficiencies and challenges in the current operations of KHCC-IRB. For example; to address the issue of IRB members' training, a budget has been allocated to ensure continuous training of IRB members through the organization of an annual local workshop to address the various issues in research ethics.
2. Additional efforts are planned to enhance the awareness among research subjects and investigators regarding the important roles of IRB and the need for ethical review of any study.
3. We are developing a glossary for the most commonly used and encountered terms in the ICF. This might help to decrease the review time for the ICF, especially those of interventional sponsored studies.

Conclusion

Since its inception in 2003, the KHCC- IRB has been perceived as a major facilitator of ethical research conduct, which was reflected by the survey we conducted in 2009, as well as personal communications received from the JFDA and from the various staff at KHCC, including the higher administration.

The KHCC-IRB represents one of the main stakeholders of research website at King Hussein Cancer Foundation (KHCF)/KHCC, where a summary of the mission, role, composition and contact details are well visualized, reiterating its important role at KHCC (available at: http://www.khcc.jo/section/institutional-review-board).

Although the KHCC-IRB serves as an example of a well-established research ethics committee, it still faces many challenges that can potentially jeopardize its function. Working with other research stakeholders at KHCC should help address these issues. Support from the institution is still needed to further enhance functioning and better acceptance from the staff regarding the roles of the IRB. Such support would include allocation of more resources for training and education. There is also a need for amending the current available local laws to be more in alignment with international regulations and to address new international research paradigms, e.g., research involving genetic testing, biobanks and stem cell research.

References

Ahmed, A.H., and K.G. Nicholson. 1996. Delays and diversity in the practice of local research ethics committees. *Journal of Medical Ethics* 22 (5): 263–266. Retrieved from http://www.ncbi.nlm.nih.gov/pubmed/8910776.

Al-Hussaini, M., and A. Abu-Hmaidan. 2014. Use of human surplus biospecimens in research: A survey from a cancer centre. *Eastern Mediterranean Health Journal* 20 (6): 378–384. Retrieved from http://www.ncbi.nlm.nih.gov/pubmed/24960514.

Alahmad, G., M. Al-Jumah, and K. Dierickx. 2012. Review of national research ethics regulations and guidelines in Middle Eastern Arab countries. *BMC Medical Ethics* 13: 34. https://doi.org/10.1186/1472-6939-13-34.

Bhutta, A.Z. 2004. Beyond informed consent. *Bulletin of the World Health Organization* 82: 771–777.

Hyder, A.A., S.A. Wali, A.N. Khan, N.B. Teoh, N.E. Kass, and L. Dawson. 2004. Ethical review of health research: A perspective from developing country researchers. *Journal of Medical Ethics* 38: 68–72.

Jordan Food & Drug Administration. 2001. Law of clinical studies provisional law no. 97 for the year 2001. Available at: http://www.menareti.net/uploadfiles/Mereti/Clinical_trial_law_jordan_provisional_law_97_2001.pdf.

Jordan Food and Drug Administration. 2011. Law no. 2 of clinical studies for the year 2011. Available at: http://www.jfda.jo/Default.aspx.

King Hussein Cancer Center – IRB. Five year summary. Annual report 2009–2013.

Klitzman, R. 2012. From anonymity to "open doors": IRB responses to tensions with researchers. *BMC Research Notes* 5: 347. https://doi.org/10.1186/1756-0500-5-347.

Lansang, M.A., and R. Dennis. 2004. Building capacity in health research in the developing world. *Bulletin of the World Health Organization* 82 (10): 764–770. Retrieved from http://www.ncbi.nlm.nih.gov/pubmed/15643798.

Menikoff, J. 2010. The paradoxical problem with multiple-IRB review. *The New England Journal of Medicine* 363 (17): 1591–1593. https://doi.org/10.1056/NEJMp1005101.

Ramahi, I., and H. Silverman. 2009. Clinical research law in Jordan: An ethical analysis. *Developing World Bioethics* 9 (1): 26–33. https://doi.org/10.1111/j.1471-8847.2007.00221.x.

Guidance for the Management and Administrative Operations of Research Ethics Committees (REC)

Farida Lada

Introduction

Several authors in this compendium have analyzed the ethical issues reviewed by the RECs. I aim to describe the management and administrative operations of RECs in an effort to provide guidance on the establishment of these committees.

Organizational Structure

Institutional Official

The Institutional Official (IO) is the most senior-level administrator at an institution. The IO promotes an institutional culture of research that is ethical and compliant with the policies of the institution and with the national regulations. Essentially, the IO is responsible for creating a culture that is committed to the protection of human subjects of research. Where applicable, the IO has the authority to legally or contractually bind the institution and take legal or contractual actions on behalf of the institution. As such, the IO serves as the point of contact for all legal and contractual matters.

The IO is responsible for providing adequate resources to the REC in order for it to function effectively. This includes an adequate budget to support the REC's daily operations, sufficient space, and the required competent staff. Finally, the IO is responsible for extending training and education opportunities for all members of the human subject research enterprise, i.e., all members of the research team and members of the REC.

F. Lada (✉)
The City University of New York, New York, NY, USA
e-mail: farida.lada@cuny.edu

H. Silverman (ed.), *Research Ethics in the Arab Region*, Research Ethics Forum 5,
https://doi.org/10.1007/978-3-319-65266-5_32

REC Chair and Vice Chair

The REC Chair and Vice Chair provide leadership to the REC panel. Thus, they are responsible for directing the REC meeting proceedings and discussions so as to ensure compliance with the REC's and Institutional policies and applicable national regulations. The REC Chair and Vice Chair also ensure that the meetings run efficiently and effectively. They are expected to be familiar with the expertise of each of the members on their panel to ensure that the expertise to review specific protocols is present and to request outside consultation as necessary. Finally, the REC Chair and Vice Chair represent the REC in discussions and communications with researchers, institutional leaders and other external parties as needed.

REC Members

REC members, including the Chairs and Vice Chairs, are expected to attend all meetings, review materials related to agenda items for the specific meetings, and participate in the discussion and review of all agenda items, except where they have a conflict. All members of the REC are expected to treat all materials related to proposed research confidentially. Suggestions regarding the process of selecting the type of members are described below.

REC Support Staff

Depending on the size of an institution and its research portfolio, the REC may or may not be supported by an administrative staff. In smaller institutions, it is common for the IRB Chair or Vice Chair to serve in this capacity. Whereas the REC members provide scientific expertise and community-based cultural expertise, the REC administrative staff provide regulatory and policy expertise in addition to administrative support. Thus, the staff provide regulatory and policy guidance to the REC, the researchers and the institutional administration. The administrative responsibilities may include receipt of proposals, preliminary analysis to ensure completeness and compliance with applicable regulations or policies, preparing meeting agendas, ensuring quorum during REC meetings, taking meeting minutes, communicating the REC's decisions to the researchers, and retaining records confidentially. For an example of a model of administrative support staff, one can refer to the roles and responsibilities of the support staff at the American University of Beirut (Al Kassar 2010).

Scope of Reviewed Research

Regarding the scope of the type of research that the REC reviews, an analysis of the current and anticipated research portfolio of the institution should be done, both in terms of volume and types of research. Factors that determine the scope of research reviewed include:

- Should the REC review all types of human subject research performed in the institution (e.g., biomedical and social behavioral research) or only those required by the regulations (e.g., biomedical)?
- Where permitted by the local regulations, should the REC exclude low risk studies (e.g., masters and PhD thesis) to reduce their volume of review, especially when they are newly formed and are just beginning to gain experience?
- Should student research that is performed at the institution be under the purview of the REC, or should another entity review it? Sometimes student research may not be considered generalizable, and as such, is not considered "research" under most guidelines and regulations.

Additional Roles of the REC

Defining the roles of the REC and its scope of research review will help in identifying and securing the types and extent of resources it will need in order to accomplish the goal of promoting ethical and compliant research (see below). In addition to its role to review research (and hence, its authority to approve and disapprove research), additional roles of the REC include the following:

Education and Training

It is important to determine whether the REC will be involved with providing initial and ongoing education and training to REC members and its staff, as well as to investigators and possibly undergraduate and graduate students, This responsibility may reside within the REC office, or it may reside with another entity within the institution.

Monitoring of Research

Similar to education and training initiatives, monitoring of REC approved human subject research, sometimes referred to as quality assurance, may also be performed by either the REC, or delegated to other institutional or external entities. Before a decision on where this responsibility should reside can be made, the institution must decide upon its monitoring strategy. That is:

- Does the institution wish to conduct audits in response to identifiable problems only, or does it wish to conduct routine monitoring of ongoing research?
- If the institution decides to perform routine monitoring, what percentage of the approved research will it monitor? Or will selection of research to monitor be based on other specific criteria, such as the type of research or the type of subject population?

Quality Assurance and Quality Improvement (QA/QI) of REC Operations

QA/QI of the REC operations entails ongoing review and assessment of the effectiveness of REC policies and the efficiencies of its procedures. Effectiveness of the REC policies can be assessed by reviewing the policies for current applicability within the institution, as well as an assessment of the determinations made by the REC and their ability to ensure protection of human subjects through REC audits. Efficiencies of its procedures can be assessed through ongoing evaluation of turnaround times, changes in volume of research reviewed and effectiveness of the current work flows through the identification of any bottlenecks in the process, to ensure timely reviews. These tasks can also be performed by individual(s) within the REC office, or by other internal or external entities.

Resources

RECs cannot operate effectively in an environment that is devoid of a supporting infrastructure. The overall needs of an effective program for oversight of human subject research at an institution can be divided into four major categories: (i) protocol review; (ii) education and training; (iii) monitoring of research; and (iv) quality assurance and improvement of REC operations.

Protocol Review

At a minimum, the REC must have adequate resources to review proposed human subject research. Possible considerations for assessing the needs to support this function may include:

(i) Given the volume of human subject research requiring REC oversight, does the institution need administrative staff in addition to what the Chair and Vice Chair can provide?
    (a) How many staff are required?
    (b) How will the staff roles be differentiated?
    (c) What will be the work flow, i.e. who receives the submission, and what path does it take from submission to approval?
    (d) Is there adequate office space for the staff and/or Chair and Vice Chair?

   (e) Is there sufficient office equipment, such as computers and printers?
   (f) Is there an adequate budget and resource to maintain office equipment?
(ii) How will submissions be tracked and how will adequate record keeping be ensured?
   (a) Is there a need for a specific database or software?
   (b) Will there be paper files? If so, is there an adequately confidential file storage system?
(iii) What resources are required for effective IRB meeting proceedings?
   (a) Is there adequate space to hold confidential IRB meetings?
   (b) Will some or all of the IRB members be allowed to join by teleconference? If so, what type of equipment and/or service do we need to accomplish this?
   (c) Are there private offices/spaces for in-person meetings (e.g., between the Chair and an investigator)?

Education and Training

Regardless of who provides the education and training (the REC or some other entity), the institution must assess whether there are sufficient human and other resources available to ensure adequate initial and ongoing training related to research ethics, stakeholder responsibilities, institutional policies and procedures, and applicable regulations and laws based on an assessment of institutional risks, and education and training needs.

Monitoring of Research

As mentioned above, the institution may decide to monitor ongoing research and assign the REC or some other department to perform this function. Once this decision is made, an assessment of the resources required to accomplish the monitoring tasks can be made.

Quality Improvement and Quality Assurance Activities

The institution must ensure that there are sufficient resources to support these initiatives as described above.

Pragmatic Aspects of Starting a New REC

Starting a new REC requires efforts in several areas, including: (i) development of policies; (ii) development of standard operating procedures (ii) setting up REC panels (e.g., one for biomedical research and another one for social behavioral research); and (iii) appointing REC members.

Policies

RECs establish policies that allow them to most effectively meet their responsibilities toward the protection of human subjects of research. The process for developing policies may differ from that of developing its own procedures, as it may require the involvement of other stakeholders (e.g., top officials). Depending on the institution and the policy topic, the REC may be required to obtain approval or advice from the legal counsel and/or senior administration for the institution, or the REC may be required to obtain policy approval by a governing body such as a Board of Trustees or an Advisory Counsel in the institution. This is because policies often have a greater impact on the institution as a whole and on the institutions' relationships with other external partners. For example, the institutional leadership may require that the policy defining the roles of the REC be approved by them, but that all other polices specific to the review of human subject research can be issued without their approval; or an institution may require that the REC work with the legal counsel and/or senior administration when determining how to manage a researcher's conflict of interest, because it affects not only human subject protection but also the financial support for the research.

It is also important to consider the institutional priorities and culture when developing policies. Are the researchers within the institution more likely to respect and adhere to policies that allow for flexibility, or are they seeking directives? Rigid policies that dictate directives without much flexibility are easier to implement; whereas, more flexible policies allow the decision makers to adjust their determinations based on the specific case at hand. Are the decision-makers sufficiently trained and confident in their ability to apply flexibility where appropriate?

What type of policies should be developed? As mentioned at the beginning of this chapter, it is important that either the institution or the REC have a policy describing the roles of the REC and granting it the authority to protect the human subjects of research through well-defined methods. Other types of policies that may be needed include:

(i) Policy defining the roles and responsibilities of the various stakeholders, including the REC members, the researchers, and any other stakeholders identified as an important participant in the REC review process.
(ii) Policy requiring confidentiality of research protocols for researchers and REC members.
(iii) Policy defining any financial or non-financial conflicts of interest of researchers and REC members, and the requirements for managing such conflicts.
(iv) Policy ensuring the independence of the REC, including the following:
    (a) Membership includes a certain number of non-affiliated persons
    (b) Members and other individuals with conflicts of interest may attend the meetings, but are not present during discussions of the protocols and subsequent voting
    (c) Senior officials responsible for creating the REC or involved in the appointment process do not serve as members of the REC or its Chair

(d) REC members are protected from retaliation based on positions taken with respect to REC-related matters or review of protocols

(v) Policy defining the classification of individuals who may serve as principal investigators.

(vi) Policies outlining any ongoing monitoring by the REC or another entity.

(vii) Policy defining the responsibilities for the review and conduct of collaborative research, both domestically and internationally.

(viii) Any other policies that may be necessary given the local rules, culture, or specific types of research being conducted.

Standard Operating Procedures (SOPs)

Standard operating procedures (SOPs) describe implementation of routine processes or operations. These provide step by step instructions to individuals who are implementing the REC processes. For example, an institution with a large REC support staff with differentiated responsibilities may need an SOP to define the work flow of each of the internal processing steps required to take a submission from receipt to approval. A recent WHO publication offers an inclusive list of items for SOPs of RECs (World Health Organization 2011). An example of an SOP that details the processes for a conveyed meeting is shown in Appendix I.

Establishing or Restructuring a REC

For an institution that is either establishing the REC system for the first time or considering restructuring of its REC system, some important considerations include:

(i) What is the anticipated volume of research? Can the volume of research that is anticipated be reviewed by one REC in a timely manner, or is there a need for more than one REC?

(ii) What types of research will be reviewed? Should all RECs review all types of research or should the RECs be differentiated by type of research they review?

(iii) How frequently will the REC meet? If more than one REC, will they meet on a rotating basis (i.e. 1, 2, 3, 4...) or will each REC meet at the same intervals (i.e. each meets every 2 weeks)?

(iv) Multiple RECs often imply larger volume. This, in turn, implies that the REC will require support staff. Will the same support staff support each REC, or will the RECs have dedicated staff?

(v) If the same staff will support multiple RECs, and each of the RECs meet at the same intervals, will the staff have sufficient time to prepare for each REC meeting, and to address the issues coming out of each REC meeting?

REC Members

Appointing REC members requires attention to the below considerations:

(i) Are there any applicable regulatory requirements (e.g., national laws) for the number of members on an REC and the type of expertise required for the REC (e.g., scientists and non-scientists; types of research that is predominantly performed at the institution)?

(ii) How many members should be on the REC? This depends on the types of expertise required to ensure adequate review of the research. Would the minimal number of members required by any applicable regulations be sufficient for the types of research expected to be reviewed by the REC, or will the research be so diverse that a larger membership will be required?

(iii) From where are the members recruited? Are the majority of the members internal to the institution? This decision may require some consideration of the institutional culture. Will the institutional researchers respect internal members more so than external members or vice versa? Will an REC comprised of mostly internal members provide sufficient representation of the community from which subjects are recruited? Will an REC comprised primarily of internal members require larger numbers of recusals due to conflicts of interest?

(iv) Is there an institutional policy or unspoken rule whereby REC members should be at a certain position level or higher?

(v) What is the process by which members are identified and appointed? Is there a nomination process? Who officially appoints the members? It is important to ensure that the membership appointments are made by someone who has the authority to terminate an appointment should that be required.

(vi) What should be the duration of the member appointment? Will there be a mechanism for evaluating members on a regular basis or when considering a member for re-appointment? If so, what process will be followed to address concerns regarding individual members' contributions to the REC? How can members not in good standing be terminated?

(vii) Will the members be paid some form of compensation for their participation on the REC? If so, will the compensation differ for Chairs and Vice Chairs?

Submission Processes

The REC's SOPs should describe the requirements for investigators submitting an application for review, including submission due dates, meeting dates, the forms to be completed (paper or online), and the list of documents to be submitted (e.g., protocol, informed consent form, investigator's drug brochure, CVs of members of the research team, recruitment materials). The SOPs should also specify the process and procedure for review, process for coordinating review with other committees, process for setting up meetings, circulating materials for the meetings, inviting non-members of the REC, approving the meeting minutes, and any related process issues.

Appeals Process

The SOPs should describe any appeals process for researchers to raise concerns about the REC process or specific determinations.

Review Criteria

The REC should make clear the specific ethical requirements upon which it basis its decisions and make them readily available to researchers and the public. To aid in determining the ethical acceptability of research protocols, an REC should utilize a checklist to ensure that all relevant criteria are considered during review (see Appendix II for an example of a review checklist) and that, as a general rule, similar protocols are treated similarly. The criteria for REC approval should be based on all applicable regulatory requirements, as well as any institutional requirements. The review criteria should also include the requirements for informed consent. Key criteria for the review of research has been articulated in more detail in international ethics guidelines and other commentaries.

Decision Making Procedure

Decisions are arrived at through either a vote or consensus. Consensus does not require that all REC members support the decision, but that all members consider the decision at least acceptable and no member considers the decision unacceptable. There should be a predefined method to determine when votes will be taken and how many favorable votes will be needed for a proposed research to be approved (e.g., majority consisting of one-half the membership + one).

Meeting Dynamics

As noted above, the REC Chair is responsible for directing the REC meeting proceedings and discussions so as to ensure compliance with the REC's roles, applicable regulations, laws and policies. This starts with the following elements, which should be addressed at the beginning of each REC meeting:

(i) Declaration of any conflicts of interest of any of the REC members with respect to the agenda items;
(ii) Reminder that all REC discussions and materials are expected to be treated with strict confidentiality;
(iii) Ensuring that the there is a quorum present, as defined by the SOPs.

Review Process

(i) How will the reviewers for specific submissions be identified? Will reviewer assignments be made based on a rotation system, or based on expertise? Will the process for making reviewer assignments differ for minimal risk research versus greater than minimal risk research? Who will review amendments and continuing reviews (e.g., only the Chair or Vice-Chair)? How many reviewers will review each submission?
(ii) What will be the levels of review (e.g., full REC review, expedited review, or exempt), types of review (e.g., continuing review, amendments, etc.), and who or which entity will be responsible for reviewing the different levels of review (e.g., chairperson or a three-person subcommittee for exempt and expedited reviews).
(iii) What types of submission level decisions can the REC make?
(iv) Depending on the work flow, what will be the submission deadline for each meeting (i.e. 2 weeks prior, 1 week prior, etc.)
(v) Are there specific procedures to be followed for obtaining external consultant review of a submission?

Communicating a Decision

Once a review is complete, there needs to be processes for communicating the decision to the investigator. Items to consider include:

(i) How will REC decisions be communicated to the researchers (e.g., letter, email)?
(ii) What will be included in the letter (e.g., due date to respond for changes, if applicable, responsibilities of the investigator (e.g., reporting requirement, progress reports)).

Investigator Responsibilities

REC should establish SOPs that define the responsibilities of investigators in regards to submission requirements for initial review, continuing review and review of amendments; ethical conduct of research; reporting requirements for safety reports, adverse events, unanticipated problems, protocol violations, and other events.

Collaborative Research

Increasingly, human subject research is being conducted in collaboration amongst researchers at different institutions and in different countries. Requiring that all research projects with multiple researchers require oversight by the designated REC for each researcher's institution may become burdensome and possibly become a barrier to research. On the other hand, it is clear that the REC members should be familiar with the local context where research is being conducted and where research subjects are being recruited. How do we balance the two? There are a few models that may be considered for oversight of collaborative human subject research.

(i) In countries where the REC requirements are being developed, it may be worthwhile to have a national conversation on whether a central REC would be feasible. If so, the REC may include representatives from the various institutions. Such a set-up may address other potential issues: (i) in places with smaller institutions, it may also prevent difficulties in ensuring sufficient REC reviewers without conflicts of interest; and (ii) where there are limited resources, both financial and human, it may be beneficial to pool these resources to the advantage of the larger community.

(ii) If all researchers are based in the same country/community and the research subjects are being recruited from the researchers' community, it is safe to assume that the designated RECs of each of the researchers' institutions have sufficient local context to review and monitor the research. In such instances, it may be appropriate for the various institutions to enter into an agreement, whereby only one of the RECs has oversight of the research. Such an agreement could be specific to one research project, or it may be applicable to a group of research projects conducted within a consortium. Deciding on which REC should have oversight would require consideration of:
   (a) Whether the research is funded, and if so, which institution is the recipient of the funds. This is important to consider since the recipient of the funds is generally responsible for complying with the terms and conditions of the funding source.
   (b) At which institution(s) are the human subjects being enrolled?
   (c) Which researchers will interact with the subjects?
   (d) Which researchers will have access to identifiable private information about the subjects?
   (e) Which researchers will obtain consent from the subjects?

(iii) In instances where researchers from different countries are collaborating, it is important to assess the need for oversight based on each of the countries' regulations and their respective institutions' policies. Many countries require that, if the subjects are being recruited from their country, there must be oversight from an REC affiliated with that country. It is clear that the reviewing REC must be familiar with the local context and the local requirements. Thus, in instances of international collaborations, it may not be possible to limit the oversight to only one REC. However, it may be feasible to limit oversight to one REC per country. Again, this should be agreed upon through a formal agreement.

Appendices

Appendix I: SOPs for a Convened IRB Review meeting (From the City University of New York)

1. **Applicability**

   These procedures apply to non-exempt human subjects research that may pose greater than minimal risk to subjects. Initial review, continuing review and amendment submissions involving non-exempt research that may pose greater than minimal risk to subjects must be reviewed by a convened IRB. The convened IRB may also review and takes action on unanticipated problems, allegations of serious or continuing non-compliance, and subject complaints.

   Convened IRB also conducts initial review of research that poses no greater than minimal risk to subjects, but that does not appear in any of the categories of research that can be reviewed via an expedited review procedure. The convened IRB may determine that continuing review of such research may undergo expedited review procedures.

2. **Meeting Proceedings**

   2.1 Meeting Frequency

   An IRB meeting of the CUNY UI-IRBs is held every week throughout the year. The 4 IRBs meet on a rotation basis. Meeting dates and deadlines for submissions are available at http://www.cuny.edu/research/compliance/human-subjects-research- 1.html.

   2.2 Quorum Requirements

   The following quorum requirements must be met in order for the convened IRB to vote on any determinations:

   - Majority of the IRB members must be present (in person or via telephone)
   - At least one member whose primary concerns are in a non-scientific area must be present
   - Approval of research is by a majority of members present at the meeting
   - Should the quorum fail during a meeting, discussion of protocols may continue; however, the IRB may not make any determinations or take any votes unless the quorum is restored

   2.3 Conflict of Interest

   IRB members may not participate in the discussion or vote related to any research protocol, for which they have a conflict of interest. IRB members are responsible for recusing themselves from the discussion and the vote if they have a conflict of interest. For the purposes of IRB proceedings, a conflict of interest is defined as follows:

   - IRB member's, his/her spouse's, dependent child's or close relative's involvement in the design, conduct or reporting of the research.

- IRB member's, his/her spouse's, dependent child's or close relative's financial interest in the sponsor of the research.
- IRB member's, his/her spouse's, dependent child's or close relative's participation as an investigator or research team member of the research protocol.

3. **Primary Reviewer System**

   CUNY IRBs operate on a primary reviewer system as follows:

   - The IRB staff assigns primary and secondary reviewers to each agenda item based on the appropriate scientific and non-scientific expertise required. A tertiary reviewer may also be assigned when necessary. For the remainder of this document, primary, secondary and tertiary reviewers are collectively referred to as 'primary reviewers'.
   - For studies involving vulnerable populations, a member who is knowledgeable about and experienced in working with the subject population is assigned as a primary reviewer.

4. **IRB Staff Responsibilities**

   IRB staff is responsible for the following:

   - Perform an administrative review of all submissions to ensure completeness, to confirm that a convened IRB review is warranted and to provide relevant regulatory and policy guidance to the IRB members
   - Distribute all agenda items, including all materials required for the review of a given submission, to all IRB members a minimum of one week prior to the scheduled IRB meeting
   - Document attendance and quorum at the meeting and ensuring that quorum is maintained for each vote
   - Take minutes during the meeting, to include IRB's discussions of significant concerns; resolutions of controverted issues; regulatory determinations and votes for each agenda item; meeting attendance; and disclosures of any conflict of interest.
   - Communicate IRB's concerns, suggestions, and determinations to the PI after the meeting

5. **IRB Member Responsibilities**

   IRB members are responsible for the following:

   - All members are expected to review and be familiar with all agenda items prior to the convened IRB meeting
   - Primary reviewers provide a brief summary of the agenda item and present any concerns they have identified
   - All members participate in the discussion of significant concerns, raise additional concerns, provide necessary clarifications and/or propose resolutions

6. **Possible Outcomes of Convened IRB Review**
   - **Approval**. The submission is approved, and no changes to the submission are required. Criteria for IRB approval are met. IRB may impose specific stipulations on the approval, which are delineated on the approval notice.
   - **Conditional Acceptance**. IRB stipulates specific clarifications or non-substantive modifications to the submission. The final approval is contingent upon the reviewer's acceptance of Principal Investigator's revisions in accordance with the IRB's stipulations.
   - **Deferral**. Substantive modifications or clarifications are required in order for the IRB to determine whether the submission meets the criteria for IRB approval. Investigator's response must be reviewed by a convened IRB.
   - **Consultant Review**: IRB determined that additional expertise is necessary in order to make an adequate determination. Consultant review shall be sought. Consultant's comments will be considered during a future convened IRB meeting. Consultant comments may be received in a written form, in-person during the IRB meeting or by telephone during the IRB meeting.
   - **Disapproval**. Criteria for IRB approval are not met.
   - **Tabled**. Submission has been tabled for review at a future IRB meeting due to lack of appropriate expertise, lack of sufficient information, or loss of quorum.

References

1. Code of Federal Regulations, Title 45 – Public Welfare DHHS, Part 46 – Protection of Human Subjects
2. Code of Federal Regulations, Title 21 – Food and Drugs, Part 56 – Institutional Review Boards

Appendix II: IRB Review Checklist

Top of Form		
Criteria for IRB approval of human subjects research	Yes	No
IRB reviewer checklist		
Risks to subjects are minimized: (i) By using procedures which are consistent with sound research design and which do not unnecessarily expose subjects to risk; AND (ii) whenever appropriate, by using procedures already being performed on the subjects for diagnostic or treatment purposes.		
Risks to subjects are reasonable in relation to anticipated benefits, if any, to subjects and the importance of the knowledge that may reasonably be expected to result.		
Selection of subjects is equitable. Given the purpose of the research: (i) the research setting is appropriate; (ii) inclusion/exclusion criteria are adequate; and (iii) special considerations for vulnerable populations, if any, have been made.		
⊟ Involves children (checklist completed)		
⊟ Involves prisoners (checklist completed)		

(continued)

Recruitment of subjects is appropriate: (i) recruitment method is appropriate for the population; (ii) procedures minimize potential for coercion or undue influence; and (iii) recruitment materials are appropriate.		
Screening: (i) process is appropriate; (ii) individuals performing screening and obtaining consent (when applicable) are qualified to do so; and (iii) consent documents, if any, are appropriate (informed consent checklist completed).		
Informed consent for screening procedures, when applicable:		
⊟ Documented informed consent will be sought from each prospective subject.		
⊟ Oral or Internet based consent will be sought from each prospective subject (waiver of documented IC checklist completed)		
⊟ Waiver of informed consent to be granted (waiver of informed consent checklist completed)		
Informed consent for main study: (i) process is appropriate; (ii) individuals obtaining consent (when applicable) are qualified to do so; and (iii) consent documents, if any, are appropriate (informed consent checklist completed).		
Informed consent for main study procedures:		
⊟ Documented informed consent will be sought from each prospective subject.		
⊟ Oral or Internet based consent will be sought from each prospective subject (waiver of documented IC checklist completed)		
⊟ Waiver of informed consent to be granted (waiver of informed consent checklist completed)		
Research plan makes adequate provision for monitoring the data collected to ensure the safety of subjects. N/A		
Research plan makes adequate provisions to protect the privacy of subjects and to maintain the confidentiality of data.		

If you selected "No" for any of the criteria identified above, please provide a clear explanation of your concerns and suggestions for how these may be addressed by the PI in your reviewer comments.

Top of Form		
IRB reviewer determination (for expedited approvals, list expedited categories)	Changes required (if yes, please provide details in your comments)	Approval duration
⊟ Expedite under Category(ies) (list of categories is provided at the end of this form):	⊟ Yes	⊟ 6 months
	⊟ No	⊟ 1 year
		⊟ Other (specify):
⊟ Convened IRB review – Approval with No Changes	No	⊟ 6 months
		⊟ 1 year
		⊟ Other (specify):
⊟ Convened IRB review – approval with minor changes	Yes	⊟ 6 months
		⊟ 1 year
		⊟ Other (specify):
⊟ Convened IRB review – deferral	Yes	N/A
⊟ Convened IRB review – disapproval	N/A	N/A

IRB reviewer comments
Please clearly detail any concerns or questions you have regarding this submission. Please also provide suggestions for how the PI may address these concerns. Please provide specific references to documents included in the submission whenever possible.

EXPEDITED REVIEW CATEGORIES

Expedited Categories. In order to be considered for expedited review, all procedures involving human subjects must fall within one or more of the following categories.

Category 1: Clinical studies of drugs and medical devices ONLY when condition (a) OR (b) is met.

(a) Research on drugs for which an investigational new drug application (21 CFR Part 312) is not required.
NOTE: Research on marketed drugs that significantly increases the risks or decreases the acceptability of the risks associated with the use of the product is not eligible for expedited review.)
(b) Research on medical devices for which: (i) an investigational device exemption application (21 CFR Part 812) is not required; OR (ii) the medical device is cleared/approved for marketing and the medical device is being used in accordance with its cleared/approved labeling.

Category 2: Collection of blood samples by finger stick, heel stick, ear stick, or venipuncture as follows:

(a) From healthy, non-pregnant adults who weigh at least 110 pounds. For these subjects, the amounts drawn may not exceed 550 ml in an 8 week period and collection may not occur more frequently than 2 times per week; OR
(b) From other adults and children, considering the age, weight, and health of the subjects, the collection procedure, the amount of blood to be collected, and the frequency with which it will be collected. For these subjects, the amount drawn may not exceed the lesser of 50 ml or 3 ml per kg in an 8 week period and collection may not occur more frequently than 2 times per week.

Category 3: Prospective collection of biological specimens for research purposes by noninvasive means.
Examples:

(a) Hair and nail clippings in a non-disfiguring manner;
(b) Deciduous teeth at time of exfoliation or if routine patient care indicates a need for extraction;

(c) Permanent teeth if routine patient care indicates a need for extraction;
(d) Excreta and external secretions (including sweat);
(e) Uncannulated saliva collected either in an un-stimulated fashion or stimulated by chewing or by applying a dilute citric solution to the tongue;
(f) Placenta removed at delivery;
(g) Amniotic fluid obtained at the time of rupture of the membrane prior to or during labor;
(h) Supra- and sub gingival dental plaque and calculus, provided the collection procedure is not more invasive than routine prophylactic scaling of the teeth and the process is accomplished in accordance with accepted prophylactic techniques;
(i) Mucosal and skin cells collected by buccal scraping or swab, skin swab, or mouth washings;
(j) Sputum collected after saline mist nebulization.

Category 4: Collection of data through noninvasive procedures (not involving general anesthesia or sedation) routinely employed in clinical practice, excluding procedures involving x-rays or microwaves.
Examples:
(a) Physical sensors that are applied either to the surface of the body or at a distance and do not involve input of significant amounts of energy into the subject or an invasion of the subject's privacy;
(b) Weighing or testing sensory acuity;
(c) Magnetic resonance imaging;
(d) Electrocardiography, electroencephalography, thermography, detection of naturally occurring radioactivity, electroretinography, ultrasound, diagnostic infrared imaging, doppler blood flow, and echocardiography;
(e) Moderate exercise, muscular strength testing, body composition assessment, and flexibility testing where appropriate given the age, weight, and health of the individual.

Category 5: Research involving materials (data, documents, records, or specimens) that have been collected, or will be collected solely for non-research purposes (such as medical treatment or diagnosis).

NOTE: Some research in this category may be exempt from the HHS regulations for the protection of human subjects. 45 CFR 46.101(b) (4). This listing refers only to research that is not exempt.

Category 6: Collection of data from voice, video, digital, or image recordings made for research purposes.

Category 7: Research on individual or group characteristics or behavior (including, but not limited to, research on perception, cognition, motivation, identity, language, communication, cultural beliefs or practices, and social behavior) or research employing survey, interview, oral history, focus group, program evaluation, human factors evaluation, or quality assurance methodologies.

NOTE: Some research in this category may be exempt from the HHS regulations for the protection of human subjects. 45 CFR 46.101(b) (2) and (b)(3). This listing refers only to research that is not exempt.

References

Al Kassar, M. 2010. The IRB administrative staff and the operation process. Available at: https://www.aub.edu.lb/irb/Documents/May Al Kassar.pdf

World Health Organization. 2011. *Standards and operational guidance for ethics review of health-related research with human participants*. Available at: http://www.who.int/ethics/research/en/.

Part VI

Building Capacity for Enhancing Research Ethics

Building Capacity For Enhancing Research Ethics: Introduction

Henry Silverman

Introduction

To discharge its functions effectively, RECs must be composed of competent and well-trained members. However, many members of RECs in Arab countries lack expertise in ethics review. In Sudan, for example, Elsayed and Kass observed that 93% of ethics review members had not received any training in ethics review, nor had the committees conducted any training courses for their members (Elsayed and Kass 2007). In a study of ethics committees in Egypt, Sleem and colleagues reported that of the 12 RECs they surveyed, 11 indicated that it had only two members with training in ethics, while one REC indicated that none of its members received any training in research ethics (Sleem et al. 2010). In that same survey study, 9 of the 11 RECs who responded stated that lack of ongoing training for members in research ethics represented a barrier to the effective functioning of the REC. In the chapter in this book describing the REC at KHCC, Al Hussaini mentioned that the lack of REC training represents a challenge for the functioning of the REC.

Investigators and other members of the research team also need to receive training in research ethics. Surveys performed in the Arab region have shown that 28–62% of researchers have not received any training in ethics (Asem and Silverman 2009; El-Dessouky et al. 2011; Kandeel et al. 2011).

These data indicate a strong need for training in ethics review. Several international organizations are responding to the training needs of individuals in the area of research ethics. These include UNESCO (United Nations Educational, Scientific, & and Cultural Organization (UNESCO) 2017) and the National Institutes of Health (NIH) in the U.S., the Fogarty International Center (FIC) since 2001 has provided

H. Silverman (✉)
University of Maryland, Baltimore, MD, USA
e-mail: hsilverm@medicine.umaryland.edu

H. Silverman (ed.), *Research Ethics in the Arab Region*, Research Ethics Forum 5,
https://doi.org/10.1007/978-3-319-65266-5_33

annual grants and awards to support the ethics training of faculty members from institutions in LMICs, including those in the Arab regions (Fogarty International Center 2017). The Middle East Research Ethics Training Initiative (MERETI) represents one such program that is focused in the Arab region (Middle East Research Ethics Training Initiative (MERETI) 2017). MERETI provides certificate degree training in research ethics and non-degree training for members of research ethics committees in the Arab Region.

Such international training programs provide the necessary resources for training. But, efforts are needed to develop regional educational programs to ensure that training are sustainable and reflect the local needs and culture. Barriers to the establishment of training programs include a lack of human and financial resources. Also, there is no specific requirement for such training at the national level, although many of the national regulations mention that members of RECs should have the expertise to discharge their functions. Shaza Abass in her chapter recommends that policies need to be developed at the national and institutional levels that "mandate that all REC members require training in research ethics and have evidence of continuous training in research ethics".

In her chapter, Shaza Abass also describes the various types of research ethics training programs that can be organized for investigators and members of RECs, and these include face-to-face as well as online programs. More recently, scholars in the Arab region has organized workshops in research ethics (Egyptian Network of Research Ethics Committees (ENREC) 2015).

Training in the responsible conduct in research (RCR) is also fundamental to the research endeavor and to ensure public trust in research. To emphasize the need for this type of training, Suhail Al-Amad in his chapter describes specifically the types of research misconduct that occurs and discusses data regarding the prevalence of such misconduct in the Arab region, as well as in other LMICs.

Ethics review capacity in the Arab region could be further enhanced by the inclusion of research ethics in the curricula of medical schools and in undergraduate and post-graduate courses. Furthermore, the establishment of sustainable diploma and masters programs in research methodology and research ethics would enhance the development of leaders in research and research ethics. A blended (face-to-face and online) diploma program has been developed at Al-Neelain University in Sudan (Al-Neelain University 2017).

In addition to REC members and investigators, clinical trial sites that perform research need to have staff (e.g., clinical research coordinators (CRAs)) with training in good clinical practice (GCP). In addition to workshops, there are numerous online programs that offer training in GCP. Such clinical trials sites need to have the necessary structures and processes to ensure that the research has been properly performed in regards to the accurate collection and reporting of data, performance of the scheduled study events, and timely reporting of adverse events. A well functioning clinical trial site ensures public trust in the performance of research and enhances the protection of the rights and welfare of research participants. As such, Nadia Zaki and Amal Al-Omari concludes this section with their experiences with the establishment of their clinical research centers in Egypt and Jordan, respectively.

References

Al-Neelain University. 2017. *Diploma of research methodology and ethics*. Retrieved at: http://neelaincourses.com/diploma/.

Asem N., and H.J. Silverman. 2009. Perspectives of faculty at Cairo University towards research ethics and informed consent. Abstract Presentation at PRIM&R, Nashville.

Egyptian Network of Research Ethics Committees (ENREC). 2015. Available at: http://www.enrec.org/.

El-Dessouky, H.F., A.M. Abdel-Aziz, C. Ibrahim, M. Moni, R. Abul Fadl, and H. Silverman. 2011. Knowledge, awareness, and attitudes about research ethics among Dental Faculty in the Middle East: A pilot study. *International Journal of Dentistry* 2011: 694759. https://doi.org/10.1155/2011/694759.

Elsayed, D.E.M., and N. Kass. 2007. Assessment of the ethical review process in Sudan. *Developing World Bioethics* 7: 143–148.

Fogarty International Center. 2017. International bioethics education and career development award (Bioethics). Retrieved August 2013 at: http://www.fic.nih.gov/Grants/Search/Pages/Awards-Program-Bioethics.aspx.

Kandeel, N., A. El-Nemer, N.M. Ali, H. Kassem, M. El-Setouhy, M.E. Elgharieb,… H. J. Silverman. 2011. A multicenter study of the awareness and attitudes of Egyptian faculty towards research ethics: A pilot study. *Journal of Empirical Research on Human Research Ethics* 6(4): 99–108. doi:https://doi.org/10.1525/jer.2011.6.4.99.

Middle East Research Ethics Training Initiative (MERETI). 2017. Certificate program in research ethics: http://medschool.umaryland.edu/mereti/.

Sleem, H., S. El-Kamary, and H.J. Silverman. 2010. Identifying structures, processes, resources and needs of research ethics committees in Egypt. *BMC Medical Ethics* 11: 12.

United Nations Educational, Scientific, & and Cultural Organization (UNESCO). 2017. Ethics education programme. Retrievable at: http://www.unesco.org/new/en/social-and-human-sciences/themes/bioethics/ethics-education-programme/.

Establishing Training Programs for Research Ethics Committees

Shaza Abass

Introduction

Over the last few years there has been an increase in research activity, including clinical trials, in the Arab region (Ahmad 2003). Such activity warrants a corresponding increase in the establishment of RECs to ensure that the ethical aspects of research comply with international standards. There have been concerns, however, regarding the lack of regulatory and oversight mechanisms for RECs in low and middle income countries (Ahmad 2003; Bhutta 2002; Hyder et al. 2004). Furthermore, many RECs continue to face challenges in their capacity to review research. One challenge emanates from members with insufficient training. In a recent survey involving 15 research ethics committees in the Eastern Mediterranean region, Abou-Zeid and colleagues found that only 25% of the members and 20% of the chairs of the RECs received training in research ethics (Abou-Zeid et al. 2009). Other studies involving RECs in Egypt revealed that one of the main barriers to effective REC functioning included insufficient member training and lack of continuing education in research ethics (Matar and Silverman 2013; Sleem et al. 2010).

Proper training of REC members is an essential step towards enhancing the capacity of RECs to perform their function in protecting human subject's rights and welfare. Accordingly, there is an increased demand for establishing training programs for REC members in many countries in the Arab region. In this chapter, I will discuss varying approaches and challenges of establishing training programs for members of RECs, as well as for investigators and members of their research staff.

S. Abass (✉)
Faculty of Dentistry, University of Khartoum, Khartoum, Sudan
e-mail: skabbas@hotmail.com

H. Silverman (ed.), *Research Ethics in the Arab Region*, Research Ethics Forum 5,
https://doi.org/10.1007/978-3-319-65266-5_34

Developing Training Programs: Initial Concepts

Many international organization, including the WHO, UNESCO, and the NIH, have emphasized the importance of training for members of RECs and members of the research staff so that they can perform their role efficiently and effectively in protecting human subjects involved in research. Many training formats exist and these include workshops, courses, degree programs and online offerings. Many of these formats are used by educators from Western universities. It is essential, however, that training courses in research ethics address the cultural, social and religious context within the Arab region (Christakis 1992). Accordingly, it is essential that educators from Arab region be included in training programs.

Training programs should not only focus on enhancing knowledge in research ethics, but also on other competencies, such as critical thinking, teaching, scientific writing, and analytic skills. Although knowledge of basic principles of research ethics is essential, learning to perform ethical analysis and provide ethical justifications for decisions and actions from established principles are necessary skills to be taught in such training programs (Macklin 2015).

In the design of training programs, regardless of format, one must be guided by achievable and measurable learning objectives, include educationally sound delivery methods and activities, and provide suitable methods of assessment. The proper alignment of these critical elements; objectives, activities, and assessments; is essential to achieving the overall goal of the training program (Harden 1999).

To implement effective training programs educators should employ active learning methods that engage learners in collaborative activities (Spencer and Jordan 1999). Active learning is a student-centered approach in which the responsibility for learning is placed upon the student, often working in collaboration with classmates. In active learning approaches, teachers are facilitators rather than one-way providers of information. Examples of active learning techniques include class-based discussions, role-playing, group projects, think-pair-share, peer teaching, debates, Just-in-Time Teaching, and short demonstrations followed by class discussion. (http://serc.carleton.edu/introgeo/gallerywalk/active.html).

Developing Achievable Learning Objectives

Learning objectives include three domains of learning: the cognitive, affective and psychomotor domains (Bloom et al. 1956). When formulating learning objectives for training in research ethics, most short training programs focus on the cognitive domain. Learning objectives from other two domains (affective and psychomotor) are usually achievable only through longer programs, such as degree programs.

The learning objectives from the cognitive domain are involved with acquisition of knowledge, comprehension, and the development of analytic skills. Learners advance in this domain in sequence from the lowest order objectives (knowledge/recall) to the highest (evaluation, synthesis, and analysis). These categories are arranged in ascending levels of complexity. Thus, the lower ones must be mastered before the higher objectives can be achieved.

Writing learning objectives is crucial when designing any training programs. Learning objectives should be written in terms of what the learners will be able to achieve (i.e., what the student will be able to do by the end of the learning activity). Hence, the objectives should include action verbs that reflect observable and measurable behaviours that can be assessed at the end of the learning experience. Examples of such action verbs include: list, discuss, evaluate, and analyse. One should avoid using ambiguous action verbs such as "understand" and "know" that are very difficult to observe and measure. In addition, learning objectives should be be relevant to the overall goals of the learning program and be attainable within the specific learning situation.

The lower order cognitive learning objectives (acquisition of knowledge) are usually achieved by various methods of delivering the content, such as lectures. Higher cognitive objectives, such as the development of the proper skills for ethical analysis, which represent an important objective of training courses aimed at REC members, need to employ activities that are focused at the higher cognitive domains, such as case-based discussions and analysis of research protocols. It is believed that training in ethical reasoning and decision-making can help learners become more capable of recognizing areas of ethical conflict in research (Sachs and Siegler 1993).

Learning Activities That Address the Learning Objectives

Instructional activities are guided by the learning objectives. Such activities are most effective when they rely on a combination of lectures and active learning techniques. Lecturing is effective in delivering "knowledge", which is the basic level of Bloom's taxonomy cognitive domain. When employed, the lectures should not exceed more than 30 min and should be followed by group work involving a case study.

Active learning contrasts with lectures and other "standard" modes of instruction in which teachers do most of the talking and students are passive. In contrast, students and their learning needs are at the center of active learning. Many teaching strategies can be employed to actively engage students in the learning process. These includes group discussions, problem solving, case studies, role plays, journal writing, and structured learning groups. The benefits to using such activities include improved critical thinking skills, increased retention and transfer of new information, increased motivation, and improved interpersonal skills. (see: https://cei.umn.edu/support-services/tutorials/what-active-learning)

Regardless of the format, the content of training programs for RECs in the Arab region should be appropriate for the social, culture, and religious context in that region. The importance of considering the local context in assessing research and avoiding the insensitivity of only applying Western-based research ethics values has been well described in the literature (Benatar and Singer 2000; Benatar 2004;

Shapiro and Meslin 2001). In addition, case studies used in the training programs need to be based on the problems experienced in the local region.

Assessment Activities to Measure the Achievement of Learning Objectives

To determine whether the learning objectives have been achieved, training programs should include methods to assess what the learners have learned. Assessment methods need to be linked to the learning objectives. For example, short answer formats are usually adequate to assess the lower order objectives (i.e., assessment of content), whereas written papers and discussion forums are appropriate for the higher learning objectives.

The types of assessments will also depend on the format being used to deliver the program. For example, modes of assessment for short training programs, such as workshops, usually include multiple choice formats that assess knowledge. Longer courses that include objectives at the higher level of the cognitive domain usually include more robust methods of assessment, such as short essays, written papers, and performance on discussion forums in online programs.

Delivery Formats

Various delivery formats can be utilized in training programs in research ethics. These includes face to face and online delivery or blended formats incorporating both face-to-face and online instruction.

Face-to-Face Formats

The face-to-face format represents the traditional educational delivery method. In a recent study assessing the multiple pedagogical approaches employed in research ethics training almost all program directors rated the face-to-face component as the strongest point of their program (Matar et al. 2014).

Face to face training that use case discussions allows instructors to monitor the comprehension and the analytical skills of the trainees, highlight discussion points and give feedback. It provides a collaborative experience where trainees can learn to discuss ethical issues with their peers preparing them for their future roles as REC members. As discussed earlier, there are many advantages of using active learning techniques. For case studies and protocol review, it is better to divide participants into groups of seven to eight so that everyone can get a chance to participate in the discussion. When selecting the members of the small groups it is important to ensure that there is optimal diversity in regards to gender, age, specialty etc. Use of real case-scenarios that are relevant to actual situations in the Arab region are recommended. Face to face training formats are used in degree programs in research ethics and can also be included as a section of a research methodology course for undergraduate students (Abdelhai et al. 2014).

The Middle Eastern Research Ethics Training Initiative (MERETI) developed a comprehensive training curriculum for research ethics workshops that target REC members and investigators from the Arab region (Silverman et al. 2010). The developed curriculum is intended to be delivered in a short workshop format (1–3 days) and is divided into modular units to enable flexibility in design of the curricular needs of the learners. One advantage of the MERETI curriculum is that it was developed by participants from several Arab countries and is sensitive to ethical issues specific to that region.

Examples of agendas for 2- and 4-day workshops are included in Appendix XI. We believe that the 4 day workshop is more appropriate as an introductory course for REC members training, since more time is given to case-based discussions and analysis of research protocols, which enhances the analytic and critical thinking skills of the trainees. As such, trainees have more time to discuss ethical dilemmas and achieve higher cognitive domain levels.

Online Formats

Online learning is used widely in many low and middle income countries to overcome the limitations of the face-to- face format, which include travel time and coordination of busy professional schedules. As such, the online format enables learners to access the courses "anytime and anywhere". Also, due to the lack of skilled trainers in many countries, online training can involve trainers from different countries. Online courses can also involve larger number of trainees from various geographical locations. Although the initial cost for preparing online courses can be high, the repeated cycles of running such courses could be cost-effective when compared to travel costs to attend face to face trainings. Studies have shown that well-designed online courses have the same gain in knowledge similar to and some times better than traditional face to face teaching in many disciplines, including research ethics (Chumley-Jones et al. 2002; Curran et al. 2006; Fordis et al. 2005).

Online learning usually requires more effort from learners, as they need to be active and continually engaged every few days. Another challenge is that trainees might feel isolated leading to frustration, especially when dealing with new concepts. In many regions in the Arab region, online training is still new and learners might not have the necessary skills to adapt to it. Although it might be difficult to replicate the interaction that occurs in face-to-face workshops, a good understanding of discussion forum techniques can create meaningful collaborate learning.

Self-pace programs are the most user-friendly type of online learning, but are limited as learners only interact with the content, which achieve objectives from the lower order cognitive domain. The **T**raining and **R**esources in **R**esearch **E**thics **E**valuation (The Training and Resources in Research Ethics Evaluation (TRREE)

2016) and The Collaborative Institutional Training Initiative at the University of Miami (The Collaborative Institutional Training Initiative (CITI) 2016) are examples of self-paced program that provide basic training in research ethics. The TRREE training focus primarily on the needs of African countries with free access to its courses and content. The Family Health International, a U.S.-based international research organization, developed a Research Ethics Training Curriculum for international trainees (Family Health International 2016). The course content was designed as an interactive self-study program that employed case studies.

Another online learning format is the facilitated format involving an instructor. Learning activities in such a format include opportunities for learner-content, learner-learner, and learner-instructor interactions. Such interactions can lead to collaborative learning resulting in the achievement of higher learning outcomes when compared to self-paced learning. Examples of such online programs include the Certificate Degree in Research Ethics at the University of Maryland (Certificate Degree Program in Research Ethics 2016). Also, some degree programs in Health Professions Education includes a segment on research ethics. An example is the joint program of the Universiteit Maastrich (Netherlands) and Faculty of Medicine, Suez Canal University (Egypt).

Blended Learning Programs: Combination of Face-to-Face and Online Formats

Blended programs offer the best qualities of face-to-face training and online training, providing flexibility and interpersonal communication and interaction. Many training programs in research ethics employs a blended pedagogy in which the face-to-face segment usually precedes the online learning experience in an effort to help trainees overcome isolation and build a sense of community that facilitates inquiry and discussion (Silverman et al. 2013).

Evaluation of the Training Program

Program evaluation is defined as a "systematic collection and analysis of information related to the design, implementation, and outcomes of a program, for the purpose of monitoring and improving the quality and effectiveness of the program" (Accreditation Council for Graduate Medical Education (ACGME) 2016). There are many models of program evaluation, each has its own advantages and limitations and they can be used alone or in combinations (Frye and Hemmer 2012).

Training program in research ethics should be evaluated thoroughly. A popular approach for training evaluation is the Kirkpatrick model (Kirkpatrick and Kirkpatrick 2006). In this evaluation method, data are gathered to evaluate the program outcomes in four hierarchical levels; (1) Reaction of trainees to the program and their level of satisfaction, (2) Learning, which involves measuring changes in knowledge, skills and attitude that can be assessed through a retest method, (3) Behaviour, which assesses how the trainees have applied the new knowledge and skills gained in the training program and (4) Results and outcomes in terms of how the training had affected the efficacy of the trainees jobs, for example improved REC functionality. The first two domains in the Kirkpatrick evaluation model can be performed by the end of each training program. The other higher level learning domains need long term evaluation of the impact of a training program. One major advantage of the Kirkpatrick model is the clear focus on program outcomes that are described beyond simple learner satisfaction.

Evaluating a program helps to make a judgement about effectiveness. Such an evaluation is important to improve delivery methods and to respond to any dissatisfaction. During program evaluation, it is important to evaluate the input, the process and the outcome of the training. The logic model, which is currently required by some U.S funding agencies, focuses on the program components and their relationship with the program context and impact which gives this model the flexibility to support a rational evaluation plan (McCawley 1997).

Challenges in Establishing Training Programs for RECs

There are several challenges with developing training programs for REC members. For example, in many countries RECs are established with members in high positions at the academic institution with little regards about their previous training in research ethics. Many such REC members are not motivated to join training programs in research ethics, because of time constraints and concerns about their ego.

Additionally, the scarcity of financial resources that are directed to capacity building of RECs make establishment of proper training programs for REC members difficult. Many health professional prefer to spend their money and time in clinical training rather than in ethics training. Furthermore, guidelines that govern the educational requirements of RECs are not well established in the Arab Region.

Finally, policies need to be developed at the national and institutional level that mandate that all REC members and investigators obtain training in research ethics and have evidence of continuous training in research ethics.

Appendix XI

Provisional timetable for a two day workshop for training in research ethics

Day one		Day two	
08:00–08:30	Registration & inauguration	08:00–08:30	Ethics of clinical trials
08:30–9:00	Ice breaking session	08:30–9:00	Case study
9:00–9:30	Pre-test	9:00–9:30	Vulnerability
9:30–10:00	Introduction to research ethics	9:30–10:00	Coercion and undue inducement
10:00–10:30	What makes research ethical?	10:00–10:30	Responsible conduct of research
10:30–11:00	Risks and benefits	10:30–11:00	Therapeutic misconception
11:00–11:15	Break	11:00–11:15	Break
11:15–11:45	Categories of research review	11:15–11:45	Reviewing national guidelines for research in human subjects
11:45–12:15	Research ethics committees; functions and operations	11:15–12:45	Protocol review
12:15–12:45	Informed consent	12:45–1:30	Break
12:45–1:30	Break	1:30–2:30	Protocol review
1:30–2:30	Protocol review	2:30–3:00	Open discussion
2:30–3:00	Waiver of informed consents	3:00–4:00	Post-test and certificates
3:00–4:00	Protocol review		

Provisional time table for a four day workshop

Day one		Day two	
08:00–08:30	Registration & inauguration	8:00–8:30	Informed consent
08:30–9:00	Ice breaking session	8:30–9:00	Case study on informed consent
9:00–9:30	Pre-test	9:00–9:30	Waiver of informed consent
9:30–10:00	Introduction to research ethics	9:30–10:30	Protocol review
10:00–10:30	What makes research ethical?	10:30–11:00	Research designs
10:30–11:00	Risks and benefits	11:00–11:30	Break
11:00–11:30	Break	11:30–12:00	Vulnerability
11:30–12:00	Case on risk and benefit	12:00—12:30	Case study
12:00–12:30	Categories of research review	12:30–1:00	Coercion and undueinducement
12:30–1:00	Exercises on categories of research review	1:00–1:30	Break
1:00–1:30	Break	1:30–2:30	Protocol review
1:30–2:30	Protocol review	2:30–3:00	Discussion
2:30–3:00	Discussion		

Day three		Day four	
8:00–8:30	Informed consent	8:00–8:30	Responsible conduct of research
8:30–9:00	Case study on informed consent	8:30–9:00	Case study
9:00–9:30	Waiver of informed consent	9:00–9:30	Research on human tissues and stored samples
9:30–10:30	Protocol review	9:30–10:30	Protocol review
10:30–11:00	Research designs	10:30–11:00	Ethics of genetic research
11:00–11:30	Break	11:00–11:30	Break
11:30–12:00	Vulnerability	11:30–12:00	Ethics of globalization of research
12:00—12:30	Case study	12:00–1:00	Protocol review
12:30–1:00	Coercion and undueinducement	1:00–1:30	Break
1:00–1:30	Break	1:30–2:00	Reviewing national guidelines that govern human subjects research
1:30–2:30	Protocol review	2:00– 3:00	Wrap up and certificates
2:30–3:00	Discussion		

References

Abdelhai, R., M.H. Hussien, and H. Silverman. 2014. Implementing a post-graduate course on medical research ethics; results of a pilot study from Cairo University. *International Public Health Forum* 1: 1–5. Available at: http://researchpub.org/journal/iphf/number/vol1-no2/vol1-no2-1.pdf.

Abou-Zeid, A., M. Afzal, and H.J. Silverman. 2009. Capacity mapping of national ethics committees in the Eastern Mediterranean Region. *BMC Medical Ethics* 4: 8.

Accreditation Council for Graduate Medical Education (ACGME). 2016. Available at: http://www.acgme.org/acgmeweb/.

Ahmad, K. 2003. Developing countries need effective ethics review committees. *Lancet* 362 (9384): 627. https://doi.org/10.1016/S0140-6736(03)14203-1.

Benatar, S.R. 2004. Towards progress in resolving dilemmas in international research ethics. *The Journal of Law, Medicine & Ethics: A Journal of the American Society of Law, Medicine & Ethics* 32 (4): 574–582.

Benatar, S., and P. Singer. 2000. A new look at international research ethics. *British Medical Journal* 321: 824–826.

Bhutta, A.Z. 2002. Ethics in international health research: A perspective from the developing world. *Bulletin of the World Health Organization* 80: 114–120.

Bloom, B.S., M.D. Engelhart, E.J. Furst, W.H. Hill, and D.R. Drathwohl. 1956. *Taxonomy of educational objectives: Handbook I: Cognitive domain*. New York: David McKay.

Certificate Degree Program in Research Ethics. 2016. Available 1 at: https://graduate.umaryland.edu/research-ethics/.

Christakis, N.A. 1992. Ethics are local: Engaging cross-cultural variation in the ethics for clinical research. *Social Science & Medicine* 35: 1079–1091.

Chumley-Jones, H.S., A. Dobbie, and C.L. Alford. 2002. Web-based learning: Sound educational method or hype? A review of the evaluation literature. *Academic Medicine* 77 (10 Suppl): S86–S93.

Curran, V., J. Lockyer, J. Sargeant, and L. Fleet. 2006. Evaluation of learning outcomes in web-based continuing medical education. *Academic Medicine* 81 (10 Suppl): S30–S34. https://doi.org/10.1097/01.ACM.0000236509.32699.f5.

Family Health International. 2016. Research ethics training curriculum: Available at: http://www.fhi360.org/sites/all/libraries/webpages/fhi-retc2/.

Fordis, M., King, J.E., Ballantyne, C.M., Jones, P.H., Schneider, K.H., Spann, S.J.,... Greisinger, A.J. 2005. Comparison of the instructional efficacy of Internet-based CME with live interactive CME workshops: A randomized controlled trial. *JAMA*, 294 (9), 1043–1051. doi:https://doi.org/10.1001/jama.294.9.1043.

Frye, A.W., and P.A. Hemmer. 2012. Program evaluation models and related theories: AMEE guide no. 67. *Medical Teacher* 34 (5): e288–e299. https://doi.org/10.3109/0142159X.2012.668637.

Harden, R.M. 1999. AMEE Guide No. 14: Outcome-based education: Part 1-An introduction to outcome-based education. *Medical Teacher* 21 (1): 7–14.

Hyder, A.A., S.A. Wali, A.N. Khan, N.B. Teoh, N.E. Kass, and L. Dawson. 2004. Ethical review of health research: A perspective from developing country researchers. *Journal of Medical Ethics* 38: 68–72.

Kirkpatrick, D.L., and J.D. Kirkpatrick. 2006. *Evaluation training programs: The four levels*. 3rd ed. San Francisco: Berrett-Koehler.

Macklin, R. 2015. Can one do good medical ethics without principles? *Journal of Medical Ethics* 41 (1): 75–78. https://doi.org/10.1136/medethics-2014-102354.

Matar, A., and H. Silverman. 2013. Perspectives of Egyptian research ethics committees regarding their effective functioning. *Journal of Empirical Research on Human Research Ethics* 8 (1): 32–44.

Matar, A., S. Garner, J. Millum, B. Sina, and H. Silverman. 2014. Curricular aspects of the Fogarty bioethics international training programs. *Journal of Empirical Research on Human Research Ethics* 9 (2): 12–23. https://doi.org/10.1525/jer.2014.9.2.12.

McCawley, P. 1997. The logic model for planning and evaluation. http://www.uiweb.uidaho.edu/extension/LogicModel.pdf (Ed.).

Sachs, G.A., and M. Siegler. 1993. Teaching scientific integrity and the responsible conduct of research. *Academic Medicine* 68 (12): 871–875.

Shapiro, H.T., and E.M. Meslin. 2001. Ethical issues in the design and conduct of clinical trials in developing countries. *The New England Journal of Medicine* 345: 139–142.

Silverman, H., Ahmed, B., Ajeilet, S., Al-Fadil, S., Al-Amad, S., El-Dessouky, H.,... Saleh, A. 2010. Curriculum guide for research ethics workshops for countries in the Middle East. *Developing World Bioethics*, 10 (2), 70–77. doi:https://doi.org/10.1111/j.1471-8847.2009.00261.x.

Silverman, H., M. Strosberg, F. Luna, S. Philpott, and C.A. Hemmerle. 2013. An analysis of online courses in research ethics in the Fogarty-sponsored bioethics training programs. *Journal of Empirical Research on Human Research Ethics* 8 (5): 59–74. https://doi.org/10.1525/jer.2013.8.5.59.

Sleem, H., S. El-Kamary, and H.J. Silverman. 2010. Identifying structures, processes, resources and needs of research ethics committees in Egypt. *BMC Medical Ethics* 11: 12.

Spencer, J., and R. Jordan. 1999. Learner centred approaches in medical education. *BMJ Open* 318 (318).

The Collaborative Institutional Training Initiative (CITI). 2016. Available at: https://www.citiprogram.org/.

The Training and Resources in Research Ethics Evaluation (TRREE). 2016. Available at: http://elearning.trree.org/.

Responsible Conduct of Research

Suhail Al-Amad

Introduction

As academic institutions, governmental regulatory agencies and pharmaceutical companies enhance capacity in research in the Arab region, appropriate attention has been placed towards training in ethics that enhances the functions of research ethics committees. However, training is also needed in responsible conduct in research (RCR), as studies have shown a high prevalence of research misconduct (Errami and Garner 2008).

This chapter aims to highlight several facets of research misconduct, including what constitutes misconduct in research, the differences in the prevalence of misconduct in various regions of the world, the reasons that might motivate investigators to commit research misconduct, and the type of measures that can be instituted to enhance the responsible conduct in research.

What Is Research Misconduct?

The Office of Research Integrity of the U.S. Department of Health and Human Services defines research misconduct as "*fabrication, falsification, or plagiarism in proposing, performing, or reviewing research, or in reporting research results*" (The Office of Research Integrity). This definition is commonly abbreviated as FFP. Despite being a widely accepted definition, the triad FFP does not cover all forms of research misconduct. For example, overlooking research data that do not support the researcher's hypothesis, designing research inappropriately to obtain results that are specifically desired by the researchers, and attributing authorship to

S. Al-Amad (✉)
College of Dental Medicine, University of Sharjah, Sharjah, UAE

Monash University, Melbourne, Australia
e-mail: salamad@sharjah.ac.ae

H. Silverman (ed.), *Research Ethics in the Arab Region*, Research Ethics Forum 5,
https://doi.org/10.1007/978-3-319-65266-5_35

individuals who are not contributors (Martinson et al. 2005). This chapter will review these additional types of research misconduct in addition to FFP.

Fabrication and Falsification

Fabrication is commonly defined as "*making up data or results and recording or reporting them*" and falsification is defined as "*manipulating research materials, equipment, or processes, or changing or omitting data or results such that the research is not accurately represented in the research record*" (The Office of Research Integrity 2016). Fabrication and falsification represent fraudulent activities if its occurrences were intended.

Detrimental Consequences of Fraud in Research

In order to understand the impact that research fraud has on the research community, three notorious cases are reviewed (see boxes at the end of this chapter). These three cases differ in their severity, but are similar in showing the actual and potential damage a scientist can cause from a single fraudulent study, and the length of time it would take to rectify the public mistrust generated from such actions.

When fraudulent research is exposed, the published papers linked to the research are retracted from the literature, an action that is publically noted. Such occurrences can be damaging to the reputation of researchers, their institutions, and science as a whole. Public skepticism in scientific findings can last for quite some time after research fraud is revealed. Additionally, research fraud means that public funds spent on that research were meaninglessly wasted and subjects participating in the fraudulent research were unnecessarily exposed to risks and their altruistic intentions in participating in research are unrealized.

Retractions due to fraud are commonly associated with: (1) appearing in journals with higher impact factor and (2) being authored by researchers from academically advanced countries, such as the United States, Germany, Japan and China (Fang et al. 2012). The large number of retracted papers from high impact journals may be due to the ability of such journals to detect and investigate suspected fraud and take firm actions against misconduct compared with lower impact journals. This also infers that we are only looking at the tip of the iceberg.

The effect of fraudulent research appearing in high impact journals and from academically advance countries is that the research (before being exposed) would be more likely to be broadly acknowledged and its findings used as a basis of further research studies. Accordingly, fraudulent research can have a "multiplier" effect if left unexposed. For example, Steen reviewed 180 retracted papers over a period of 10 years and found that these papers were cited in 851 consecutive publications before the fraudulent papers were retracted (Steen 2011). As such, a large number of research participants were enrolled in research projects that were fully or partly designed based on fraudulent papers (see Table 1). The COOPERATE study for

Table 1 Number of papers and research subjects involved in the research described in the retracted papers and secondary publications that cited the retracted papers

	Number of publications	Number of research subjects
Retracted publications	180	28,783
Publications based on the retracted papers	851	445,064

Source: Steen (2011)

example, had enrolled 263 patients, but 35,929 patients were recruited in subsequent trials that were directly or indirectly designed based on the COPPERATE study (Steen 2011). As the COOPERATE study was fraudulent, subsequent investigations that were designed based on its findings unnecessarily exposed further subjects to research-related risks. The number of secondary research participation is directly related to the time between publication and retraction (Fang et al. 2012).

Plagiarism: Inappropriate Referencing of Published Literature

Plagiarism is defined as "*the appropriation of another person's ideas, processes, results, or words without giving appropriate credit*" (Stretton et al. 2012). Plagiarism is a serious ethical misconduct that represents intellectual stealing. The proper attributing of text to its original source is important for maintaining the integrity of science. The rapidly evolving technology is making information instantly available to those who are searching for it. This makes copying material from an article, a book or a website both tempting and easy. But technology has also been assisting teachers and journal editors in discovering plagiarism with the use of software that can detect it.

Historically, Islamic scholars have set a standard of attribution during the years following death of the Prophet of Islam Mohammed (PBUH). When such scholars wanted to document and archive the words and actions of Prophet Mohammed, known as *Hadith*, they formulated a strict system in which they would only registered the *Hadith* when a chain of trustworthy narrators leading back to the Prophet or to his close companions was established. The chain of narrators, which precedes every *Hadith*, is called *Sanad* or *Isnad.* This is equivalent to today's referencing.

Common Knowledge Versus Plagiarism

When ideas or concepts become common knowledge, the borrowing of these ideas would not usually be considered plagiarism. For example, if one writes "*milk is a rich source of calcium*" and this happens to appear exactly as such in a given reference, the reuse of this statement would not constitute plagiarism, because this sentence is considered to be "common knowledge". Common knowledge is an established fact that is attributed to no one, and which cannot be paraphrased in any other meaningful way. But the concept of "*common knowledge*" is rather subjective and can be interpreted differently depending on the readership's depth of knowledge and on the extent of formality of the writing.

Furthermore, the time it takes for *proprietary* knowledge to become *common* knowledge is not well-established, which adds further ambiguity to deciding the scope of common knowledge. For example, when one writes "*DNA consists of two helical chains*", should one reference this sentence to Watson and Crick (1953), or consider this as common knowledge without the need for referencing?

There is no definitive answer for this issue. What is advisable is that when in doubt whether a statement that refers to existing or common knowledge is to be duly cited, it is always better to avoid plagiarism by making sure that text, concepts and ideas are appropriately attributed to their original sources.

Direct Copying (Verbatim) Versus Paraphrasing

Plagiarism is avoided by making attributions to the sources. This can either be done with using quotation marks (verbatim text), or by paraphrasing the original text. In both cases, the references should be stated. The following are examples on what would constitute plagiarism in a variety of scenarios representing student's assignments (adapted from: Frick 2016).

The Original Source

Surgeon Abu Al-Qasim Al-Zahrawi wrote the *Tasrif* which, translated into Latin, became the leading medical text in European universities during the later Middle Ages. Al-Zahrawi was also a noted pathologist, describing hydrocephalus and other congenital diseases as well as developing new surgical technologies such as catgut sutures (Majeed 2005).

> Scenario 1
> The student writes the following:
> Many Islamic scholars left significant inputs to science and medicine during the Islamic Golden Age. For example, Surgeon Abu Al-Qasim Al-Zahrawi wrote the *Tasrif* which, translated into Latin, became the leading medical text in European universities during the later Middle Ages. Al-Zahrawi was also a noted pathologist, describing hydrocephalus and other congenital diseases as well as developing new surgical technologies such as catgut sutures (Majeed 2007).
>
> Majeed A. How Islam changed medicine. BMJ (2005) 24;331(7531):1486–7.

This is plagiarism because the student copied the text from the source as is, which gives the reader the wrong impression that the text is the student's. The text presented should have been re-written in the student's own words (i.e. paraphrasing) with the information attributed to the original course.

Scenario 2:
The student writes the following:
Many Islamic scholars left significant inputs to science and medicine during the Islamic Golden Age. In his editorial, Majeed describes the contributions of some of those scholars, such as Abu Al-Qasim Al-Zahrawi, whom he portrayed as "a noted pathologist, describing hydrocephalus and other congenital diseases as well as developing new surgical technologies such as catgut sutures" (Majeed 2007).

Majeed A. How Islam changed medicine. BMJ (2005) 24;331(7531):1486–7.

In this scenario, the student used quotation marks when Majeed's text was copied word-for-word. This is not plagiarism since the quoted text had been put between quotation marks, and was later referenced to the author.

Scenario 3:
The student writes the following:
Many Islamic scholars left significant inputs to science and medicine during the Islamic Golden Age. In his editorial, Majeed spoke about Surgeon Abu Al-Qasim Al-Zahrawi who wrote the *Tasrif* which, translated into Latin, became the leading medical text in European universities during the later Middle Ages. Majeed also described how Al-Zahrawi was a noted pathologist, describing hydrocephalus and other congenital diseases as well as developing new surgical technologies such as catgut sutures (Majeed 2007).

Majeed A. How Islam changed medicine. BMJ (2005) 24;331(7531):1486–7.

This is plagiarism because, even though the student attributes the text to the author (Majeed spoke about…etc.), the student performed very minor paraphrasing and copied the rest of the text word-for-word without using quotation marks to indicate that the words were those of Majeed.

Scenario 4:
The student writes the following:
Many Islamic scholars left significant inputs to science and medicine during the Islamic Golden Age, such as Ibn Al Nafis who discovered the pulmonary circulation, Ibn Sina who articulated the holistic approach to patient care and Abu Al-Qasim Al-Zahrawi, who was a renowned surgical pathologist and who introduced new surgical tools, such as the well-known catgut suture (Majeed 2007).

Majeed A. How Islam changed medicine. BMJ (2005) 24;331(7531):1486–7.

The student in this scenario wrote information which he attributes to the source. The information have been paraphrased by the student, and have been written in the student's own words. This is not plagiarism.

Prevalence of Research Misconduct

Measuring the prevalence of research misconduct is difficult because it represents behavior that is professionally and socially unacceptable. As such, reporting bias serves as a constant limitation to obtaining an accurate measure of its prevalence. Roberts and St. John found that the frequency of reporting research misconduct is inversely related to its seriousness, i.e., researchers who self-report misconducts would be less likely to do so if those misconducts represented significant immoral acts (Roberts and St John 2014).

Regardless, prevalence of research misconduct is measured either by surveying researchers own acts of misconduct, reporting of researchers' knowledge of their colleagues' misbehaviors, or by reviewing cases investigated by a centralized authority for research integrity.

Fanelli examined 21 published surveys (mostly from the US and the UK) that investigated research misconduct admitted by the researchers themselves and by observation and knowledge of their colleagues' activities (Fanelli 2009). In this systemic review, Fanelli found an overall average of 1.97% of researchers who admitted to committing fraud (fabrication and falsification), while a pooled estimate of 14.12% knew about a colleague who had falsified or fabricated research. The authors also assessed from the surveys the prevalence of other "questionable research practices" (Martinson et al. 2005; Titus et al. 2008) and showed that an average of 33.7% admitted to committing one type of such practices, while between 6.2 and 72% knew about a colleague who had committed any one of these questionable research practices. Questionable research practices included the following: (Martinson et al. 2005; Titus et al 2008)

1. Omitting data which contradicts the researcher's hypothesis.
2. Modifying results to strengthen the research outcomes and conclusions.
3. Overlooking questionable data or data interpretation produced by co-investigators.
4. Insufficiently detailing methodology in research publications so that other can replicate.
5. Insufficiently detailing results published in prior researches when writing research proposals.
6. Not disclosing potential or actual conflict of interest.
7. Duplicate publications (known as *salami slicing*).
8. Inappropriately crediting authorship.
9. Negligence related to research record keeping.
10. Having a power relationship with the research subjects.
11. Concealing or overlooking research limitations.
12. Deliberately overlooking contradictory research findings.
13. Choosing a specific statistical method to prove a theory or avoid specific outcomes.
14. Selectively reporting significant findings, and deliberately ignoring others.

Ranstam et al. measured the prevalence of research misconduct from a different perspective by surveying biostatisticians rather than directly from the researchers (Ranstam et al. 2000). Their findings showed that 51% of statisticians knew of at least one fraudulent project during the previous 10 years. Alarmingly, 31% stated that they were involved in a project in which "*fraud took place or was about to take place*", and 13% "*had been requested to support fraud themselves*", a finding that reflects the relatively high tolerability to make-up or manipulate data.

Prevalence of Research Misconduct in Low and Middle Income Countries

Data about the prevalence of misconduct in low and middle income countries is scarce. Okonta and Rossouw found that more than two-thirds of Nigerian researchers had committed some form of research misconduct and approximately 27% had falsified data (Okonta and Rossouw 2013). They also found that the most common form of misconduct was related to authorship. Similarly, Adeleye and Adebamowo found 54.6% of medical and dental researchers had committed some form of misconduct (FFP and other questionable research practices), and 14.4% and 9.8% committed fabrication and falsification, respectively (Adeleye and Adebamowo 2012).

A recent survey involving researchers from Egypt, Bahrain, Saudi Arabia, and Lebanon showed that more than half admitted to committing some form of misconduct, while 20% admitted to committing fabrication or falsification (Marwan Felaefel et al. 2017). Approximately 10% admitted to acts involving plagiarism and 18% said they gave authorship credit when it was undeserved. The results of this survey also showed that respondents who had prior training in research ethics and those who were established academic faculty were less likely to report committing research misconduct compared to those who didn't have training or who were postgraduate students. Overall, training in research ethics was associated with certain positive attitudes by the researchers regarding responsible conduct in research.

Causes of Misconduct in Research

Misconduct in research can be attributed to several factors. Qiu described the situation in China and opined that the pressure to publish and academia's focus on quantity rather than quality in its evaluation of academic achievement facilitated misconduct (Qiu 2010). Fanelli et al. believed that the main reasons for misconduct in research are related to absence of policies defining and governing research integrity rather than the pressure to publish (Fanelli 2009). Ana et al., on the other hand, emphasized the importance of establishing national regulatory bodies in low and middle income countries, particularly as these countries have witnessed a recent growth in research activities, and hence, might lack a research culture that emphasizes responsible conduct in research (Ana et al. 2013).

In regards to plagiarism, commentators offer three main reasons as to why researchers commit this act (Debnath 2016). First, researchers may not regard that such practices are wrong, as they view the word-for-word copying as an acceptable behavior, as long as the reference is mentioned in the bibliography. Second, they have difficulties writing effectively in a different language for publication purposes. This is particularly pronounced for the English language, as the majority of scientific journals publish in English, a language that many researchers from low and middle-income countries are deficient. Thirdly, some researchers are careless and are under time pressure to complete the writing tasks and hence, do not take the time to proof-read their papers to avoid plagiarism.

Davis et al. recently classified the causes of misconduct in the following categories: individual, situational, organizational, structural, and cultural (Davis et al. 2007).

Individual: Personality traits of ego, vanity, and a sense of entitlement may cause individuals to commit various questionable research practices. The mental or emotional state of the individual may also play a role.

Situational: Personal stressors (e.g., divorces and financial pressures) can test the most fundamentally honest researchers to conform to acceptable academic practices.

Organizational: The research culture and ethical climate of organizations can also be conducive to research misconduct and include factors such as lack of appropriate modeling behavior by senior academics, the absence of penalties for misbehavior, absence of policies that enforces behaviors related to responsible conduct of research, and limited training programs in research ethics.

Structural: Certain characteristics of the scientific enterprise within academia may cause departures from responsible conduct and include "publish or perish" pressures related to academic promotions in which publication quantity is more important than quality and pressures from research sponsors to embellish and/or overlook certain findings.

Cultural: Researchers from different cultures may harbor different norms of behaviors, such as honorary (gift) authorship for senior professors (Al-Adaw et al. 2016) and the view that word-for-word copying is an acceptable behavior. As mentioned above for causes of plagiarism, lack of familiarity with the English language may prompt individuals to copy without appropriate attribution.

Methods to Address Research Misconduct

Enhancing responsible conduct in research requires a multi-faceted approach, which can be summarized in three domains: regulation, training, and monitoring.

Regulating the Research Environment

The accelerated research production requires a parallel process of regulation. The vague definitions of what constitutes a research misconduct, and the inability to appropriately handle allegations of wrongdoings are viewed to be the major cause of research misconduct (Fanelli et al. 2015). National governments (Rosenberg 2016) should work towards establishing a regulatory agency that will develop the necessary policies to;

1. Define the types and scope of research misconduct
2. Set the pathways to report allegations of misconduct
3. Determine the steps to follow when investigating a misconduct
4. Determine the range of penalties that will be imposed on researchers (and their institutes) when a misconduct in research has been established.

Training in Responsible Conduct in Research

The relationship between research misconduct and the researchers' knowledge in this field has been investigated. Adeleye and Adebamowo found that researchers with inadequate knowledge in research ethics were significantly more likely to admit research wrongdoings than those who felt their knowledge in this regard was adequate (Adeleye and Adebamowo 2012). Martinson et al. also found a significant increase in questionable research practices between early-career and mid-career researchers (Martinson et al. 2005). Finally, Felaefel and colleagues found a positive association between previous training in ethics and responsible conduct in research in their study involving researchers from countries in the Arab region (Marwan Felaefel et al. 2017). These studies highlight the importance of instituting academic programs design to build the capacity of students and young researchers in the field of research ethics.

Monitoring Activities

Investigating an incident of research misconduct is a process that can be damaging to the reputation of researchers, as well as to their institutions. The corrective process is commonly associated with severe detrimental consequences (Roberts and St John 2014). In order to avoid these consequences, research misconduct need to be monitored both internally (by the academic or research institute) and externally by journal editors (Marusic et al. 2007). The monitoring process should be guided by written policies that determine the extent of monitoring and the circumstances under which intervention would be necessary. Studies have shown, however, that many academic medical centers in the U.S. lack clear policies regarding authorship practices (Lacasse and Leo 2010). Also, editors of small medical journals may not consider authorship problems to be serious (Marusic 2011). Finally, there is software to detect plagiarism that is well tested, widely available and is becoming economically affordable (Masic 2014); although it may still be beyond the economic reach of several countries in the Arabic region.

Conclusion

The growth in research infrastructure in the Arab region is encouraging, but should be coupled with a parallel process in which scientific honesty and integrity are enforced by regulations, training, and monitoring of researchers' conduct.

The soundness of medical research can easily and severely be undermined when research misconduct is detected. Previous incidents of misconduct show how vulnerable the entirety of science is to the dishonesty of few individuals. The severity of research misconduct varies from a negative impact on individual researchers and their institutions to very harmful consequences on science and humanity.

Three Notorious Cases

Case 1: Jon Sudbö's Work on Oral Cancer Chemo-Prevention

In 2005, Jon Sudbö and his colleagues published a paper in the Lancet titled "Non-steroidal anti-inflammatory drugs and the risk of oral cancer: a nested case-control study". In that paper, Sudbö and his team found a protective effect of non-steroidal anti-inflammatory drugs (NSAIDs) against oral cancer. Skepticism of fabrication of Sudbö's data was soon raised when it was found that the cancer patient database (the core base for Sudbö's study) was never used. An investigation revealed that Sudbö had fabricated data of more than 900 subjects in his study. The paper was very soon retracted from the Lancet (Pincock 2006). Should this paper not have been promptly retracted, NSAIDs would have become accepted as a recommended chemo-protective agent against oral cancer that might have resulted in providing false assurances to heavy smokers who might have quite smoking otherwise and also the design of futile clinical trials to provide prospective evidence of a chemo-protective effect. The Lancet's prompt retraction aborted those potential consequences.

Case 2: Naoyuki Nakao and the COOPERATE Study

In 2003, a team of researchers led by Naoyuki Nakao published their clinical trial, named the COOPERATE trial, in the Lancet. The paper showed that when a dual-drug therapy consisting of angiotensin-II receptor blocker (losartan) and angiotensin converting enzyme inhibitor (trandolapril) is given to patients, renal disease was delayed compared with single-drug therapy. Consequently, many clinicians modified the treatment protocols for their hypertensive patients and started to prescribe the dual-drug therapy. However, in 2006, concerns surfaced over the validity of the COOPERATE trial (e.g., claims regarding a reduction in protein loss by the kidneys using the dual therapy was viewed as being unrealistic (Bidani 2006) and skepticism arose over the integrity of the methodology and data management as a whole).

Following repeated concerns, the Lancet made a request to undertake an investigation into the integrity of the COOPERATE trial. The results of the investigation concluded that the study had been fabricated. Consequently, the Lancet retracted the paper in 2009 due to several ethical breathes ("*Retraction. Combination treatment of angiotensin-II receptor blocker and angiotensin-converting-enzyme inhibitor in non-diabetic renal disease (COOPERATE): a*

(continued)

randomised controlled trial" 2009). However, by that time, an estimated 140,000 patients in the US alone were receiving this combination instead of the traditional mono-therapy, and over a considerable amount of time. The length of time between publication and retraction had exposed a large number of patients to a scientifically foundationless therapy.

Case 3: Andrew Wakefield and the MMR Vaccine

In 1998, Andrew Wakefield and his colleagues reported a case series of 12 children with reactive intestinal changes and pervasive developmental disorder (mostly autism) that followed MMR vaccination. Those findings created a worldwide scare from what the authors called in their paper the "MMR syndrome (Wakefield et al. 1998). The years following Wakefield's publication witnessed greater reluctance by parents to using vaccines for their children that lead to outbreaks in measles and mumps in various countries (McBrien 2003; Pugh 2002), and recently in the USA (Centers for Disease Control and Prevention n.d.). These outbreaks were seen in non-immunized children, and in some cases were linked with parental attitude towards children's vaccination. Other studies investigating the link between MMR vaccine and autism failed to prove Wakefield's findings. In 2010, following intensive investigations, the results of the 1998 paper were found to have been falsified with substantial tampering of children's histories (Deer 2011).The Lancet eventually retracted the paper in 2010 based on ethical violations related to children's recruitment process and the reviews by the research ethics committee ("*Retraction – Ileal-lymphoid-nodular hyperplasia, non-specific colitis, and pervasive developmental disorder in children*" 2010). Further ethical violations were also revealed when Wakefield had a financial conflict of interest and did not disclose it to his colleagues nor to the journal. Wakefield, whose name has been erased from the General Medical Council Register, continues to deny any wrongdoing and insists on the association he had found between MMR vaccine and autism (Ziv 2015).

References

Adeleye, O.A., and C.A. Adebamowo. 2012. Factors associated with research wrongdoing in Nigeria. *Journal of Empirical Research on Human Research Ethics* 7 (5): 15–24. https://doi.org/10.1525/jer.2012.7.5.15.

Al-Adawi, S., B.H. Ali, and I. Al-Zakwani. 2016. Research misconduct: The Peril of publish or perish. *Oman Medical Journal* 31: 5–11.

Ana, J., T. Koehlmoos, R. Smith, and L.L. Yan. 2013. Research misconduct in low- and middle-income countries. *PLoS Medicine* 10 (3): e1001315. https://doi.org/10.1371/journal.pmed.1001315.

Bidani, A. 2006. Controversy about COOPERATE ABPM trial data. *American Journal of Nephrology* 26 (6): 629–632. 629, 632; author reply Retrieved from http://www.ncbi.nlm.nih.gov/pubmed/17236263.

Centers for Disease Control and Prevention. n.d.. Measles cases and outbreaks. Available at: http://www.cdc.gov/measles/cases-outbreaks.html.

Davis, M.S., M. Riske-Morris, and S.R. Diaz. 2007. Causal factors implicated in research misconduct: evidence from ORI case files. *Science and Engineering Ethics* 13 (4): 395–414. https://doi.org/10.1007/s11948-007-9045-2.

Debnath, J. 2016. Plagiarism: A silent epidemic in scientific writing – reasons, recognition and remedies. *Medical Journal Armed Forces India* 72 (2): 164–167. https://doi.org/10.1016/j.mjafi.2016.03.010.

Deer, B. 2011. How the case against the MMR vaccine was fixed. *BMJ* 342: c5347. https://doi.org/10.1136/bmj.c5347.

Errami, M., and H. Garner. 2008. A tale of two citations. *Nature* 451 (7177): 397–399. https://doi.org/10.1038/451397a.

Fanelli, D. 2009. How many scientists fabricate and falsify research? A systematic review and meta-analysis of survey data. *PLoS One* 4: e5738.

Fang, F.C., R.G. Steen, and A. Casadevall. 2012. Misconduct accounts for the majority of retracted scientific publications. *Proceedings of the National Academy of Sciences of the United States of America* 109 (42): 17028–17033. https://doi.org/10.1073/pnas.1212247109.

Frick, T. 2016. Plagiarism lesson: Retrieved from: https://www.indiana.edu/~tedfrick/plagiarism/index2.html

Lacasse, J.R., and J. Leo. 2010. Ghostwriting at elite academic medical centers in the United States. *PLoS Medicine* 7 (2): e1000230. https://doi.org/10.1371/journal.pmed.1000230.

Majeed A. How Islam changed medicine. BMJ (2005) 24;331(7531):1486–7.

Martinson, B.C., M.S. Anderson, and R. de Vries. 2005. Scientists behaving badly. *Nature* 435: 737–748.

Marusic, A. 2011. Problems of editors with authorship in small medical journals. *International Journal of Occupational Environmental Medicine* 2 (3): 130–132. Retrieved from http://www.ncbi.nlm.nih.gov/pubmed/23022829.

Marusic, A., V. Katavic, and M. Marusic. 2007. Role of editors and journals in detecting and preventing scientific misconduct: Strengths, weaknesses, opportunities, and threats. *Medicine and Law* 26 (3): 545–566. Retrieved from http://www.ncbi.nlm.nih.gov/pubmed/17970252.

Marwan Felaefel, M., M. Salem, R. Jaafar, G. Jassim, H. Edwards, F. Rashid-Doubell, R. Yousri, N. Ali, and H. Silverman. 2017. A cross-sectional survey study to assess prevalence and attitudes regarding research misconduct among investigators in the Middle East. *Journal of Academic Ethics*: 1–17. Retrievable at: https://link.springer.com/article/10.1007/s10805-017-9295-9.

Masic, I. 2014. Plagiarism in scientific research and publications and how to prevent it. *Materials Sociomedical* 26 (2): 141–146. https://doi.org/10.5455/msm.2014.26.141-146.

McBrien, J., J. Murphy, D. Gill, M. Cronin, C. O'Donovan, and M.T. Cafferkey. 2003. Measles outbreak in Dublin, 2000. *The Pediatric Infectious Disease Journal* 22 (7): 580–584. https://doi.org/10.1097/01.inf.0000073059.57867.36.

Okonta, P., and T. Rossouw. 2013. Prevalence of scientific misconduct among a group of researchers in Nigeria. *Developing World Bioethics* 13 (3): 149–157. https://doi.org/10.1111/j.1471-8847.2012.00339.x.

Pincock, S. 2006. Lancet study faked. The Scientist. Available at: http://www.the-scientist.com/?articles.list/categoryNo/2884/pageNo/184/.

Pugh, R.N., B. Akinosi, S. Pooransingh, J. Kumar, S. Grant, E. Livesley, and S. Ramaiah. 2002. An outbreak of mumps in the metropolitan area of Walsall, UK. *International Journal of Infectious Diseases* 6 (4): 283–287. http://www.ncbi.nlm.nih.gov/pubmed/12718822.

Qiu, J. 2010. Publish or perish in China. *Nature* 463 (7278): 142–143. https://doi.org/10.1038/463142a.

Ranstam, J., M. Buyse, S.L. George, S. Evans, N.L. Geller, B. Scherrer, and P. Lachenbruch. 2000. Fraud in medical research: an interntional survey of biostatisticians. ISCB Subcommittee on Fraud. *Controlled Clinical Trials* 21: 415–427.

Retraction--Ileal-lymphoid-nodular hyperplasia, non-specific colitis, and pervasive developmental disorder in children. 2010. *Lancet, 375*(9713), 445. doi:10.1016/S0140-6736(10)60175-4.

Roberts, D.L., and F.A. St John. 2014. Estimating the prevalence of researcher misconduct: A study of UK academics within biological sciences. *PeerJ* 2: e562. https://doi.org/10.7717/peerj.562.

Rosenberg, J. 2016. Approaches to increasing ethical compliance in China with drug trial standards of practice. *Journal of Alzheimer's Disease* 52 (3): 825–827. https://doi.org/10.3233/JAD-151196.

Steen, R.G. 2011. Retractions in the medical literature: how many patients are put at risk by flawed research? *Journal of Medical Ethics* 37 (11): 688–92. https://doi.org/10.1136/jme.2011.043133.

Stretton, S., N.J. Bramich, J.R. Keys, J.A. Monk, J.A. Ely, C. Haley, and K.L. Woolley. 2012. Publication misconduct and plagiarism retractions: A systematic, retrospective study. *Current Medical Research and Opinion* 28 (10): 1575–1583. https://doi.org/10.1185/03007995.2012.728131.

The Editors of the Lancet. 2009. Retraction—Combination treatment of angiotensin-II receptor blocker and angiotensin-converting-enzyme inhibitor in non-diabetic renal disease (COOPERATE): A randomised controlled trial. *The Lancet* 374 (9697):1226

The Office of Research Integrity. 2016. Definition of research misconduct.

Titus, S.L., J.A. Wells, and L.J. Rhoades. 2008. Repairing research integrity. *Nature* 453 (7198): 980–982. https://doi.org/10.1038/453980a.

Wakefield, A.J., S.H. Murch, A. Anthony, J. Linnell, D.M. Casson, M. Malik, and J.A. Walker-Smith. 1998. Ileal-lymphoid-nodular hyperplasia, non-specific colitis, and pervasive developmental disorder in children. *Lancet* 351 (9103): 637–641. http://www.ncbi.nlm.nih.gov/pubmed/9500320.

Watson, J.D., and F.H.C. Crick. 1953. A structure for deoxyribose nucleic acid. *Nature* 171: 737–738.

Ziv S. 2015. Andrew Wakefield, Father of the anti-vaccine movement, responds to the current measles outbreak for the first time: Newsweek. Available at: http://www.newsweek.com/2015/02/20/andrew-wakefield-father-anti-vaccine-movement-sticks-his-story-305836.html.

Clinical Research Management at the King Hussein Cancer Center, Amman, Jordan

Amal Al-Omari

Introduction

Cancer is the second leading cause of death in Jordan after cardiovascular diseases (Ministry of Health 2009). Cancer mortality and morbidity are expected to increase with the projected increase in life expectancy, which will be coupled with prolonged exposure to risk factors such as tobacco use, consumption of unhealthy foods and limited physical activity. The number of new cancer cases diagnosed among Jordanians has increased by about 40%, from 3362 cases in 2000 to 4675 in 2011. The crude incidence rate of all cancers among Jordanians is 74.8 per 100,000 (68.1 for males and 81.9 for females) (Ministry of Health 2011).

During the 1990s, cancer care in Jordan was weak and fragmented. Coordination in the plan of care between pathologists, radiologists, surgeons, and medical oncologists was severely deficient. There was much variation in the availability of treatments at private and public hospitals, including the Ministry of Health hospitals and the Royal Medical Services of the military. Some patients who could afford the costs traveled outside Jordan for treatment. There was severe deficiency in patient support services, such as palliative care, nutrition, psychosocial support and rehabilitation.

The need for high-quality cancer care in the country was evident, and high-level relationships between the royal court of Jordan and the U.S. government led to a cooperative agreement with the National Cancer Institute of the United States (National Institutes of Health) to transform Al-Amal hospital, which was dedicated since its inception for cancer care, into a "U.S. model" comprehensive center for cancer care, training and education as well as research. In 2003, the King Hussein Cancer Center (KHCC) was inaugurated (Moe et al. 2007). Following intense efforts, KHCC gained accreditation from the Joint Commission International (JCI)

A. Al-Omari (✉)
Office of Scientific Affairs and Research, King Hussein Cancer Center, Amman, Jordan
e-mail: asomari@khcc.jo

H. Silverman (ed.), *Research Ethics in the Arab Region*, Research Ethics Forum 5,
https://doi.org/10.1007/978-3-319-65266-5_36

in 2006, followed by JCI accreditation in 2008 for the cancer care program as an oncology center equipped to treat all types of adult and pediatric cancers. Currently, KHCC treats approximately 60% of cancer cases in Jordan, in addition to patients from neighboring countries and the region (Abdel-Razeq et al. 2015).

Research is a core component in the center's operations. The 2015–2017 strategic plan of KHCC is built around three main priorities: (1) fostering safe and effective patient-centered care, (2) improving and sustaining institutional core competencies, and (3) positioning KHCC as a leading regional oncology center as well as a leading regional research center. The Office of Scientific Affairs and Research is the administrative body responsible for the administration and management of all research operations at KHCC.

Scope of Research

KHCC medical staff conducts retrospective and prospective clinical and translational research projects in addition to clinical trials. The first clinical trial sponsored by a pharmaceutical company was initiated in 2006. Since then the number of clinical trials conducted at the center has increased steadily (Fig. 1). As of November 2015, the Clinical Trials Unit at KHCC supported 24 clinical studies that encompassed phase II, III and IV trials. These trials covered different disease types, including breast cancer, lung cancer, colorectal cancer and leukemia. Other types of research include investigator – initiated clinical trials and academic research by students to meet the requirements of their master's or Ph.D. degrees. Studies initiated by KHCC researchers consist mainly of retrospective chart reviews of existing patients' data, some prospective studies and psychosocial studies. Survey-type of research started gaining popularity after the activation of the survey-research unit at

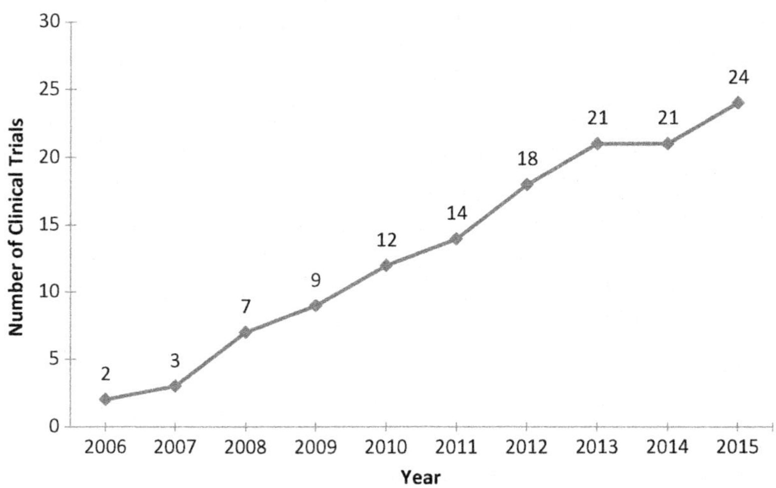

Fig. 1 Clinical trials conducted at KHCC, data as of November, 2015

the Office of Scientific Affairs and Research (OSAR) in 2014. Furthermore, the support of the Intramural Research Grants (IMG) program (see below) that started in 2012 motivated researchers to conduct investigator-initiated protocols.

Research Governance at KHCC

The Office of Scientific Affairs and Research (OSAR) was established in 2006; its current structure is shown in Fig. 2. OSAR is responsible for research administration and management at KHCC and oversees the Center of Research Shared Resources, the Center for Grants and Contracts Management and the Cancer Registry. It also supports the two other governing bodies for research; the Institutional Review Board (IRB) and the Research Council (RC).

Center of Research Shared Resources

Center of Research Shared Resources was established to provide researchers with services required to advance their clinical and translational cancer research projects. This center is managed through the following units:

(a) *The Clinical Trials Unit (CTU):* This unit manages and supports all clinical trials at the center in compliance with institutional, local, and international regulations governing the conduct of clinical trials. It works closely with all departments to investigate the feasibility of each clinical trial and its importance to KHCC patients. The CTU also works to develop, implement, and improve

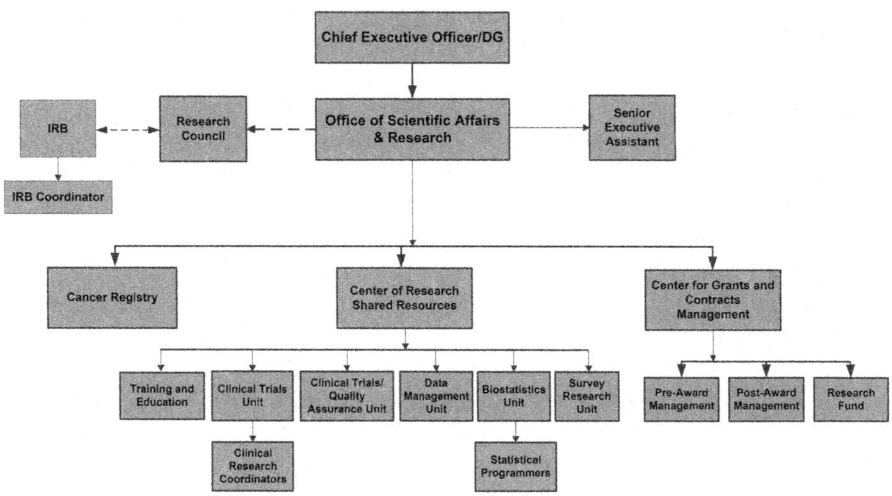

Fig. 2 Organizational structure of the Office of Scientific Affairs and Research

policies and procedures related to the conduct and management of clinical trials at KHCC in compliance with Good Clinical Practice (GCP) guidelines.

The CTU also facilitates interdepartmental communication between members of the trial team. In addition, the CTU supports communication with the sponsor, local regulatory bodies, and IRB. It oversees audits and inspections on ongoing clinical trials. The unit has a dedicated archive space for closed clinical trials. Moreover, there is a dedicated pharmacy storage area for investigational medicinal products. The unit has a history of meeting 100% of commitments with sponsors.

Clinical Research Coordinators (CRCs) at the CTU organize and coordinate the implementation of clinical trial protocols by supporting patient accrual, follow up visits, management of investigational products (shipment, storage, dispensing, retention, return, or destruction), collection and shipment of study-related samples, handling of trial samples and products, maintenance of trial master file, archiving, and reporting including adverse events. They are engaged in continuous education programs at KHCC and are required to sit for the Association of Clinical Research Professionals certification exam after 2 years of work at KHCC to become certified clinical research coordinators.

(b) *Biostatistics Unit:* This unit includes statistical programmers and biostatisticians, who can provide consultation and statistical resources to all IRB-approved research projects. The team helps researchers in their experimental design, such as sample size, study design and planning of statistical methodology. In addition, the staff helps researchers in data analysis, reporting and writing of statistical methodology in publications. The biostatistics unit works closely with the Cancer Registry to produce KHCC cancer registry annual report.

(c) *Clinical Research Quality Assurance Unit:* This unit ensures compliance of clinical research conducted at KHCC to local and international requirements for good clinical practice. It provides monitoring, auditing, continuous improvements, and education services. The unit assists with the development, implementation, communication, and review of policies and procedures that promote compliance and excellence in clinical research, as well as leads quality improvement initiatives. It is also responsible for contact with regulatory authorities for up-to-date follow up and compliance with regulations governing clinical research.

(d) *Survey Research Unit:* The Survey Research Unit was activated in 2014 to initiate and support qualitative research and population-based surveys. The unit assists in designing and implementing new initiatives, evaluating proposals, providing support services and education in qualitative survey research methodology and ensures that this type of research (commonly mistaken to be easy and quick) is conducted according to sound scientific principles.

(e) *Data Management Unit (DMU):* Establishment of the DMU in 2015 was motivated by the belief that data represent a core element in clinical research and that the validity of data reflects on the integrity of the entire research process and research site. Research data management activities were previously handled by the CRCs and the biostatistics unit. Currently, the DMU supports development of data management plans both for investigator-initiated and sponsored clinical research including clinical trials managed through the CTU, as well as designs and develops data collection tools such as case report forms (CRFs) and customized electronic databases for each CRF. The DMU ensures that reportable data are accurate and verifiable, extracts documented clinical results and completes the study CRFs, as well as ensures the data is ready for statistical analysis.

(f) *Training and Education Unit:* This unit surveys the needs of KHCC staff and develops training programs on research methodology, protocol development, cancer statistics, cancer registration as well as good clinical practice (GCP). As of January 2015, GCP training and certification became mandated by the IRB as part of the submission checklist of any clinical study. Training is coordinated with the Academic Affairs Office at KHCC and is delivered through lectures, webinars, workshops as well as one to one consultations. Initiatives toward public outreach and education have included the development of a patient booklet on medical research and clinical studies, in which definition of terms commonly used in clinical research as well as the different phases and procedures of research are explained in simple layman language.

Center of Grants and Contracts Management

The Center of Grants and Contracts Management (CGM) was established to respond to the increasing demand for assistance in obtaining and managing research grants, and to ensure proper accounting and financial compliance of sponsored projects. The CGM manages the pre-award and post-award administration of research grants and contracts funded by KHCC through the IMG program, or other national or international agencies.

Pre-award functions include all stages from finding and disseminating funding opportunities, assisting in preparation of grant applications and budgets, negotiating and preparing research agreements, to the submission of proposals to funding agencies. The Center is also responsible for the management of other types of research agreements such as memorandum of understandings, collaborative agreements, partnership agreements, consultation agreements, non-disclosure agreements, and material transfer agreements. Post-award functions include the administration of grants, e.g., preparation of subcontracting agreements, preparation of renewals, requesting cost and no cost extensions, following up on and submission of progress reports, and closing out of projects in close coordination with the Finance Department and the Research Council.

Grants specialists are available to assist established investigators, junior faculty, and other researchers in identifying funding opportunities and in obtaining support for their research projects. Grants specialists help with the preparation, review, and submission of applications. Grants and Contracts staff works closely with administrators and investigators to ensure that proposals and awards comply with KHCC's policies and procedures, and the funding agency's instructions, guidelines, and regulations.

Cancer Registry

The Cancer Registry at King Hussein Cancer Center is a hospital-based cancer registry that systematically collects data about cancer patients treated at KHCC. Its database includes over 35,000 cases accessioned since July 2006. Patients' information is abstracted directly from the patient medical files by Certified Tumor Registrars (CTRs). The Cancer Registry regularly reports to the Jordanian National Cancer Registry/Ministry of Health. The staff and management of KHCC cancer registry are dedicated to guarantee the completeness, timeliness, and accuracy of the data, and are involved in several initiatives for improving the use of this quality data to better understand and enhance cancer care.

The functions and responsibilities of the *Institutional Review Board (IRB)* at KHCC are discussed in a different chapter.

The Research Council (RC) is the newest addition to the research governing bodies at KHCC. It is a standing committee established in 2012 to oversee the promotion, regulation, and monitoring of all aspects of research activities undertaken by members of, or within KHCC. It is responsible for developing KHCC research strategic plan and research priority areas and sets and monitors the research performance indicators in collaboration with KHCC's Quality Council. The RC receives applications of research projects for scientific evaluation in accordance with its internal policies and procedures which is then coordinated with the IRB review for final approval. In addition, the RC recommends the allocation of capital in the research fund on annual basis and makes decisions on funding of research projects based on scientific merit through the Intramural Research Grants (IMG) program.

The IMG program is supported by KHCC Research Fund, which receives a designated annual contribution from KHCC as part of its operational budget for each fiscal year. This amount is determined each year based on multiple factors including overall operational budget for KHCC and the estimated demand from KHCC researchers. The Research Fund budget is approved by KHCC's Board of Trustees as part of KHCC's overall annual budget. There are two application cycles annually (Spring and Fall) for the IMG program. Deadline for the spring funding cycle is March and the deadline for the fall funding cycle is September of each calendar year. The exact deadline dates are announced by the Center for Grants and Contracts Management at least 1 month before the deadlines. The Research Council announces decisions for funding by May for the March funding cycle and by November for the September funding cycle.

Clinical Research Challenges at KHCC

Despite a strong infrastructure and funding for research at KHCC, the extent and type of research, especially clinical trials, needs to be enhanced. This belief is reflected by the type of proposals submitted to the IRB in 2014. Specifically, of the 80 submitted proposals, 65 were of the Exempt category (mostly retrospective chart reviews and questionnaire-based studies) and only 8 (10%) were full-board reviewed proposals. Furthermore, only 47 manuscripts representing research performed at the KHCC was published in 2014 (KHCC unpublished data). Understanding the challenges that impede clinical research is essential to advance research at KHCC. These challenges occur at the institutional and the investigator levels.

Institutional Level: Research is integral to KHCC mission, therefore resources have been dedicated since its inception to advance and promote a clinical research culture. However, other types of institutional support are needed. This includes providing the overwhelmingly busy clinical staff the required research protected time, instituting a faculty incentive plan that provides financial rewards and recognition for investigators, and addressing the current brain drain in which the more experienced, foreign-trained clinical investigators are migrating to GCC countries, EU and the US.

Investigator Level: Balancing between the demands of clinical care and research activities remains a main challenge. Defining a system for research protected time as explained above is needed to support active investigators in their research endeavors. In addition, there is a knowledge gap in research methodology due to lack of research education in the curricula of medical schools. This is currently being addressed by the educational activities conducted by OSAR, as described in a previous section.

Knowledge, Attitudes, and Practices (KAP) Towards Clinical Research: Physicians and Public

Physicians face several barriers in the conduct of clinical research that deter them from actively pursuing a research career. In addition, public awareness and understanding are key in conducting effective clinical research, but the nature of the recruitment obstacles in Jordan are not specifically known. Therefore, the Office of Scientific Affairs and Research (OSAR) at KHCC conducted in 2015 a needs assessment project to explore the knowledge, attitudes, and practices (KAP) towards clinical research among KHCC physicians and the general public (KHCC patients, companions and visitors).

Physicians KAP

A self-administered questionnaire was distributed to KHCC physicians in different departments. The questionnaire was based on a literature review and consisted of three sections: demographics, clinical research knowledge (ten questions; five on epidemiology and five on biostatistics) and attitudes/practices towards clinical research. The questions on statistics were based on the list of the most often used statistical methods (Novak et al. 2006). Only 55 physicians completed the questionnaire with a response rate of 37%. The mean total knowledge score was 3.33 (out of 10) and only 32.7% of respondents scored 5.0 and above. The mean knowledge score of epidemiology was higher than biostatistics (2.13 vs. 1.2) (unpublished data). This finding of low level of knowledge in the basic principles of study methods and data analysis among doctors was not totally unexpected due to the lack of courses on research methodology in the curriculum of medical schools in Jordan and the region. It is also in agreement with previous studies reporting a serious gap in knowledge of medical research methods among physicians (Novak et al. 2006). This knowledge gap not only negatively affects the doctors' ability to conduct research, but also their ability to practice in a modern healthcare environment with its emphasis on self-directed learning and evidence-based medicine. Therefore, there is a clear need for clinical research training and education among physicians as well as collaborating with key stakeholders to include clinical research education in the curricula of medical schools.

The responses on the attitudes and practices section of the survey were generally positive. The majority of respondents were interested in attending training on clinical research methodology (90.6%) as well as referring patients to clinical trials (86.8%).

Leading barriers towards clinical research as reported by responding physicians included unavailability of time (32.7% of respondents) followed by lack of training on clinical research methodology during formal medical education (30.9%) and unfamiliarity with the application process (16.4%). Top management is in support of dedicating protected time for research and initiatives are currently underway to define a system and create a clear incentive plan that will further encourage and advance research at KHCC.

Public KAP

A self-administered questionnaire was distributed to a convenient sample of adult visitors in the waiting areas of KHCC. Questions assessed KAP towards clinical research and barriers hindering participation. Four hundred and thirty-five questionnaires were returned with a response rate of 90%.

More than half of the surveyed sample claimed to understand the definition of clinical research and approximately one third identified it as "trials where sick patients are given different forms of medicines/drugs". Most of the respondents (92.9%) had never participated in clinical research before and 97.7% of those were never offered to participate. These results are consistent with previous studies reporting lack of awareness of clinical trials as the chief barrier to participation in clinical studies among cancer patients (Fenton et al. 2009). While 56% had heard about the IRB, none were able to identify its role in clinical research, thus highlighting deficiencies in knowledge about clinical research ethical principles and rights of participants.

General perception and attitudes towards clinical research were positive. A majority of 81.1% and 86.5% believed that clinical research offered participants superior care and is important to advance treatment, respectively (Fig. 3) (unpublished data).

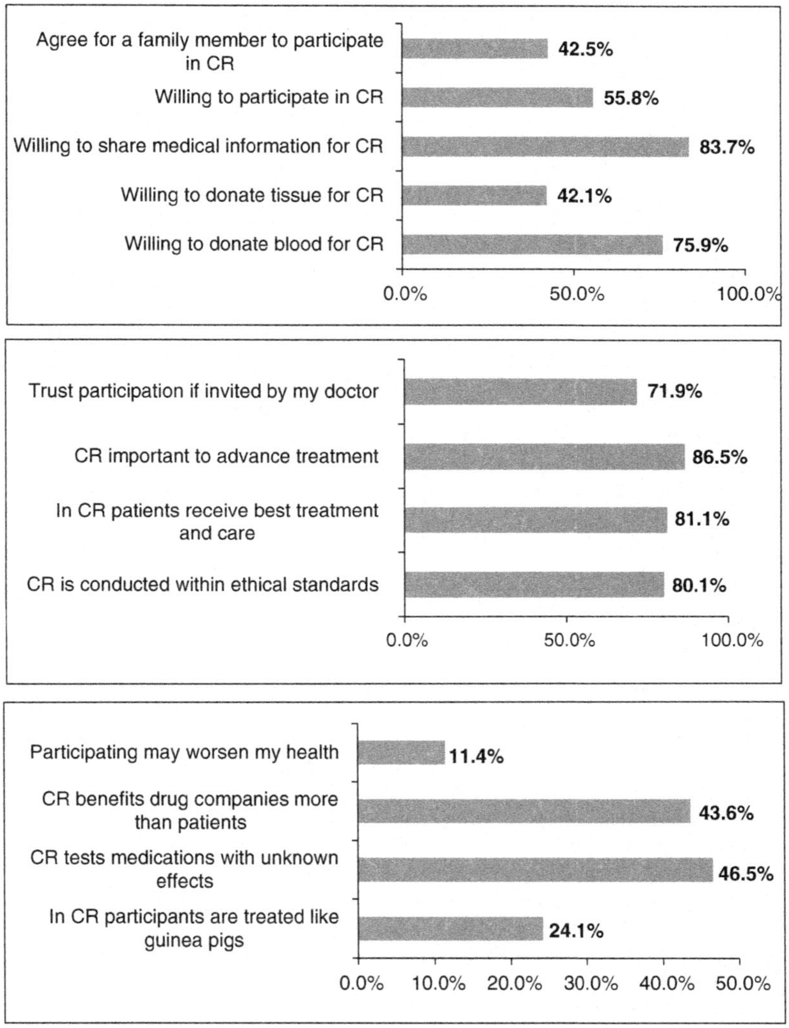

Fig. 3 Public perception and attitudes towards clinical research, KHCC unpublished data. *CR* Clinical research

Participants younger than 41 years (mean age of sample) were more inclined to participate in clinical research compared to older individuals (61.4% vs. 48.5%, $p = .028$). The young age group was also more willing to donate blood and tissue for research. The majority of participants (84.3%) stated they preferred to be invited to participate in clinical research by their physician, thus stressing the role of the physician in determining a patient's enrollment in a clinical trial, consistent with what had previously been reported in the literature (Fenton et al. 2009; Mannel et al. 2003). Almost 70% of participants was unaware of any clinical research conducted in Jordan. This result demonstrated a need for public outreach campaigns and media-based educational programs to advertise clinical research and its importance to advance medicine and cancer treatments.

Next Steps

King Hussein Cancer Center follows a continuous journey to improve healthcare services through evidence-based practices and research studies. There is a progressive endeavor to increase the number of clinical trials and research projects to add to the research experience and allow patients access to novel treatments that are not available in Jordan otherwise. KHCC is continuously building and promoting a culture of clinical research at the institution. For example, KHCC is seeking AAHRPP accreditation (Association for the Accreditation of Human Research Protection Programs), the gold standard of quality in clinical research that will further advance clinical research operations and increase KHCC's credibility as a clinical site of excellence among sponsors, peers and the public. The future of clinical research is bright at KHCC and in Jordan.

References

Abdel-Razeq, H., A. Attiga, and A. Mansour. 2015. Cancer care in Jordan. *Hematology/Oncology and Stem Cell Therapy* 8: 64–70.

Fenton, L., M. Rigney, and R.S. Herbst. 2009. Clinical trial awareness, attitudes, and participation among patients with cancer and oncologists. *Community Oncology* 6: 207–213.

Mannel, R.S., J.L. Walker, N. Gould, D.R.J. Scribner, S. Kannelle, T. Tillmanns,... M.A. Gold. 2003. Impact of individual physicians on enrollment of patients into clinical trials. *American Journal of Clinical Oncology* 26: 171–173.

Ministry of Health. 2011. Jordan cancer registry cancer incidence in Jordan-2011: Available at: http://www.moh.gov.jo/AR/Pages/Periodic-Newsletters.aspx.

Misik, V. 2011. Shifting sands. Euro Pharma Contract, September, 66–70.

Moe, J.L., G. Pappas, and A. Murray. 2007. Transformational leadership, transnational culture and political competence in globalizing health care services: A case study of Jordan's King Hussein Cancer Center. *Globalization and Health* 3: 11.

Novak, L., A. Jotkowitz, B. Knyazer, and V. Novak. 2006. Evidence-based medicine: Assessment of knowledge of basic epidemiological and research methods among medical doctors. *Postgraduate Medical Journal* 82: 817–822.

The Ministry of Health. 2009. Mortality data in Jordan, available at http://apps.moh.gov.jo/MOH/En/publications.php.

Establishing a Clinical Research Center in Egypt

Nadia Zaki

Introduction

The Clinical Research Center (CRC) at Alexandria University in Alexandria, Egypt was established in July 2006 and was the first center for clinical trials in Egypt. The vision of the CRC is to become a Center of Scientific Excellence in Clinical Research. Its mission is to enhance and expand the magnitude of high-quality and ethical clinical research. Our objectives include: (1) to foster innovative, high-impact clinical trials that will enhance drug development activities; and (2) to train regional researchers to conduct multinational trials and other health research.

Accordingly, our activities include both research and educational. Research activities comprise of investigator-initiated and industry-sponsored phase II, III and IV multicenter international clinical trials. Educational activities include training courses on Good Clinical Practice (GCP) and research ethics for investigators, research coordinators, members of research ethics committees (RECs), post-graduate and under-graduate students. The CRC provides a full range of resources and services directly or in coordination with the institutional resources of Alexandria University Hospital: trained research personnel to conduct clinical trials, lab facilities, statistical consultation, and computer and data management support.

Development of the Clinical Trial Center at Alexandria

The motivation for establishing a clinical trials center was prompted by several Egyptian-American doctors, all graduates of the Alexandria School of Medicine, during their visit at the University in March 2006. At that time, the concept of

N. Zaki (✉)
Faculty of Medicine, Alexandria University, Alexandria, Egypt
e-mail: nadiazaki65@yahoo.com

H. Silverman (ed.), *Research Ethics in the Arab Region*, Research Ethics Forum 5,
https://doi.org/10.1007/978-3-319-65266-5_37

clinical trials was new and only a handful of trials were being conducted by several professors. Such trials were phase IV, performed either on the wards or in their private clinics without the application of strict ethical guidelines toward informed consent and ethical approval. Three major items were discussed to implement the idea of the CRC: the location of the center, funding, and staff training.

Regarding location, at that time the New Alexandria University Hospital was in the final stages of completion and as such, space on the eighth floor of the hospital was able to be allocated for the CRC. Regarding funding, Alexandria University provided the funds for computer and lab equipment. The issue of training was accomplished by sending five Egyptian physicians to the University of Maryland Baltimore to receive training on the principles of clinical trials, good clinical practice and clinical research coordination through support from an NIH training grant.

Initial Activities

Enhancing Awareness: Our first activity was to present to the faculty an introductory lecture that gave an overview on clinical trials, the importance of conduction of clinical trials in the faculty, and the value of the CRC for the ethical conduct of research. At that time, we faced large resistance from several professors who accused us of exploiting the Egyptian patients and using them as guinea pigs. We explained to them that trials will be conducted under strict ethical international guidelines and GCP, which was a new concept to the faculty at that time.

Development of Standard Operating Procedures: We developed our Standard Operating Procedures (SOPs) in 2011 followed by a revision 2012. It is exclusively for professionals involved in clinical trials at the CRC. All clinical trials at the CRC are conducted according to International Conference on Harmonization (ICH)/Good Clinical Practice (GCP) standards, regulatory authorities (Ministry of Health-Egypt) requirements and CRC- Standard Operating Procedures (SOPs).

All CRC investigators have an obligation to adhere to the established CRC- Site Specific SOPs. When a clinical trial is sponsored by another agency/pharmaceutical company, the investigator may also be requested to comply with company's requirements. Consensus between any differences is achieved between all parties before initiating the trial.

The SOPs include chapters on investigator and delegated trial's staff SOPs, communication flow with the sponsor to the site, and audit process, and references. The most important parts of the SOPs are those involved with: management and control of informed consent procedure within the clinical research center, investigational product handling SOPs within clinical research center, and management and control of adverse event reporting procedures within clinical research center.

Governance

The CRC reports to the REC of the Alexandria School of Medicine. Accordingly, we prepare annual reports to the REC regarding the current status of each study conducted at the CRC. Specific information includes the study status (active recruiting, active non-recruiting, suspended, terminated, etc.), number of subjects recruited, number of adverse events and how they were managed, and requests for annual renewal. Simultaneously, we report to the MOH (usually through the international sponsor). For investigator-initiated trials funded by the University or international funding agencies, we report to the involved sponsor on quarterly/year basis.

Resources of the Clinical Research Center

The physical space of the CRC consists of

1. Eight inpatient rooms, each with 2 beds to accommodate a total of 16 patients
2. An examination room for outpatients' follow-up visits
3. Rooms (2) for storage of essential documents (e.g., study files, source documents, case report forms, etc.)
4. Pharmacy unit
5. A small laboratory for blood sampling
6. Meeting rooms for CRC staff, investigators' teams, CRC visitors, site selection visits, sponsor monitor visits and audit visits

The staff consists of two directors, six pharmacists/study coordinators, three site coordinators, two secretaries, and an accountant.

Research Activities

Research activities comprise of investigator-initiated and industry-sponsored phase II, III and IV multicenter international clinical trials.

Investigator-initiated clinical trials: Research projects funded by national or international sponsors, e.g., Science and Technology Development Fund (STDF), University of Maryland, and Alexandria University Research Enhancement Program. There have been four completed projects and three are ongoing.

Industry-sponsored clinical trials: The CRC provides on-site resources for the conduct of Phase II, III and IV multicenter clinical trials in collaboration with inter-

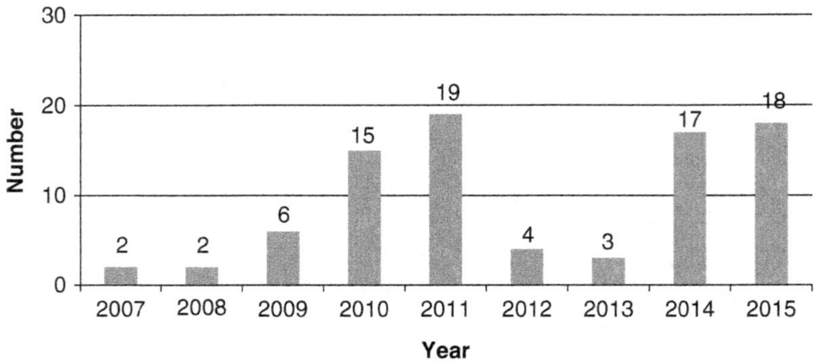

Fig. 1 Number of clinical trials at the Clinical Research Center

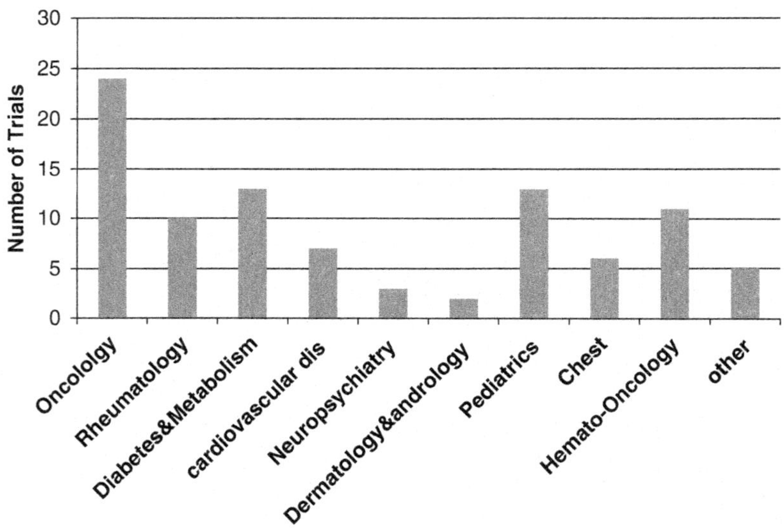

Fig. 2 Disease conditions studied in clinical trials performed at The Clinical Research Center

national pharmaceutical companies. Since its opening the CRC has been involved with 86 clinical trials. Currently, there are approximately 1,500 subjects recruited in different studies. Figure 1 shows the number of clinical trials performed on a yearly basis. Figure 2 shows the most common disease types that are the focus of the clinical trials. These are as follows: Oncology (35%), Diabetes Mellitus (12%), Hematology (12%), Cardiovascular (10%), Rheumatology (7%), Chest (7%), Hepatology (5%), Neuropsychiatry (5%), Pediatrics (4%), Andrology and Dermatology (2%), and Endocrinology (1%).

Financial Management

All financial issues are discussed during the site selection visit between sponsor representative(s) and the director of the CRC in the presence of the principal investigator/study coordinator. Currently, a specific research office that handles contracts does not exist. Review of the technical issues is the responsibility of the directors and the site coordinator. We negotiate with sponsors in conjunction with the PIs of the studies to develop the budget. According to our SOPs, the sponsor shall pay to the CRC 30–40% of the investigator fee (as hospital overhead) and 30% of coordinator fee.

Processes Involved with Initiating a Clinical Trial at the CRC

1. Study Site Visit: Before any trial begins, representatives from the Contract Research Organization (CRO) conduct a study site visit at the CRC. The entails inspecting the facilities (pharmacy space, refrigerator to store samples, etc.), and meeting with the directors of the CRC, clinical coordinators, pharmacists and the Principle Investigators. Discussions are held regarding expected monthly recruitment (as detailed in a previously completed feasibility questionnaire), turnaround time for the REC to review the protocol, turnaround time to approve the contract, and time needed to import the drug.
2. Study submission to the Alexandria REC: the protocol is submitted to the REC at Faculty of Medicine, Alexandria University.
3. Ministry of Health (MOH) Submission: Following REC approval of the clinical trial protocol, the study documents are submitted to the National Scientific and Research Ethics Committee at the Egyptian MOH for approval.
4. Egyptian National Security Approval: If the study involves shipment of biological samples to central laboratories outside Egypt, approval from the Egyptian National Security office is required.

Challenges

We have experienced the following challenges in the conduct of clinical trials:

Workload: There is a high volume of effort required to prepare for each clinical trial, which includes completion of required feasibility questionnaires and forms required for submission to the REC and the MOH for approvals. The number of submissions prepared compared with the actual number of studies eventually conducted in the CRC is in the ratio of approximately 7:1. Such a high ratio leads to a large amount of uncompensated effort for the study staff in their preparation of submission documents. Common reasons for not initiating a clinical trial include the following:

(a) The political status in Egypt during the last few years have markedly affected the Egyptian MOH approval process, although this has improved recently and now the maximum time for obtaining REC opinion is 60 days from submission.
(b) Delayed approvals from the Egyptian National Security Office for trials involving the export of biological samples to central laboratories outside Egypt.
(c) Delayed import of investigational products and/or lab equipment/kits that are required to initiate the study.
(d) Initially, the Alexandria REC disapproved several phase II trials even when these studies were low-risk and were approved by the MOH committee. After providing more data regarding Phase II trials, this issue was resolved.

Human Resources: Initially, we had a shortage of experienced and GCP-trained full – time PIs and sub-PIs, experienced full – time clinical research coordinators, pharmacists and nurses to conduct the clinical trials. Also, we initially experienced a high turnover rate, which necessitated much time devoted to training.

Another major challenge involved low salaries for the staff affiliated with the CRC, which is part of the Faculty. We are trying to improve salaries according to our budget and the university limits. Another issue is that the majority of the PIs are not able to devote much time to their clinical trials due to their busy schedules. Hence, it becomes difficult to contact them when issues arise with the conduct of the studies. Accordingly, we attempt to select the most committed PIs.

Recruitment Issues: Maintaining acceptable enrollment numbers to satisfy the requirements of the CROs and to reach the targets we set for ourselves in our submitted feasibility questionnaires has sometimes proved difficult. We have encountered an imperfect referral system between the investigators and treating physicians and also confusion regarding study criteria, which results in increased rate of screening failures. To resolve those issues, we hold regular meetings with each study team in the CRC and with the referring physicians.

In one hypertension study, the eligibility criteria were very restrictive, such that the investigator was unable to find an eligible subject. Recruitment was about to close without achievement of the target. To help the PI, the CRC team participated in a health campaign organized by Alexandria Medical Syndicate in a village outside of Alexandria. The team was able to refer a considerable number of hypertensive patients to the CRC to meet with the PI next morning. After approaching them, recruitment of eligible subjects increased.

Informed Consent Issues: Many patients and their families have inadequate knowledge of clinical trials, which at times makes obtaining informed consent problematic. For example, some patients would refuse to sign although they had agreed to participate in the study. Additionally, the presence of the therapeutic misconception represents a concern, as research subjects tend to conflate research studies with clinical care. We conducted a study in collaboration with investigators at the University of Maryland to determine the extent of this issue. The study was a cross-sectional qualitative pilot study in which 103 participants in 10 clinical trials responded to a questionnaire regarding the quality of informed consent and the presence of the therapeutic misconception. Several best practices in informed consent practices were followed, as over 90% agreed they had time to ask questions and received adequate information about the risks prior to their providing consent. However, all participants held a misperception regarding benefit, as they thought the experimental drug would improve their condition; only 46.1% were aware of receiving a non-approved experimental drug and only 21.3% realized that they were being randomized to one of the two study drugs (Mansour et al. 2015). On the basis of this study, we recommended to the investigators to provide more time for discussions with potential research participants regarding the distinction between research and clinical care before signing the ICF.

Finally, several investigators would not give a copy of the ICF to the study participants due to their fear that the participants might change their mind or withdraw their consent after showing the ICF to their treating physicians, who would sometimes advise them not to participate in the experimental study. We held sessions with such investigators to convince them that participants have a right to receive a copy of the ICF.

Lack of an Accredited Local Laboratory: One of the requirements of international clinical trials is that the local laboratory performing study laboratory tests with research subjects should have a certificate of accreditation to provide assurances of accurate and reliable results. This problem was initially overcome by contracting accredited labs outside the Faculty through separate contracts with the sponsor. Finally, the Faculty lab was accredited by the end of 2013.

Challenges with the onsite clinical pharmacy: A major challenge involved designating an appropriate area in the CRC pharmacy to prepare cytotoxic drugs, which is a requirement of international clinical trials in order to ensure the safety of the patients and protect the pharmacists handling the drugs. As such, we would perform this task in the clinical pharmacy at the Alexandria Main University Hospital, which consumed much time and effort. Finally, we were able to receive the financial funds necessary to build such a pharmacy unit in the CRC.

Another issue regarded adequate space for storage of study drugs. This issue was solved by prior agreement with the sponsors to provide/donate refrigerators and cupboards for storage of investigational products (IPs) used in their studies. However, we faced the problems of electricity cutting off during temperature excursions, which frequently resulted in suspension of the current study until additional samples of stored drugs could be obtained.

Finally, we had a problem with the destruction of unused investigational drugs at the end of studies due to lack of an established drug destruction policy in our hospital. As such, we would frequently return unused drugs to the sponsor, which sometimes resulted in unnecessary inconvenience. Finally, our hospital developed its own drug destruction policy. The sponsor shall pay a specific fee for local destruction of unused study medications, as agreed initially in the CTA.

Document Storage Space: Inadequate facility for storage and archiving of study documents became an obstacle when dealing with international pharmaceuticals. As per E6 GCP (4.9.5), "Essential documents should be retained until at least 2 years after the last approval of a marketing application in an ICH region or longer if required by regulatory authorities or sponsor." We solved this issue by expanding the place for document storage and archiving. We also established an archiving fee, which is included in all clinical trial agreements.

Access to Source Documents: As per E6 GCP (4.9.7), "Upon request of the monitor, IRB/REC, or regulatory authority, the PI/institution should make available for direct access all requested trial-related records." At the beginning of our work, we faced difficulties to obtain the source documents (especially those related to admissions prior to enrolment in clinical trials) that were archived in the hospital. After discussions with the hospital administration, they agreed to provide us with certified copies of those documents upon our request. All source documents related to subjects during conduction of the trial are kept in the CRC and nobody can access them except the PIs and their delegated personnel.

Challenges with Pharmaceutical Companies: We face many challenges with pharmaceutical companies and CROs. These include interacting with poorly trained monitors and CRAs, especially with newly developing research offices in the pharmaceutical companies. Most of those CRAs were originally working in sales as medical representatives and were new in the field of clinical research.

We also encountered problems with the sponsors and CROs in regards to delayed payments, inadequate fees, underestimation of time devoted to follow up of study subjects, delayed notifications regarding site-selection and monitoring visits, and insufficient post-trial availability of drugs. Also, there is sometimes lack of fairness regarding the budgets between Middle East sites and European/US sites. Partnership agreements with several of the CROs and pharmaceutical companies helped resolve several of these issues.

Educational Activities

The CRC have organized the following educational activities:

1. Workshops on GCP and research ethics for investigators, research coordinators, REC members and post-graduate students.
2. We provide advice on the establishment of clinical trial centers for other universities, e.g., Cairo University, Beni Suif University, and the National Research Institute.
3. Collaboration with the WHO and MOH on several workshop involving "GCP and Research Ethics".

4. Collaboration on an International Inter-University course of Clinical Research in French between Alexandria Clinical Research Center and Université Senghor in Alexandria.
5. Hands-on training opportunities for house officers.
6. Organization of "Clinical Trials Awareness Days" for undergraduate students.

The CRC has given input on the following activities:

- Drafting of the Egyptian law for Clinical Trials
- Establishing a National data base registry for clinical trials
- Developing a clinical trial center to officials at other Egyptian universities

Achievements

The following represents several of our achievements:

1. In September 2014, we received the First EMA (European Medical Agency) inspection in the Middle East for a hematology trial in which the PI was among the highest recruiters in the world. EMA reported no major critical findings.
2. Publications and Presentations at International Conferences: We have given oral and poster presentations at regional and international meetings as well as publications in peer-reviewed journals representing the results of the clinical trials performed at the CRC.
3. The Science and Technology Development Fund (STDF) project: In January 2013, we submitted a 3-year project to the Science and Technology Development Fund (STDF) offered by the Egyptian Ministry of Scientific Research entitled "Upgrading of Alexandria Clinical Research Center into a Center of Scientific Excellence in Clinical Research".

The project was accepted and obtained funding of approximately 5 million Egyptian pounds distributed over 3 years to build capacity and upgrade the CRC. The objectives are to foster more innovative, high-impact clinical trials and to streamline drug development activities enabling Egyptian patients to access the best medical care and new treatment, to coordinate multidisciplinary research, conduct state of- the-art clinical research, assume leadership in clinical research within the Middle East region, to train and educate local/regional researchers to conduct multinational clinical trials and other health research projects and to integrate all parties involved in clinical trials such as MOH, WHO, Academia, pharmaceuticals, CROs and RECs in Egypt into one extensive network for clinical trials.

The most important achievements from this grant included the organization of the "First Alex Clinical Research Networking Forum" held at Alexandria University on the twenty-first of February 2017 and attended by representatives of many of the Egyptian Universities, Research Centers, Ministry of Health, Regulatory

Authorities, Research Ethics Committees, Armed Forces, Alexandria Medical Syndicate, Pharmaceutical Companies and CRO's. The broad aim of this event was to establish a national network to promote training and collaboration in clinical research through building an effective network that will support academic teaching and research across multiple disciplines. It also provides a forum for sharing the best practice and sustainable collaboration. Though based on local priorities, this research network is able of being internationally competitive and could expand into multinational collaborative research groups.

Future Steps

The following represents our plans for the future to enhance our clinical trial center:

- Establish a dedicated Intensive Care Unit (ICU) to perform trials involving critically ill patients.
- Conduct phase I studies.
- Establish a database registry for clinical trials in Egyptian Universities.
- Expand training and educational services.
- Train local and regional researchers in conducting multinational clinical trials (English and French courses).
- Help foster other local and regional clinical research centers.
- Establish a Quality Assurance Unit in collaboration with Alexandria Faculty of Medicine Research Ethics Committee. The Quality Assurance Unit aims at ensuring that all clinical trials conducted in the CRC follow the international guidelines including ICH/GCP, the local regulatory (Ministry of Health-Egypt) requirements, the CRC- Standard Operating Procedures (SOPs) and pharmaceutical company obligations (if applicable). This unit will provide local oversight for the trials. Oversight extends from pre-study procedures through study conduction steps to post-study procedures. It includes but-not limited to ensuring that clinical trial staff are well-trained on GCP, ethical principles and specific study-related procedures, granting requested approvals are obtained for all clinical trial supplies (investigational product, lab kits, etc.) and are delivered to the site prior to study initiation, written informed consents are taken in the proper time and copies of the ICF are given to study subjects before any screening procedure is performed, adequate rates of recruitment and retention of study subjects, accurate and proper handling and storage of essential documents of each study and ensuring that access occurs only to authorized personnel, including REC members, monitors, auditors, accurate and timely reporting of adverse events and ensuring proper management of serious adverse events, and investigating causes of delayed recruitment, repeated screening failures, and frequent subject withdrawal of consent.

- Collaboration with our REC to achieve the aims of the Quality Assurance Unit. This will result in direct involvement of the REC in the oversight of the trials to further augment protection of subjects participating in research studies.
- Collaborate with the Clinical Genomic Center at Alexandria Faculty of Medicine.
- Reduce the need for transporting genetic tissue samples to International Labs for performing genetic studies. We plan to accomplish this goal by obtaining international accreditation of the already existing Clinical Genomic Center in the Faculty of Medicine, so that we can perform genetic testing locally according to international standards that would be approved by the sponsor.

Conclusion

We continue to expand the activities of the Clinical Research Center, as we have become successful with representing the benefits of clinical trials to our stakeholders. These benefits include (a) contribution to science; (b) fostering international collaborations; (c) creation of job opportunities to those involved in research; (d) patient access to novel therapeutics;(e) provision of research opportunities to medical faculty and students; (f) enhancement of training opportunities in GCP, research ethics, and conduct of clinical trials.

Reference

Mansour, H., N. Zaki, R. Abdelhai, N. Sabry, H. Silverman, and S.S. El-Kamary. 2015. Investigating the informed consent process, therapeutic misconception and motivations of Egyptian research participants: A qualitative pilot study. *Eastern Mediterranean Health Journal* 21 (3): 155–163. Available at: http://www.ncbi.nlm.nih.gov/pubmed/26074215.

Concluding Remarks

Henry Silverman

Several themes shape the significance of this book. One entails the practice of research ethics that should govern the resolution of dilemmas occurring in research in the Arab region, both at the micro level – interactions between researchers and research participants, and at the macro level – interactions between international collaborators of research, i.e., sponsors, investigators, and governments. Regarding the macro level, major points to consider is that international actors need to recognize the potential effects of colonialism, discover new paradigms to work collaboratively, and ensure that research achieves social justice. Regarding the micro level, Part I described the various ethical issues and demonstrated that while determining whether ethics principles are universal or relative remains elusive, how ethical issues are deliberated and resolved at the local level will depend on the social, cultural, economic, and political domains that exist in the Arab region.

Parts II–IV reviewed important aspects of research governance systems and provided examples of those that exist in several Arab countries. These sections showed that several countries have developed sophisticated frameworks for the regulation and oversight of research that are comparable to those in western countries. Specifically, in the past 10 years, Jordan and Saudi Arabia have developed regulatory systems to protect human subjects of research by promoting scientifically and ethically sound research. Their regulatory systems include the presence of comprehensive national regulations, an extensive oversight system, and properly constituted, functional and multi-disciplinary ethics review committees. Several other countries are making major efforts to achieve similar results, notably Egypt, which currently has draft national regulations and through a series of ministerial decrees has put in place the building blocks of a functioning oversight system for research and ethics review systems. These efforts challenge what might be a current belief

H. Silverman (✉)
University of Maryland, Baltimore, MD, USA
e-mail: hsilverm@medicine.umaryland.edu

H. Silverman (ed.), *Research Ethics in the Arab Region*, Research Ethics Forum 5,
https://doi.org/10.1007/978-3-319-65266-5_38

that countries in the Arab region uniformally have weak regulatory systems regarding the oversight of research. Parts II–V also described the national regulations existing in the Arab region as well as the current landscape of research ethics committees, which are major aspects of a research governance system.

While Parts II–V demonstrate that much progress has been made in the last two decades in establishing research ethics capacity in many parts of the Arab region, several countries have evolving research governance systems that rely on international research guidelines that are not responsive to the local context, depend on voluntary non-legally enforceable regulations, and lack a robust oversight mechanism for their ethics review systems. Such regulatory systems potentially expose their citizens to avoidable or unnecessary research risk and makes the possibility of exploitation in international research more likely.

A final theme represents current challenges, with regards to fostering sustainable educational programs, including degree programs in research and research ethics. Several efforts are ongoing to meet these educational challenges.

To conclude, by showing what has been accomplished in several countries and emphasizing the current gaps in research ethics capacity, a roadmap for developing and achieving scientifically credible and ethical research in the Arab region is now clearer. Presenting such a roadmap represents a major accomplishment of this book.

Index

H. Silverman (ed.), *Research Ethics in the Arab Region*, Research Ethics Forum 5,
https://doi.org/10.1007/978-3-319-65266-5

CPSIA information can be obtained
at www.ICGtesting.com
Printed in the USA
LVOW13*1952260118
564149LV00007B/181/P

9 783319 652641